the baby sleep book

Also by the same authors:

The Baby Book
The Good Behaviour Book
The Fussy Baby Book

the baby sleep book

How to help your baby to sleep
and have a restful night

Dr William Sears, Dr Robert Sears and Martha Sears, R.N.

Edited by Caroline Deacon

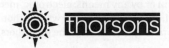

thorsons

Please consult our website, AskDrSears.com,
for updates on any of the products mentioned in this book.

Thorsons
An Imprint of HarperCollins*Publishers*
77–85 Fulham Palace Road,
Hammersmith, London W6 8JB

The website address is: www.thorsonselement.com

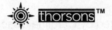

and *Thorsons* are trademarks of
HarperCollins*Publishers* Ltd

First published by Thorsons 2005

1 3 5 7 9 10 8 6 4 2

© 2005 William, Robert and Martha Sears

William, Robert and Martha Sears assert the moral right to
be identified as the authors of this work

Illustrations by Melanie Vandevelde

A catalogue record of this book
is available from the British Library

ISBN 0 00 719822 1

Printed and bound in Thailand
by Imago

to our children – who now all sleep through the night

James
Robert
Peter
Hayden
Erin
Matthew
Stephen
Lauren

and dr bob's

Andrew
Alex
Joshua

contents

A Restful Word from Dr Bill xi

a restful word
from dr bill

Each day in our pediatric practice we hear tired parents sigh, "If only our baby would sleep more." In all our years of writing books and of practising pediatrics, our goal has been to do good things for babies and make life easier for parents. We believe that helping babies sleep better is not only good for them, but good for parents. Parents who get enough sleep at night will be happier during the day.

Over the years, we have devoted a lot of time and energy to the sleep problems parents in our practice share with us. We have offered these tired parents many suggestions for helping their baby sleep longer, and we have asked them to report back to us about which worked and what didn't. We have also asked parents who have visited our website (www.askdrsears.com) to share their sleep problems and solutions with us. As a result, much of the advice in this book comes from parents like yourselves who have struggled to help their babies sleep, found solutions, and willingly shared them with us. You will find quotes (the ones in italics) from these parents sprinkled throughout the book. We've also taken the advice of these parents on how to write a book about

sleep. They told us, "Cut right to the plan." This is why the first two chapters of this book contain our step-by-step approach to help your infant and toddler sleep healthier and happier.

As authors we lose sleep reading many of the baby sleep books currently on bookstore shelves, since most of them are yet another variation on the tired old theme: "Just let your baby cry it out." This tough love for babies is like training a pet, and taking this approach to parenting babies at night puts families in a lose-lose situation. Babies may eventually give up crying and go to sleep, but they lose their trust in their parents to meet their nighttime needs. This can't be good for a baby. Parents lose because this quick ticket to the promised land of sleep keeps them from learning about their baby's individual sleep needs along the way. Most baby sleep books preach the extremes: either *cry it out* (forcing baby to sleep) or *tough it out* (just hang in there). Neither of these approaches is fair to tiny babies or tired parents. Instead, ours is a *sleep tools* approach.

If babies could talk, they would say: "Please don't *force* me to sleep; instead, *teach* me to sleep. After all, I'm just a baby!" Sleep is not a

how to read this book

In response to our "advisers" (sleepless parents) we begin this book by giving you steps and tools to help your baby sleep so you can begin our sleep plan right away. But, nighttime parenting is not just a list of sleep tools, it's a *relationship* with your baby. So, if you're not too tired, you may want to *read chapter 3 first.* It will help you understand how babies sleep – or don't! After you've read the first three chapters then you are ready to put all these sleep tools together into your baby's individual sleep plan (ISP), which we show you how to do in chapter 4. The rest of the book takes you to a deeper understanding of all the sleep tools listed in the first four chapters. Promise you'll read the *whole book!*

We could have just written a booklet in cookbook fashion with a catchy title such as *Two Weeks to Sleeping through the Night – Twenty Tips.* This has never been our way of writing. Parenting is too precious to be cheapened by such gimmicks. Instead, in this book we have taken our usual approach: giving you the tools to become *your* own expert in *your* baby and to help you work out your own style of nighttime parenting.

state you should try to force a baby into. It's better to set conditions that allow sleep to overtake baby and that make self-settling and sleeping longer, easier and more attractive to baby. Yes, you read it correctly – self-settling, which does not imply selfish parenting. While newborns and young babies need help from parents to relax and fall asleep, older babies will eventually learn to settle themselves. Depending on their temperaments and need levels, different babies will master self-settling skills at different ages, but parents can do a lot to help them along. It requires commitment, time, and sensitivity to teach your baby how to sleep and how to go back to sleep. In this book, we'll show you how.

This is a book of options, not "should do's". There is no one-bed-fits-all approach to helping babies sleep. We will give you tools and help you select the ones which fit the sleep temperament of your child so that you can create an individual sleep plan. Helping your baby learn to sleep better is not like following a diet or exercise regimen. There's a lot of give and take, and the options you choose to try will depend on your baby's personality. Just as there are quiet and more active babies in the daytime, there are sound sleepers and frequent wakers during the night. Some high-strung babies are not fans of sleep in general and will need an extra set of tools to help them want to sleep longer.

This is also a book about options for different family lifestyles and different philosophies of nighttime parenting. Realistically, many parents juggle many different sleeping arrangements during the years their children are small. There are co-sleepers, cot sleepers, and families who play musical beds. One baby may start out as a cot sleeper and then upgrade to being a co-sleeper, and then back to a cot sleeper. There is no right arrangement for every family. The one that gets all family members the best night's sleep is the right arrangement for your family. Yet, the key is to be open to trying various sleeping arrangements at various stages of your child's development until you arrive at one that works for your family. The important thing is to keep working at it. Sleep is important. Higher quality sleep is associated with happier and healthier babies – and parents.

Nighttime parenting is a season of child rearing. Yes, your baby will eventually sleep through the night. Now, you may wonder how to get your infants down to sleep at night. In a few years, you'll be wondering how to get them up in the morning. Remember, the nights of baby in your arms, at your breasts and in your bed is a very short while in the total life of your child. Yet the memories of your love and availability last a lifetime.

We wish you and your child years of restful sleep.

William, Robert and Martha Sears
San Clemente, California
February 2005

chapter 1

five steps to get your baby to sleep better

You are probably thinking, "Wow, it's only the first chapter and we're getting right to the point!" That's because we assume you're too tired to wade through a lot of the sleep facts and theories which we've placed in chapter 3. You just need to get your baby to sleep longer stretches.

But, here's the bargain. In order to make these five steps work best, you still need to learn a lot about how and why infants sleep differently than adults, and how to develop a realistic attitude about nighttime parenting. So, promise to read the rest of the book as soon as your whole family is more rested. Do we have a deal? This chapter is designed to help a baby of any age sleep longer, and more importantly, to get you a better night's sleep. After you read this first chapter we hope you and your baby will be ready to sleep soundly the whole night through. Maybe *you'll* be ready, but unfortunately your baby won't just yet. But trust us. We'll help you all get there soon.

Here's a preview of the five steps you will now learn:

- Find out where you and baby sleep best.
- Learn baby's tired times.
- Create a safe and comfortable environment conducive to sleep.
- Enjoy a variety of bedtime rituals.
- Help baby stay asleep longer.

We also call this plan:

- *Ready:* Work out when, where, and how baby goes to sleep.
- *Set:* Use consistent bedtime rituals at predictable tired times.
- *Go:* Use various strategies to teach baby to go to sleep and resettle back to sleep.

First we offer some precautions:

- If your baby is a newborn, do not jump into this plan (or any other plan) in the early weeks. Get to know your baby first, before you introduce a sleep plan into your parenting life.

- Be aware that not everything we suggest will be right for *your* baby. We don't like parenting books that tell parents "this is how you have to do it. This is the only right way. Tough luck if it doesn't fit your own ideas or your baby's personality." We believe that parents who know and love their baby are the best judges of how to care for that baby. This is why it's so important to first get attached to your baby – so that you have the wisdom to know what's best for your baby. In this book we will give you lots of strategies to help your baby learn healthy sleep habits. Which ones you choose depends on your baby's unique sleep temperament.

So let's get started, and here's to a good night's sleep … finally!

step 1: find out where you and your baby sleep best

Where will your baby sleep best? With you in your bed? In a co-sleeper, Moses basket cradle, or cot next to your bed? In a cot in your room, or in his own room? Where do you sleep best? Where do *you* want your baby to sleep?

Realistically, be prepared to play musical beds with all of these sleeping arrangements as you try to work out where all of you get the best night's sleep. Expect these sleeping arrangements to change at various stages of your baby's development. The only people who can answer the question "Where should baby sleep?" are Mum and Dad. Listen to what your

baby and your inner voice are trying to tell you! Perhaps you have a new baby (or you will soon) and you are trying to decide where baby will sleep. Or, if your current sleeping arrangement is one of the reasons why you or your baby are not getting a restful night's sleep, let's explore your three options:

1. Sleeping alone in baby's own room. This is the traditional picture that many first-time parents envision for their babies. As you flip through baby magazines and furniture catalogues you see pictures of smiling parents (who look like they've had plenty of sleep) placing their baby into a cot or cradle in the corner of a beautifully decorated nursery with the evening sunset filtering through the curtains. Parents gaze happily at their baby, who smiles up at them. You dream that this is how your baby will go to sleep, too. You'll pat her little tummy, kiss her on the cheek and say "night-night". She closes her eyes, you tiptoe out of the room, and you and your partner enjoy a nice quiet evening together. Your baby sleeps peacefully the whole night through.

Sounds like a fairy tale, doesn't it? Will it all come true? Eventually, but not in the early months. Most, if not all, younger babies need more out of their parents at bedtime than this magazine picture. This is "quality time" for babies. They often do not willingly succumb to quick-to-sleep methods.

Will this sleeping arrangement work? It may work for easy-going babies. Mellow babies tend to fall asleep more easily and awaken less often at night regardless of where they sleep. Some of you parents-to-be are nodding your head, "Yeah, that's the kind of baby we are going to have, right sweetheart?" Yet many of you have discovered that you have been blessed with a baby who is already letting you know that she's going to need more nighttime closeness than this distant arrangement offers.

Those of you with cot sleepers are probably in one of two situations right now: either your baby had been sleeping well in a cot for months, and is now waking up too often, or you have been trying to get your baby to sleep in a cot for months, but he has never really slept well in the other room and you (and he) are tired.

You have two choices. You can either continue to try to get baby to learn to sleep well in the cot using the rest of the steps in our plan, or you can explore some other options of where baby can sleep.

Why won't your baby sleep well in a cot in his own room? It may be that teething or a temporary medical cause of night waking is suddenly rousing your baby at night. We discuss many such causes of night waking in chapters 3 and 11. But there may be much more to this picture. If your baby has never really slept well alone, and nights of stumbling down the hallway to rescue your crying baby every two hours have taken their toll, it may be that your baby is trying to tell you that he needs more nighttime comfort and closeness.

"But our neighbour's baby sleeps just fine through the night in her own room", you may hear. Every baby has a different personality. Some needier babies simply need more of you day and night. On page 70 we discuss infant personalities and temperaments and how these relate to nighttime needs. It's time to lose the magazine fantasy and work out on your own what is best for you and your baby. If we had to pick the single most important message of this book, it would be: trust your own instincts and make your own decisions about what is best for your individual baby and you.

2. Sleeping in your room, but not in your bed. This is a common sleep set up for two types of families: those who are living in a one-bedroom apartment (like medical resident Dr Bob was when his second son was born – four people sleeping in one room!), and those who want their baby close by (but not so close that baby's tiny feet are kicking them in the ribs). Maybe you want baby close by simply for convenient breastfeeding, because baby wakes up several times each night. Or, perhaps your baby is a great sleeper, yet you prefer having baby sleep near you for your own peace of mind.

Having baby in your room has these advantages:

- When baby wakes he is within arm's reach or just a step away from you.
- You can get to baby quickly and rock or feed him back to sleep before he fully wakens.
- If you wake up, you can easily check on baby to reassure yourself all is well.
- You feel close to baby, yet you and your partner have the bed to yourselves.
- Baby enjoys a sense of security.
- You can easily bring baby into your bed to feed back to sleep so your comfort is less interrupted.

Of course, there are possible disadvantages as well:

- If you are a light sleeper, you may find yourself disturbed by every sound that baby makes.
- Baby may grow accustomed to your proximity and may wake up *more often* because there is something to wake up for (feeding) and someone to wake up to.

Here are some common options for finding a safe place for baby to sleep in your room:

- *The Arm's Reach Co-sleeper.* This is about as close as you can get to having baby nearby but not technically in your bed. With the co-sleeper, you can truthfully tell your in-laws, "No, our baby is *not* sleeping in our bed with us." Since baby is on a separate mattress, he won't feel your every movement, and you won't feel his. You and your partner can enjoy your intimate space. It also gives you instant access to baby when he wakes (he's within arm's reach) so you can move close to him and feed or pat him back to sleep before he fully wakes up and cries. (See page 123 for illustration of the Co-sleeper).
- *Cradle or Moses basket.* These baby beds have the advantage of being right next to your bed, but don't offer the convenience of easy-access feeding like the co-sleeper. Cradles and Moses baskets are portable, however, so you have the flexibility of seeing if baby would sleep well in his own room, too.
- *Swinging hammock bed.* This baby bed is like a soft-bottomed cradle, and it hangs from a spring inside a steel frame, so every time baby moves, the spring gently moves and often lulls baby back to sleep. It too has the advantage of being portable, so baby can sleep in any room

of the house. It can sit right next to your bed for easy access to baby at night.

Some of you reading this book may be finding that your baby thinks being in the same room with you just isn't close enough. Baby needs to feel you right next to him, and if he doesn't, he wakes up. So, what do you do? Co-sleep!

3. Sleeping with baby in your bed. Perhaps your baby isn't even born yet, but you've decided that you want to sleep with your baby right from the start. You may feel: "after all, she's a baby. She's been close to me for nine months." Or maybe you are just getting to know your newborn, and you aren't yet sure what you want to do. Or, you may encounter this situation. "When I put our baby in the cot he wakes up a lot, but as soon as I bring him into our bed he sleeps better – and so do we." Baby is trying to tell you something: "For my well-being I need to sleep closer to you." Listen to your baby!

Sleeping with your baby has some unique advantages:

- You can feed baby back to sleep while you fall easily back to sleep.
- Baby can fall back to sleep more quickly because you can comfort him before he fully wakes up, and you fully wake up.
- Baby may sleep longer and better because you are nearby.
- Baby benefits from eight extra hours of closeness each night.
- Working parents get extra "touch" time with baby.

Studies have shown that even though sleep-sharing babies wake up more to feed, co-sleeping mothers actually get more restful sleep compared to mums who don't sleep with their babies.

These very advantages can also turn out to be disadvantages (depending on how you look at it):

- Baby may actually wake *more* frequently *because* he feels you nearby.
- Some parents don't sleep well with a baby in their bed. They want their baby close, but not that close.
- If Mum sleeps well with the baby, but Dad is a light sleeper and can't get used to the extra presence in his bed, Dad may not sleep well. This may prompt Dad to find another room to sleep in, such as the pastel-coloured nursery that he painted for the baby.
- Once baby gets used to sleeping with you, he may not want to give it up. For some of you, this is an advantage because you welcome this long-term bonding arrangement. For others, co-sleeping may go on longer than you would have liked.

You may have enjoyed sharing sleep with your baby, but now one or all of these disadvantages are interfering with your sleep. If your co-sleeping baby is waking up too much, you can choose either to keep baby in your bed and work through the other steps in our plan, or you can look at the other options for where baby may sleep.

Deciding about co-sleeping isn't as simple as weighing a short list of pros and cons. Co-sleeping is part of an Attachment Parenting style that can be rewarding for families in many ways. (See the "Baby B's of Attachment Parenting", page 66.) Because most parents sleep with their baby at some time in the first couple of years, in chapter 5 we will go into detail about sharing sleep with your baby and how to decide if it is the right arrangement for you.

4. All of the above. Most families play musical beds during their child's early years and juggle bits and pieces of all of these sleeping arrangements. For example, baby may start off in a separate bed or room, then move closer to Mum sometime during the night. Remember, it's about what's best for you and your baby, and adapting to everyone's changing nighttime needs.

Now let's move on to step two.

step 2: learn baby's tired times

When opportunity comes yawning, don't miss it! Watch for drowsy signs. Try to catch her by the third yawn. Observe your baby's need-to-go-to-sleep signs as you do her hunger cues. When babies begin to show signs of being tired, there is a 10–15 minute window of opportunity in which they will fall asleep fairly easily. If you miss this window of opportunity, the tired baby may get progressively more cranky and revved up (the proverbial "second wind"). Even though baby is growing more tired by the minute, this cranky

sleepy signs

Get to know your baby's "I need to go to sleep – NOW!" signals. Here are the usual ones:

- Change in mood. Baby starts to fuss. Some babies become quieter when they are tired or they get less coordinated and their limbs get more "floppy". A great deal of fussing may mean baby is *overtired* and you missed the earlier signals.
- Drooping eyelids
- Nodding head

- Glazed look, "zoning out"
- Yawning
- Whimpering

Toddler signs:
- Rubbing eyes
- Lies on floor
- Grabs favourite sleep prop or "cuddly"

mood makes it harder for him to relax and fall asleep.

The reason for figuring out when your baby is most likely to be tired is so that you can work out when to begin your baby's bedtime ritual (more about bedtime rituals below). If you wait until baby is actually showing signs of being tired and then you give him a bath, put on his pyjamas, feed him, and rock him to sleep, the tired time will be over and baby will be revved up and ready to rock and roll for another hour. A better strategy is to begin the bedtime routine twenty or thirty minutes before the expected tired time. That way, baby will be feeling sleepy just as you get to the part of the bedtime routine when he is supposed to fall asleep. What's more, since sleepy feelings begin to creep over baby as you go through the bedtime ritual, he will eventually learn to associate these drowsy feelings with his usual bedtime ritual.

A prompt response at tired times is especially important in energetic, alert babies and toddlers who fight sleep. The baby or child who is tired but who is resisting going to sleep is trying to tell you, "I don't know how to relax. Please help me!" The longer he fights it, the harder it gets. If you can jump in and ease baby off to sleep before he starts to put up a fight, he will go to sleep more easily and stay asleep longer. He will also learn to associate these first signs of being tired with going to sleep immediately – both at naptime and at nighttime.

As soon as he seems tired, I pick up on his cues. I talk very softly, hold him, feed him, rub him (but not in a stimulating way), and gradually lower my voice and slow down my lullaby. This is his cue that sleep is expected to follow.

Charting your baby's tired times. On the chart below, write down baby's tired time every evening for one or two weeks. Do you see a pattern? Does your baby get sleepy around the same time every night, give or take 15–30 minutes? In our experience, most babies have their natural sleepy time between 6:30 and 7:30pm if they routinely take a nap in the early afternoon, or around 8:30 or 9 if a late afternoon nap is the norm.

Or does your baby get sleepy at times that vary by more than an hour? Your baby's internal clock may not yet have developed a routine sleepy time, especially if he's still quite young. Or, this may be because baby's naptimes are not yet consistent. It may also be

tired time chart

Write down your baby's natural tired times over one week. Tired times are not the times when baby actually falls asleep. They are the times of day when you observe tired behaviour, regardless of whether or not you get baby to sleep at that time.

	Naptimes	Nighttimes
Day 1	_____	_____
Day 2	_____	_____
Day 3	_____	_____
Day 4	_____	_____
Day 5	_____	_____
Day 6	_____	_____
Day 7	_____	_____

If five out of seven of these times are all within 30 minutes of each other at naptimes and bedtime, then you have likely found a predictable sleepy time.

Your baby's predictable Tired Times at this age are:

_____ for naps and _____ for bedtime.

because your family's day-to-day schedule is not predictable.

If your chart is not showing you a predictable evening sleepy time after one week of observation, continue charting for another week. Be sure baby's naps are on a fairly routine schedule. If you still don't find a routine evening sleepy time, you may need to focus more on nap scheduling. In that case, read "Naptime Parenting", chapter 9, now. It takes effort to get baby on a nap schedule. It may be easier to let baby nap whenever he happens to, but in order to get a predictable sleepy time in the evening baby needs to take naps at predictable times as well, most of the time.

Changing your baby's tired time. If you have determined your baby's tired time is around 7:30pm, and you want baby to have an early bedtime, then you're all set. But what if your baby is happily wide awake at 7:30pm, at 8:30pm, even at 9pm? What if your baby doesn't act tired until 10pm? You can either accept this and help baby fall asleep at his natural time, or you can try to change it. If you want your baby to be in bed earlier in the evening (for whatever reasons), put baby down for a nap earlier in the afternoon. You may enjoy having baby's company at night, especially if you are away from your baby during the day. In this case, don't worry about working on an earlier bedtime. What if you would rather have your baby stay up late with you, but baby is always tired by 7:30pm? Again, you can adjust baby's afternoon naps. We'll show you how in chapter 9.

To summarize: find your baby's predictable tired time, schedule your baby's naps if needed to get a more predictable bedtime, start your bedtime ritual about 30 minutes before tired time, and baby will eventually learn to fall asleep easily and predictably.

to schedule or not to schedule?

A week or two of charting baby's tired times may show you that your baby's tired times are more predictable than you thought. Or it may show you that your baby's naptimes and bedtimes depend a great deal on what else is going on in your household. At this point you may have to make some choices: *put yourself on a predictable schedule,* so that baby can take predictable naps and go to bed at the same time every night, or continue to "go with the flow" during the day and give up the idea of baby having a set, early bedtime. You may not be able to have it both ways.

step 3: create a safe and comfortable environment conducive to sleep

If baby's bedroom (or your bedroom) is too light, too dark, too noisy, too quiet, too scary, or too stimulating, your baby may have difficulty going to sleep or staying asleep. Some babies are more sensitive to their sleeping environment than others. What kind of environment is best for your sleeping baby depends on her sleep temperament. For example, some are "subway sleepers", meaning they can sleep through loud noises as long as the noise is always there. Others need a relatively noiseless environment. Here are some ideas to help you set the stage for your baby to sleep.

Quiet the bedroom. Most babies can block out disturbing noise, so you don't have to create a noiseless sleeping environment for your baby. Yet, some babies do startle and awaken easily with sudden noises. For noise-sensitive babies, oil the joints and springs of a squeaky cot or the door hinges, put the dog outside before he barks, and shut the windows.

Quiet the house. Quieting the house down at tired time will give your baby the message that it's time to transition into sleep and also programme her to associate this quiet routine with sleepy time. Lower your voice, close the doors, turn off the phone ringer, slow down your movements, and minimize any other distractions. Turn off the TV and put on some calming music. Let your baby sense that the general mood is changing from one of activity to one of quiet. Don't bounce or jiggle baby. Remember, he's already over stimulated.

I made sure he knew the difference between day and night. During the day I did not try to keep a very quiet house. The phone rang, the dog barked. I kept it dark and quiet at night. I would feed him by nightlight, change him by nightlight, and everything would be calm. During the day we would sing at the changing table, at night we wouldn't sing. Now he understands that when the lights go out it's time for bed and not playtime.

Darken the bedroom. Help your baby learn to associate darkness with sleep. Don't turn on any bright lights during the night, as this can trick baby's internal sleep clock into thinking it's daytime (and wake time!). You can use a nightlight, or install a dimmer switch on the bedroom lights, so that you can keep the light level low during nighttime nappy changes. If necessary, close the curtains to keep out the morning (or evening) light. Use opaque shades to block out the light. This may get you an extra hour of sleep if you have one of those little early birds who wakes with the first ray of sunlight entering the bedroom.

We used a room-darkening temporary shade, a heavy black-pleated fibre paper shade which quickly sticks to the top of the window as a temporary solution.

Warm the bed. Always make sure baby's bed (or yours) is warm. Laying baby down onto cold sheets is a sure way to shock baby awake. One creative dad told us he used to lie in bed with baby snuggled on his chest for five minutes before scooting over and laying baby down in the warm spot. Before laying baby into a cold cot or cradle, warm the sheets with a warm towel from the tumble dryer, a hot water bottle, a heating pad, or an electric blanket (any of which you remove before laying baby down, of course, for safety reasons). Use flannel sheets in cold weather.

Lessen physical discomforts. A baby who itches, hurts, or has difficulty breathing is going to wake up. Here are some tonsil-to-toe tips on helping your baby sleep more comfortably:

- *Clear the nose.* Babies need clear nasal passages to breathe. Bedroom inhalant allergies are a common cause of stuffy noses and consequent night waking.
- *Remove airborne irritants.* Environmental irritants can cause congested breathing passages and awaken baby. Common household examples are cigarette smoke, baby powder, paint fumes, hair spray, animal dander (keep animals out of an allergic child's bedroom), plants, clothing (especially wool), stuffed animals, dust from a bed canopy, feather pillows, blankets, and fuzzy toys that collect lint and dust. If your baby consistently awakens with a stuffy nose, suspect irritants or allergens in the bedroom.
- *Make your baby's bedroom as dust-free as possible.* Besides dusting regularly, remove fuzzy blankets, down comforters, dust-collecting fuzzy toys, etc. If your baby is particularly allergy-prone, a HEPA-type air filter will help. As an added nighttime perk, the "white noise" from the hum of the air filter may help baby stay asleep longer.
- *Relieve teething pain.* Teething discomfort may start as early as three months and continue off and on all the way through the two-year molars. A wet bed sheet under baby's head, a drool rash on the cheeks and chin, swollen and tender gums, and a slight fever are telltale clues that teething is what's disturbing your baby's slumber. If the teething pain seems really bad, with your doctor's advice, give appropriate doses of paracetemol just before parenting your baby to sleep and again in four hours if baby awakens. (See "Teething", page 226).
- *Change wet or soiled nappies.* Wet nappies bother some babies at night. Most are not. If your baby sleeps through wet nappies, there is no need to awaken her for a change – unless you're trying to get rid of a persistent nappy rash. Nighttime bowel movements necessitate a change. Here's a nighttime changing tip: if possible, change the nappy just before a feed, as baby is likely to fall asleep during or after feeding. Some breastfed babies, however, have a bowel movement during or immediately after a feeding and will need changing again. If you are using cloth nappies, putting two or three nappies on your baby before bedtime will decrease the sensation of wetness. Also, if baby is prone to nappy rash, slather on a hefty layer of barrier cream to protect baby's sensitive skin from the sensation and irritation of wetness. Cold nappy wipes are sure to startle baby awake. Run wipes under warm water (a great job for Dad!).
- *Remove irritating sleepwear.* Many infants cannot settle in synthetic sleepwear (some adults, too!). A mother in our practice went through our whole checklist of night waking causes until she discovered her baby was sensitive to polyester sleep suits. Once she changed to 100 per cent cotton clothing, her baby slept better. Besides being restless, some babies show skin allergies to new clothing, detergents and fabric softeners by breaking out in a rash. (See "Sleepwear – How to Dress Your Baby Safely and Comfortably for Sleep", page 72.)

Create a comfortable bedroom temperature.
Try these temperature tips. A consistent
bedroom temperature of around 21°C is
preferable. Also, a relative humidity of around 50
per cent is most conducive to sleep. Dry air may
leave baby with a stuffy nose that awakens him.
Yet humidity that's too high fosters allergy-
producing moulds. A warm-mist vaporizer can
act as a heater in your baby's sleeping area, and
it helps maintain an adequate level of humidity
in homes with central heating (and the "white
noise" of the consistent hum can help baby sleep
longer.)

Fill tiny tummies. The tinier the tummy, the
more frequently babies need to be fed – both day
and night. Babies have tiny tummies – about the
size of their fist – which is why babies under six
months of age need one or two night feedings.
Some babies (especially breastfed) continue to
need night feedings even in the second six
months of life. You can maximize the amount of
time baby will sleep after a feeding by being sure
that baby fills his tummy as he feeds off to sleep
and again when you feed him in the middle of
the night. (See "Night Feedings", pages 131–52
for how to comfortably fill tiny tummies for
longer sleep.)

Swaddle your baby. Swaddling recreates the
womb environment. In the early months, many
babies like to "sleep tight", securely swaddled in
a cotton baby blanket. Older infants like to sleep
"loose", and may sleep longer stretches with
loose coverings that allow them more freedom of
movement. Often, dressing a baby loosely
during the day, but swaddling him at night,
conditions the baby to associate sleep with
swaddling. Make sure baby doesn't get too
warm.

*Once I started swaddling her, she slept through
the night. At about three months she got too
strong to swaddle in the traditional way. She
would get her arms out and rub her face and
startle herself awake. I took a larger thin blanket
and wrapped the sides individually over each
arm and under her back so she couldn't get loose.
It may sound cruel, but she smiles as I do it and
nods off peacefully all night long.*

Babies usually start squirming out of the
swaddling wraps by six months. Another
possible problem with swaddling is that once
babies get used to it, they have a hard time

caution about over swaddling

Dr Robert Salter, Professor of Orthopedics at
the largest children's hospital in the world, the
Hospital for Sick Children in Toronto, Canada,
literally wrote the book on infant hip
development. He wrote me a long letter after
the publication of the first edition of *The Baby
Book*, in which we extolled the merits of
swaddling and showed parents how to swaddle
a baby. He believes leaving babies swaddled
too long, especially in the early months, can
interfere with the development of the ball-and-
socket hip joint. For this reason, we
recommend parents only swaddle babies
during sleep time. Give baby plenty of time to
"let loose" when awake.

sleeping without being swaddled. The movement of their arms and legs wakes them up.

step 4: create a variety of bedtime rituals

You are learning where baby sleeps, when baby sleeps, and how to create a comfortable sleepy environment, and now we come to the next step in our plan: helping you work out what bedtime rituals work best for your baby. As you use these same routines night after night (or alternate through several routines consistently) baby will learn to fall asleep easily and stay asleep longer.

Creating healthy and relaxing sleep associations

A sleep "association" is not a naptime playgroup or a group of sleepy parents who gather to yawn and complain about their baby's sleep habits. A *sleep association* refers to a connection in baby's mind between falling asleep and the various activities, places, experiences, and feelings that precede his nodding off into slumber. The wiring in baby's brain is full of *patterns of association*. For example, if you usually feed and sing your baby to sleep in a rocking chair, this setting will become programmed into your baby's mind as a sleep-inducing routine. He will remember the calm and drowsy feelings he gets from rocking and feeding, and this will help him fall asleep.

What kind of sleep associations do you want to teach your baby? Do you want to create *attachment-based* sleep associations or *independence-based* sleep associations?

- *Attachment-based sleep associations.* Many parents like to "parent" their babies to sleep; rocking, feeding, or snuggling while baby drifts off to sleep. Baby learns to associate falling asleep with a parent's presence. The advantage? Closer bond between parent and baby. The disadvantage? Mum or Dad must be involved with baby falling asleep for months or years. Depending on your own instinctive parenting style, you may actually view this as an advantage; certainly your baby would.
- *Independence-based sleep associations.* Other parents strive to help baby learn a more independent way of falling asleep, without the need for parent involvement. The most popular method for learning to fall asleep independently is the cry it out method. The disadvantage? You don't *teach* baby to fall asleep, you *force* him to. Medical research has shown that excessive crying creates stress for a baby. So a baby learns to associate falling asleep with fear, stress, and worry. This is not healthy in the long run.

(We will discuss sleep anxiety more on page 100 and the harmful effects of crying it out on page 204.) We all want our babies to eventually learn to fall asleep independently by their own self-soothing strategies at an appropriate age. Our sleep plan teaches them how, rather than forcing them to sleep independently.

As parents ourselves, we chose to create attachment-based sleep associations in our kids.

But we know that not all parents will make the same choice. Is there a middle ground? Is there a way to help a baby learn to fall asleep independently but without excessive crying or stress? Is there a way to create attachment-based sleep associations that meet baby's need and at the same time aren't overly demanding on parents? We believe the answer to these questions is YES!

Why is it necessary for you to help your baby develop healthy sleep associations? Why not just put baby down in her cot, walk out of the room, and let her fall asleep on her own? Won't she learn that being in the cot means there's nothing to do now but sleep? Well, yes, she will begin to associate being left alone in the cot with sleep. Her developing brain is busy building patterns of association all the time. That's what brains do. But in the early months, babies do not have the developmental capacity to transition themselves from the state of being awake to being asleep without help. A tiny baby left alone in her cot to fall asleep on her own is likely to cry fearfully and then *sleep anxiously.* Going to sleep anxiously defeats one of the goals of your sleep plan: *to teach baby a healthy attitude about sleep; that sleep is a pleasant state to enter and a happy state to remain in.*

Babies need to be parented to sleep so that they can form pleasant sleep associations. So what kind of activities, experiences, and feelings do you want your baby to associate with going to sleep? Babies who fall asleep while breast- or bottle-feeding will learn to associate warm milk, rhythmic sucking, and being cuddled close to Mum with sleep. Babies who are carried around or rocked to sleep will learn that motion and comfort, as well as contact with Mum or Dad, are what send them into dreamland. Babies who are put in a cot to cry themselves to sleep learn that sleep is a lonely time when they need to comfort themselves.

Remember, you not only want your baby to sleep *longer,* but to sleep *happier.* So, in considering any advice about sleep, including the advice in this book, ask yourself:

"If I were my baby, how would I want to go to sleep?"

Getting behind the eyes of your baby and imagining how you would want your parents to act in a certain situation is one of the most important parenting tools we have learned over our years as parents and pediatricians. You will nearly always make wise decisions about how to parent your children if you begin your decision process by trying to understand the situation from your child's point of view. If you were a baby, would you rather be parented to sleep at the breast of mother or in the arms of father, or just put down in a lonely cot and left to cry off to sleep?

We are now going to show you ways to create sleep associations that have one goal in mind – to help baby learn that sleep is a pleasant state to enter and a happy state to remain in.

Primary and secondary sleep associations

Another concept we want you to understand is primary and secondary sleep associations. Think of your baby's primary sleep association as whatever usually turns on the sleep switch.

and the sleep association winners are:

Primary

- Feeding to sleep (breast or bottle)
- Rocking
- Wearing down in a sling
- Falling asleep independently

Secondary

- Soft music
- Singing lullabies
- Dimmed light
- White noise
- Dummy or "cuddly"
- Patting
- Being walked
- Stroking (massage)
- Swinging
- Dancing in arms
- Scent of mother
- Verbal sleep cues (i.e. "nighty, night" …)
- Stories
- A combination of several

Secondary associations are things such as soft music, dim lights, or stories that may help to calm a child and prepare her for sleep. Some parents will choose one primary sleep association as the foundation, and use several secondary associations to help. Others like to get baby used to several different primary associations for sleep so that they have more options for bedtime.

Choosing sleep associations that fit your baby best

Which primary sleep association is going to work best for your baby? You won't know until you've tried them all. We suggest you go through a trial period of a few weeks to see what primary method of putting baby to sleep works the best. Try feeding baby to sleep a few nights, then try rocking or walking. Try snuggling with baby but not feeding to sleep. Involve Dad in the routine as well. Try a variety of methods until you learn what works best. Here are the main primary associations to consider as you decide what will work best in your family: feeding baby to sleep, feeding baby almost to sleep, lulling baby to sleep without feeding, and laying baby down to fall asleep independently.

1. Breastfeeding or bottle-feeding your baby to sleep. Breastfeeding mums often find the easiest way to get their baby to sleep is by breastfeeding.

In fact, in the first few weeks it is almost impossible to keep a baby awake at the breast for more than ten minutes. Baby is inevitably going to fall asleep feeding. Young babies also fall asleep very easily while bottle-feeding. Breastfeeding seems to be nature's plan for comforting babies and helping them fall asleep. In fact, breast milk contains a sleep-inducing protein that helps lull baby into dreamland. As baby relaxes, so does mother, thanks to the hormones released when baby sucks at the breast.

We recommend that you not place any limitations on your baby feeding to sleep during the early weeks of breastfeeding. In the first four to six weeks after birth, you are learning to read your baby's hunger cues, your baby is learning to tell you when he is hungry, and your milk supply is adjusting to baby's needs. Relax and enjoy the breastfeeding experience.

A smart baby will get to love this feeding-to-sleep association and come to enjoy and expect it for as long as you breastfeed or use bottles. On the one hand, this means that you will be able to count on feeding as an easy way to get baby off to sleep. Even a baby who is fighting sleep will eventually succumb to the relaxing feelings that come from feeding. On the other hand, Mum's breasts have to be there at bedtime, and again, when baby awakens in the middle of the night. Even if breastfeeding is your baby's number one primary sleep association, you may want to help him learn other associations so you have other ways to put him to bed.

In developing our sleep plan, we asked mothers of frequent night wakers, "For your next baby, what will you do differently?" The following answer, from our daughter Hayden (formerly the star of our *Fussy Baby* book and now a new mother), is representative of what many mums told us:

I cherish those precious times of feeding Ashton to sleep, as I realize they will pass all too soon. Yet, for our next baby, I will not use just one way of putting her to sleep. I'll do a variety of things so she's not so set in only one way of falling asleep. This will include my husband, Jason, putting her to sleep now and then, so that when she's older he can put her to sleep in his own way.

Many parents tell us that feeding baby at bedtime and a couple more times during the night works very well for them. Baby is content, and mother manages to get enough sleep, because baby is sleeping close by and she can feed baby back to sleep without waking up completely herself. Maybe Mum wakes a little more often, but she feels that the benefits outweigh any inconvenience for her.

Some mums, however, have told us that at age six months, twelve months, even eighteen months, their babies continue to wake up several times (or more!) each night to feed, and that they can no longer cope with this much night-feeding. They wish that their babies would learn that there is more than one way to fall asleep. Well, babies *can* learn other ways to sleep, and we will share ways to teach a baby new sleep associations later in this book. For now, we want you to know that many mothers breastfeed their babies to sleep for many months, feed them during the night, and still manage to get enough rest. If you currently enjoy breastfeeding your baby to sleep, we don't want to get in the way of a good thing. One of the lessons we want you to learn about parenting is to *enjoy the moment.* We want you to get attached to your baby without worrying about a lot of what-ifs. (If frequent night feeding is a top concern, you will welcome the tips offered in chapter 6.)

2. Feeding baby ALMOST to sleep. Breastfeeding parents who want Dad to be able to put baby to sleep, as well as Mum, often teach their baby sleep associations beyond breastfeeding. Baby breastfeeds at bedtime, settles down, and starts to feel drowsy. Then Dad takes over while baby drifts off to sleep, using walking or rocking while patting baby's back, and other methods, for easing the transition into sleep. (See "Try Our Favourite Nighttime Fathering Strategies", page 176). Bottle-feeding parents can use this approach, too, if they don't want their baby falling asleep with a bottle in her mouth. This approach helps baby learn that there are other ways to fall asleep besides relying on the comfort of sucking. When you use this approach with an older infant who no longer needs two or three nighttime feedings, baby may be less likely to wake up at night and she may be more willing to go back to sleep with just some gentle patting or snuggling from either Mum or Dad.

The main reason for getting baby used to other sleep associations is to avoid mother burnout from frequent night feeding of the older infant (the most frequent sleep concern we encounter in our pediatric practice). In the wonderful world of night feeding, babies absolutely love going fully to sleep at mother's breast and having instant access to this warm and cosy prop when they awake, and if it's working for you please don't change. Yet, it often helps to add the finishing touch of another prop after feeding to help baby go from being awake, but drowsy, through light sleep into a state of deep sleep. Try these finishing touches:

- *Feed, then pat, sing, or rock to sleep.* Instead of feeding baby completely to sleep, breastfeed until she starts to slow down her sucking and closes her eyelids, but she's not yet asleep. Ease your nipple out of her mouth (see Martha's de-latching trick, page 137), and then rock, pat, or sing her down until she is completely asleep.
- *Mother nurse, plus father nurse.* Near the end of the feeding, ease baby gently into father's arms to add the finishing touch (see a complete discussion of how fathers can do this, page 179). Then, hopefully, when baby wakes up, she is more likely to accept Dad or another caregiver putting her back to sleep using the same finishing touch.
- *Add a variety of secondary sleep associations.* You can use any of the tools listed on page 28 to lull your baby to sleep. If these techniques are not working and baby insists on feeding to sleep, consider that a baby who is not willing is not yet ready. Give your baby a few weeks for her sleep patterns to mature and then try again.

3. Putting baby to sleep without feeding. Easier said than done. Because of the sleep association principle discussed above, if baby always falls fully asleep the same way, especially at the breast, she will expect, demand, or even scream for the same prop – usually the breast – to put her back to sleep. Occasionally try putting your baby down when he is sleepy, but not totally asleep (or feeding *almost* to sleep as mentioned in tip number two). Learning to fall asleep without feeding teaches him that it's okay to go to sleep in other ways. Expect that your baby might fuss when you try to use some of these sleep-inducing tools listed on page 28. If he does fuss more than just a little, remember the parenting principle: *don't persist with a bad experiment.* Yet, even if just once or twice a week you try to put your baby down partially asleep, at least you've planted a bit of the "I can do it" association.

4. Putting baby down to sleep independently. Some parents like to set up a more independent sleep arrangement early on, in which, hopefully, baby learns to settle himself down to sleep without much parental interaction. They reason that a baby who learns to fall asleep on his own will also be able to settle himself back to sleep on his own when he wakes during the night. This type of sleep training has become popular with some parents because it results in a "low maintenance" baby at night. It has also received a great deal of criticism because of the amount of crying that baby experiences during the training phase. Babies are born with an innate need for comfort and security while falling asleep, upon waking, while going *back* to sleep, and in some cases even while sleeping.

Ideally, a human caregiver supplies this comfort. Babies who sleep independently

varying baby's sleep associations

Get baby used to a variety of sleep associations at bedtime. The way your baby goes to sleep is the way she expects to go back to sleep when she awakens. When baby is older, you and your partner may want to take turns putting baby to sleep. Baby will learn Mum's way of getting her to sleep (probably feeding) and Dad's way of getting her to sleep (walking, "wearing down" in the baby sling, rocking and humming, and so on). For example, you may decide that you want to have your baby sleep in bed with you, but you are going to vary what you do to help her fall asleep. Some nights Mum will feed baby to sleep. Other nights Dad will soothe baby to sleep. You both can vary your soothing techniques. Some nights wear baby down to sleep by walking her around in a baby sling carrier. Other nights lull her to sleep in a baby swing. Mum has the option of *not* feeding baby to sleep and instead using Dad's "wearing down" technique. You can even vary *where* baby sleeps. Some nights put baby in her cradle. On other nights put her in a cot and bring her into bed with you when she wakes. Or, share the whole night in your big bed together.

usually need to have some sort of secondary sleep association handy to calm them when they are falling asleep and when they awaken. They may need motion, such as rocking, swinging or bouncing movements of a cradle, swing, or baby hammock. They may depend on a dummy. Perhaps they learn to associate soft music or other sounds with sleep. Parents develop a routine around this sleep association that lulls baby into dreamland.

To train babies to fall asleep lying in a cot by themselves without any comforting sleep associations would be very tough on them. In chapter 10 you will learn why we discourage this "tough-love" approach to sleep training when it involves crying it out.

Research shows that a sleep-training method that involves extended crying *alone* (without parent comforting) is not emotionally or physically healthy for babies – or for parents. Very easy-going babies may be able to learn to fall asleep independently with only minimal fuss, and we will offer suggestions on how this can be done in an appropriately sensitive way later in the book. Remember, our goal is for you to create stress-free sleep associations that result in a happy, healthy sleeper.

We'll now go through a list of favourite sleep associations to help your baby fall asleep happier.

Laying baby down to sleep – transitioning tips

Babies don't come equipped with the type of sleep switch that you can suddenly turn off at naptime and bedtime. Yet, a transitioning-to-sleep ritual can be like a *dimmer switch* that gradually tunes out and turns down stimulation in baby's environment. In sleep psychology, this is known as "fading" (like what happens when you are listening to a dull talk). You can't expect a baby to go from his exciting waking life right into sleep. (You don't fall asleep this way, do you?) There has to be a transition time. Here are some favourites that have worked in our families:

Feeding down. If babies could vote, going off to sleep the *warm way* would win the Best Transition Award. A high-touch continuum from warm bath, to warm arms, to warm breast, to warm bed is a winning recipe for sleep. Nestle up next to your baby on your bed and feed her off to sleep. If you feed baby to sleep in your arms, be sure to wait until she is fully asleep before you try to transfer into her own bed. Once baby is asleep, try Martha's de-latch technique (page 137) to learn how to ease away. (For related strategies, see "Night Feeding", page 131, to learn why night feeding is such a special and effective sleep-inducer. See also "Try Our Favourite Nighttime Fathering Strategies" where Dad adds the finishing touch to mother nursing, page 176).

Fathering down. "Nursing" implies comforting, not only breastfeeding. Fathers can and should "nurse" their babies down to sleep. Place baby in the neck nestle position (see illustration, page 177) and "dance" or rock your baby to sleep.

One day after explaining the concept of sleep associations to a tired mother, she replied, "My baby has only one sleep association – ME!" If this is you, read – with your partner – chapter 8, "Twenty-three Nighttime Fathering Tips".

Nestling down. Transferring the sleeping baby from your arms to his bed may prove to be tricky. An abrupt change from being nestled next to a parent's body to lying alone on a mattress will awaken some babies. To ease your baby through this transition, try the intermediate step of lying down on your bed with your sleeping baby still in your arms. We call this the "teddy bear snuggle". Once he's sound asleep (see limp-limb sign opposite), you can ease yourself away and maybe even move him to his own bed.

Sucking down. Sucking is soothing, yet the human pacifier can wear out. Besides the breast or bottle, try your finger or teach baby to find his own hand to suck on.

Patting down. As you are easing baby into her bed, pat her chest or tummy gently and rhythmically, around 60 pats per minute (like your heartbeat). Gradually lighten and slow the patting as she succumbs to sleep. Add some verbal sleep cues (listed on page 36).

As she was just about to sleep, I'd run my fingers across her face, over her eyes, and down her nose so that her eyes would close.

Touching down. Oh, how babies love to be touched as they fall asleep. Here are some ideas for soothing, loving touches:

- Patting – gentle, rhythmic patting on baby's back or bottom while she is being held in your arms. Gentle patting on her tummy can also be used to soothe a baby who is lying in bed,

sears' sleep tip for dads:

Avoid the quick release in getting your baby to sleep. Have patience. Sometimes a too-quick release of the feeling of being securely attached to a parent can bother babies and cause them to jerk back awake. If baby continues to wake up when you try to transition him from your arms into his bed or is not falling completely asleep in your arms while rocking or walking, try putting him down on your chest in the neck nestle position or next to you. Once he is fully asleep (you can tell by observing the *limp-limb sign* – hands unclenched, arms dangling loosely at his side, facial muscles still), then ease yourself away. If baby's hands are fisted and limbs flexed, chances are he is still in the state of light sleep and will awaken if you try to put him down too quickly.

especially when picking her up might be too stimulating.
- Massage – light stroking of baby's head and back is a favourite.
- Skin-to-skin – young babies especially love the familiar feel of your skin on theirs.

Wearing down. Place your baby in a baby sling and wear her around the house for a half-hour or so before the designated bedtime. When she is fully asleep in the sling, ease her out of the sling onto your bed. Or, if she's not fully asleep, lie down with her in the neck nestle or snuggle hold position on your chest. When baby is fully asleep, roll over on your side, slip yourself out of

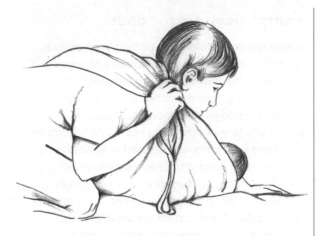

Wearing down in a sling.

the sling, and let baby lie on the bed on her back using the sling as a cover. Wearing down (or what we also dub "slinging down") is particularly useful for the reluctant napper. When baby falls asleep in the sling you can both lie down and enjoy a much-needed mutual nap.

Rocking or walking down. Try rocking baby to sleep in a bedside rocking chair, or walk with baby, patting her back and singing. To keep the motion going (and keep baby asleep), ease her into a cradle and continue the rocking motion at a rate of about sixty rocks per minute. This is the heartbeat rhythm your baby was used to in the womb.

Swinging down. Try a bedside baby hammock. For most babies, motion, not stillness, signals sleep. Remember how your baby used to sleep during the day when you were pregnant but kept you awake at night when you lay down to sleep.

When you were up and around, the motion of your body soothed her into sleep. When you were still, she woke up.

Wind-up swings for winding down babies are a boon to parents when their arms are wearing out. Some infants find the mechanical swing less interesting, if not downright boring, compared to being in the arms of a human being. So, off to sleep they go. Yet some babies are notoriously resistant to mechanical mother substitutes and will protest anything less than the real Mum. Before you actually spend money on a swing, you might want to borrow one for a week or two to see if the spell of the swing will work for your baby. You may discover that you are uncomfortable with mechanical mothering and decide that your baby is better off in your arms.

Driving down. If you've tried all the above transitioning techniques and baby still resists falling asleep, place baby in a car seat and drive around until he falls asleep. When you return home and baby is in a deep sleep, carry the infant car seat (with the sleeping baby) into your bedroom and let baby remain in the car seat until the first night waking. If he is in a deep sleep, you may be able to ease him out of the car seat into his own bed.

Using props. Called transitional objects or "cuddlies", these are favourite toys that help children more easily transition from the familiar and interesting waking world to the world of sleep. Transitional objects should be cuddly, but safe. (See "Sleep Safety", page 72). Rolling over on plastic toys may awaken baby.

Transitional touch. If baby starts to stir as you try to slip her out of your arms or ease away from her in bed, offer the laying on of hands. Place your hand on baby's chest or tummy and leave it there until she drifts back to sleep. This extra touch is especially important in babies who have a hard time transitioning from your arms into the Moses basket or cot. They need this *transitional touch* to stay fully asleep. It can save you a trip back to the rocking chair, to soothe an awakened baby back to sleep.

The scent of mother. Leaving in the cot a breast pad or t-shirt mother wore all day may help baby transition from the whole mother at night.

Music to sleep by. A parent softly singing a lullaby is the classic sound cue for babies to go to sleep. Quiet instrumental music is another traditional favourite. Here are some creative ways you can use sound to soothe baby to sleep:

- Mum's musical voice. The soft sounds of Mum's voice, either in song or in quiet words will mesmerize baby. That's why they're called lullabies.

I saved one song, our sleep song, for when it was time to go to sleep. She learned to associate that song with falling asleep.

need more sound advice?

- Put together a medley of easy-listening lullabies on a CD or tape, and then set the player for continuous play. You won't have to worry about running out of music and breaking the sleepy mood.
- Tape a medley of you singing baby's favourite lullabies. Your familiar voice may help baby settle when put to sleep by someone else.
- For babies in a cradle or cot, turn on a musical mobile to help baby associate the gentle movement and the sound with going to sleep. If the mobile helps to get him to sleep, restart it when he wakes to get him back to sleep.

- Besides choosing music that is easy listening to your ears, select tunes that your baby enjoys. Infants usually settle better with classical music that has slowly rising and falling tempos with lots of repetitive themes. Simple music with repetitive rhythms tends to work best. Turbulent rap or rock music is likely to be a night waker. A music box with classics, such as Brahms' Lullaby, is a proven settler. For some suggestions from the Sears' family library of music to fall asleep by, see Appendix A.

- Dad's deep tones. Some babies really take to Dad's full, rumbly tones. Besides hearing his voice, they can feel the vibrations from the voice box when held on Dad's chest. (See the neck nestle, page 177).
- Rhythmic music. Music with simple repeating words and rhythms is soothing to babies. Nursery rhymes and lullabies are the classic examples. Even quiet pop music with a steady beat can get baby into the rhythm of sleep. Peaceful classical music is another favourite. Complex classical music, on the other hand, can be over stimulating.

More sounds to sleep by. Use *white noise* – monotonous sounds that block out other noises and bore a baby to sleep. Besides the continuous monotone humming or "Shhhh" of a parent, here are some white-noise sounds that work:

- Sound of a fan, air conditioner, or even tape recordings of womb sounds or vacuum cleaner sounds. (Don't wear out your vacuum – record the sound.)
- Running water from a nearby tap or shower. (Record it to conserve water.)
- A bubbling fish tank.
- A loudly ticking clock or a metronome set at sixty beats a minute. (These can be tape-recorded too.)
- Recordings of waterfalls or ocean sounds.
- Rocking in a rocker to the hum of a small fan.

I wore my baby in a sling while vacuuming. The sounds lulled him to sleep and I got some cleaning done.

Our son loves to feed to sleep and sometimes will prolong the feed as much as 30–40 minutes. My partner realized one evening that our son had fallen asleep after only ten minutes while feeding and listening to a quiet Mummy and Daddy conversation. I decided to tape our conversation one evening. Now when our son needs to go to sleep a little faster and my partner isn't around to talk to, I just play our Mummy and Daddy tape.

If baby is restless and won't feed off to sleep, my partner turns on the dishwasher for white noise and then walks baby for a while.

Motion for sleep. What baby doesn't like motion? This is why babies fall asleep in swings, rockers, cars, and while being held and walked. Here are suggestions for slings, swings, and other things you can use to lull baby to sleep:

- Rocking. Mum or Dad's arms and the steady motion of a rocking chair have been putting babies to sleep for ages.
- Cradle. Gently rock baby's cradle to lull baby to sleep or back to sleep.
- Baby swing. Many babies will drift off to sleep in a baby swing at nap time or bedtime.
- Baby slings. "Wearing baby" in a sling or other infant carrier while you move about simulates the womb environment and will soothe baby to sleep. (See wearing down, page 148).

Dancing for all the senses. You can combine all kinds of sensory input in a dance that will envelop baby in a soothing environment. This works well for fussy babies or those that fight sleep. Snuggle baby in your arms, either in the

science says: crying it out could be harmful to babies

Is it possible that excessive crying can harm a baby's intellectual, emotional, and social development? Here is how science answers this alarming question:

- Infants who are routinely separated from parents in a stressful way have abnormally high levels of the stress hormone cortisol and lower growth hormone levels. These imbalances inhibit the growth of nerve tissue in the brain.[1, 2, 3, 4]
- Researchers at Yale University and Harvard Medical School found that intense stress early in life can alter the brain's neurotransmitters and structure in a similar way to that found in adults with depression.[5, 6]
- A study from the University of Hertfordshire, U.K., showed infants with persistent crying episodes were 10 times more likely to grow up to have ADHD, concluding this may be due to unresponsive parenting.[7]
- Research at Baylor University found when chronic stress over-stimulates an infant's brain, the child will grow up with an over-active adrenaline system, causing aggression, impulsivity, and violence later in life.[8]
- Studies at the UCLA School of Medicine found the stress hormone cortisol actually destroys nerve connections in critical portions of an infant's developing brain, and when babies are neglected, they can grow up to be violent, impulsive, and emotionally unattached children.[9, 10]
- Doctors at Case Western and Duke Universities showed prolonged crying in infants caused increased pressure in the brain, elevated stress hormones and decreased oxygenation to the brain.[11, 12]
- Researchers found babies whose cries are usually ignored will not develop healthy intellectual and social skills.[13]
- Doctors at the National Institute of Health found that infants with prolonged crying (not due to colic) in the first 3 months of life had an average IQ 9 points lower at five years of age and had poor fine motor development.[14]
- Infants with excessive crying during the early months show difficulty controlling their emotions and become even fussier when parents try to console them at 10 months.[15]

All babies cry, and most babies grow up to be emotionally and neurologically healthy children. However, this research is clear on one point: intense, extended periods of crying alone can permanently harm a baby's developing brain. What does this mean for the CIO method? A baby who only cries briefly for a few nights is probably fine. What about crying for many minutes, night after night? We can't say how many minutes and how many nights are safe, because no one has ever researched this. We urge parents to be very cautious if they decide to try this method.

cradle hold, up on your shoulder, or draped tummy down over your forearm. Move around gently in all directions – up, down, and back and forth, and pat baby's bottom as you hum, sing, or make other gentle sounds. All this gentle stimulation blocks out the anxious, fretful feelings coming from inside of baby and really takes baby back to the womb.

A box full of tricks. While most babies need a predictable routine to get to sleep, some enjoy novelty. And even your best transitioning tips may not work when baby enters a new stage of development. You need a box full of sleep strategies to see you through the first year or two of your baby's life. Keep trying new things.

Your attitude. Consider winding-down routines as an opportunity to spend *quality time* with

your child. Enjoy this peaceful time together. Don't look at your watch. Don't think about everything else you have to do. Your baby will pick up on your relaxed attitude and probably go to sleep more easily.

Trial Period

During this first week or two you will be trying to work out what primary sleep associations work for your baby.

For newborns and younger babies, you will be trying to find one (or maybe two) things that you can depend on to get your baby off to sleep. This may turn out to be feeding, rocking or walking.

For older infants and those who already have a strong primary sleep association (in other words, something you can count on to

	Primary association tried	Secondary associations	How long it took baby to fall asleep
Day 1	_____	_____	_____
Day 2	_____	_____	_____
Day 3	_____	_____	_____
Day 4	_____	_____	_____
Day 5	_____	_____	_____
Day 6	_____	_____	_____
Day 7	_____	_____	_____

What is your baby's favourite sleep-association combo? _____

nearly always turn on the sleep switch), you will be trying to find one or two new primary sleep associations either because the old ones are no longer working for you or because you want your baby to be able to fall asleep in other ways. Your baby will probably protest or fight this change and want you to go back to the tried-and-true. Keep trying different ideas, as long as you are comfortable. Use secondary sleep associations, such as music or motion, along with whatever primary sleep association you are trying to establish. Write down your observations, to help you remember what works.

Now that you have figured out a variety of ways to happily parent your baby to sleep, let's learn ways of helping baby to enjoy sleeping *longer.*

step 5: help baby stay asleep longer

Babies – and parents – enjoy a more restful night if their sleep is not cut short. As you will learn in chapter 3, babies are wired to wake up during the night, and they usually need a parent's help to settle back into sleep. As babies mature, so do their sleep patterns, so that they are able to sleep longer stretches and resettle themselves. When this blissful time happens varies greatly from baby to baby. While you can't force your baby to sleep through the night, you can provide conditions that will help your child attain sleep maturity to sleep longer stretches.

Why do babies wake up so much? Answer: they're babies! In chapter 3 and chapter 11 we'll discuss the many developmental, medical, and physical reasons babies wake up. Keeping in mind that breastfeeding babies under one year typically need to feed twice a night, and over a year sometimes at least once, here are some ideas for teaching babies how to go back to sleep.

Change where baby sleeps. In step one you chose where you want baby to sleep. Hopefully it is working for both of you. However, the bed that baby starts the night in may not necessarily be the same bed she wakes up in each morning. Consider this: is your baby waking during the night because she is alone in another room and wants to be closer to you? If you think this may be the case, try moving baby closer to you (see "Sleeping in your room, but not in your bed", page 3, or "Sleeping with baby in your bed", page 4) at the first night waking. Or is baby already in your bed, and waking up *because* you are right there? If so, try moving baby further away from you when you come to bed or at the first night waking.

"Coach" baby to sleep. Repeating cue words, sounds that baby associates with going to sleep, will often help baby get back to sleep. Offer these cues as the last sound baby hears before drifting off to sleep and use these same words again when she awakens in the middle of the night: "night-night", "sleepy-sleepy", "happy nappy", or "Shhhh". Using the sleep associations principle, baby learns to associate these sounds with both going to sleep and going back to sleep. The time-tested sound "shhhh", which mothers naturally do, has a biological basis. It is similar to the sound of uterine blood flow that baby was used to while in the womb.

When he made his first peep, we quickly issued reminders, such as: "Shhhh … sleepy-sleepy." We let him know that it wasn't time to get up yet.

Lay on hands. When baby stirs, gently lay hands on her without picking her up. Stay with her and continue laying on a comforting hand as you say or sing your favourite sleep cues, such as "night-night", "sleepy-sleepy" … Stay by her bedside until she falls asleep. If she starts to wake up right away or awakens during the night, again lay on hands and give her your "sleepy-sleepy" sleep cue. Hopefully this will be enough to soothe her back to sleep. If she just can't fall asleep, pick her up and walk around the bedroom a while holding her in a sleep-inducing position, such as the neck nestle (see this technique, page 177), or sit in a rocking chair or recliner and try to get her back to sleep.

Leave a little bit of mother behind. To help a baby stay asleep when you are not there, have something nearby that smells like you. This might be a breast pad, which has the odour of your milk, or an item of your clothing. Your bed will naturally have your scent. You can also sleep with baby's cot or cradle sheets for a night (use them for a pillow case), and then place them on baby's mattress. Your scent should last for a few days.

I feed and wear my baby a lot during the day. He actually sleeps better if I take off the shirt that I have worn all day and cover him with it before I put the blanket on him at night.

Offer a thumb or a dummy. Pacifier, the American name for dummy, literally means "peacemaker". Giving baby something to suck on will often bring peace to both baby and parents. You can actually help your baby learn to suck his thumb. Thumbs are handier than dummies. They are warm, soft, and easily available. They don't fall on the floor; they are just the right size for baby's mouth. They don't obstruct the nose or need to be clipped on with a cord. Babies feel more in control of a thumb.

As you're putting baby down to sleep, ease her thumb into her mouth, and do this again each time she wakes up. This way she learns to associate sucking her thumb with going to sleep – and back to sleep. If baby continues to suck but wakes up anyway, she's probably hungry and needs you, and not just a milk-less thumb. During a check-up when I need tiny babies to be quiet so that I can listen to their hearts, I sometimes insert their thumb in their mouth. Sometimes I notice mothers raise their eyebrows as if they didn't realize they could do this. Babies in the womb suck their thumbs. In the early months, babies who can't quite find their thumbs will suck on their wrists, or even forearms. They are born with their own natural pacifier. Take advantage of it. And don't overuse artificial pacifiers. If when baby cries you find yourself by reflex reaching for the dummy instead of baby, remember our advice: "use it, don't abuse it, and quickly try to lose it".

Some parents worry that purposely teaching baby to suck his thumb will lead to a long-term habit which will be hard to break (you can't just throw the thumb away like you can the dummy). While this can happen, if it gets you a better night's sleep for now it's probably worth it.

Try both the quick and the delayed response. Should you come running as soon as you hear your baby awaken in the night? Or should you hold off and see if baby goes back to sleep? Again, it's your decision. Some parents find it easier if they quickly get to baby and help baby back to sleep before the cries escalate and baby gets revved up. If you wait too long, it can be much harder for both mother and baby to get back to sleep. With co-sleeping babies, a half-awake mother can simply roll over and feed her half-awake baby, and the pair drift back to sleep without either one getting worked up. Other parents find that if they just let their baby squirm and fuss a bit, baby is able to resettle without intervention. This is a waking-by-waking decision. It helps to remember that not all noises that sleeping babies make are cries for help. (See "Normal Night Noises Sleeping Babies Make", page 61). If you think your baby can settle himself back to sleep, delay rushing in and picking him up. Give him a chance to work things out on his own. He will let you know if he needs help.

Sometimes in the middle of the night I would quickly offer her a breast or a "soothie" dummy and she would not fully wake up.

The trick is to never let him fully wake up and never let him cry. If he cries, he's wide awake.

learn when to let sleeping babies lie

One of the most difficult lessons for new co-sleeping/breastfeeding mothers is to develop a balance between "I feed my baby at the first whimper" and "Oh, that's just a normal sleep noise – she'll go back to sleep by herself." If you feed your baby right away, you will probably both get back to sleep sooner. Yet if you feed every time she awakens, you may end up with a baby who wants to feed all night long and doesn't know any other way of falling back to sleep. You have to try to find the balance that works best for you and your baby. We'll discuss this dilemma in detail in chapter 6.

Keep it simple and quick. No middle-of-the-night entertainment, please. You're there as a comforter, not a playmate. Nighttime is for sleeping, not for playing. If baby needs your help to resettle, try to do it quickly, calmly, and comfortably. Even though you're tired – and perhaps angry – try what we dub the *Caribbean approach* – "no problem, baby". If baby senses your anxiety and irritation, she is less likely to resettle. Try to resettle baby with a simple song or patting with your hands. If you need to pick up baby for a bit of swaying or rocking, don't make the routine too interesting. Your goal is to lull her back to sleep.

Someday your child will find the promised land of sleeping through the night. Babies will wean! This high maintenance stage of nighttime parenting will pass. The time in your arms, at your breast, and in your bed is a relatively short

your checklist of sleep tools

In helping your baby sleep happier, healthier, and longer, here's a checklist of all the topics we covered in this chapter, or will cover in subsequent chapters:

- Review sleep safety (page 72)
- Juggle different sleeping arrangements to see where baby sleeps best (page 2)
- Chart baby's tired times (page 7)
- Try a variety of sleep associations (pages 12, 17)
- Turn on sounds to sleep by (page 21)
- Try a loving touch (page 19)
- Offer a familiar scent (page 26)
- Offer a dummy (page 26)
- Try motion for sleep (page 22)
- Try feeding baby partially to sleep (page 16)
- Teach baby back-to-sleep cues (page 25)
- Enjoy bedtime rituals (page 12)
- Enjoy feeding down (page 14)
- Try wearing down (page 19)
- Try fathering down (pages 18, 176)
- Try nestling down (page 19)
- Try patting down (page 19)
- Try walking/rocking down (page 20)
- Try swinging down (page 20)
- Offer a "cuddly"(page 20)
- Quiet the bedroom (page 9)
- Quiet the house (page 9)
- Darken the room (page 9)
- Warm the bed (page 9)
- Clear stuffy noses (page 10)
- Fill tiny tummies (page 11)
- Swaddle baby (page 11)
- Create a comfortable bedroom temperature (page 11)
- Dress baby comfortably for sleep (page 72)

while in the life of a baby, yet the memories of love and availability last forever.

keep a sleep log

While most mothers would rather spend their free time resting than filling in charts, sleep logs can help in many ways. Charts give you a visual picture of your child's individual 24-hour sleep patterns. You may be surprised that he sleeps more – or less – than you thought. Sleep logs help you spot problem times and track progress to see if your sleep strategies are working. When discussing your baby's sleep concerns with your health visitor or GP, show him or her the sleep log and point out the problem areas that you've identified. In this way you can see at a glance your baby's sleep patterns and where certain sleep strategies may be applied. Photocopy the sample sleep log on the next page. As you try all the sleep-inducing strategies described in chapters 1 and 2, fill in the sleep log as you chart your baby's progress.

10 day sleep log

Directions: Colour black each hour of sleep including daytime naps. Mark ‡ for each time your baby wakes up. Mark F for each time you feed baby.

DAY	8am	9am	10am	11am	12am	1pm	2pm	3pm	4pm	5pm	6pm	7pm	8pm	9pm	10pm	11pm	12pm	1am	2am	3am	4am	5am	6am	7am	Total Hours of Sleep	No. & Time of Night-wakings	Comments
1																											
2																											
3																											
4																											
5																											
6																											
7																											
8																											
9																											
10																											

Comments: _____

chapter 2

fifteen tips to
help toddlers sleep

The five steps to happy sleeping that we described in the previous chapter apply to toddlers as well as babies. Yet, as babies turn into toddlers, their nighttime needs change and parents need to learn more sleep strategies. Toddlers still need your presence at bedtime, and their bedtime rituals will reflect their need for closeness.

Sometime between two and three years of age, children begin to form conscious memories that will stay with them for the rest of their lives. What bedtime memories do you want your child to file away?

Sears' Parenting Tip: As children learn to sleep, they learn to live.

what toddlers learn at bedtime

It's good to have goals as a parent. When you know what you want for your children in the long term, it's easier to do the things you have to do right now to reach that goal. So what are your sleep goals for your child? Two important sleep goals are:

- Children should learn that sleep is a pleasant state to enter and a peaceful state to stay in, and therefore develop healthy sleep habits.
- Children should have pleasant memories of how they were parented to sleep.

Children need to develop a pleasant attitude toward falling asleep and staying asleep. We believe that your child's ability to sleep well in the future depends on his having happy, stress-free, positive experiences at bedtime when he is young. Eventually, these positive experiences will translate into sleep independence – the ability to fall asleep and back to sleep on his own. And all these good sleep experiences will help your child grow up to be a happier, less stressed, and healthier person.

Many well-meaning parents push their kids into sleep independence too soon. After a long day at work and caring for the kids, parents need a break and want the evening for themselves. Between the ages of one and four their whole goal at bedtime is for a child to fall asleep on his own, and do so quickly and quietly. When this is achieved, parents feel they have finally succeeded in creating a "good sleeper".

But what if a child isn't quite ready for this? What happens when a child grows up feeling that bedtime is a time when she is forced to stay in a darkened room alone and told to be quiet and go to sleep? This is a child who will procrastinate because she fears or resents the isolation at bedtime. She will make up all kinds of reasons why she wants Mum or Dad's attention at bedtime. She will get up to come and find you because she's thirsty or there's a monster under the bed. She will ask you to leave the light on or the door open. She will use every stalling tactic she can think of when what she really means is she just wants *you*. This is a child who is more likely to grow up with a fear of bedtime, of the dark, and of being alone. She may feel anxious and insecure, because her parents have pushed her into nighttime independence before she was truly ready. Imagine how you, as an adult, would feel if you went to bed every night feeling stressed, scared, and unfulfilled. There is one more ingredient that parents often add to this bedtime picture without realizing it – anger or hostility. We use phrases like "Get back to bed", "If you get out of bed one more time …" "Stop your whining and go to sleep." Even if there is no anger in your voice, these negative phrases night after night over the years add up to a child who resents and fears bedtime.

Ask yourself: are you willing to put in some time now to help your kids achieve the long-term goal of a healthy attitude about sleep and a trusting, secure attitude toward life?

Remember what we said about keeping the long-term goal in mind when you are making short-term decisions about parenting? While most of what is in this chapter assumes that you are going to be close by while your toddler drifts off to sleep, one of your long-term goals is a child who goes to sleep happily on his own. So, keep in mind that while you are *parenting*, not just putting your toddler to sleep, you are also teaching him skills and attitudes that he will someday use to help himself fall asleep without you there. As he is ready, you are encouraging him to use these skills. No, you are not a victim of childish manipulation. When you rub a child's back at bedtime to help her relax or soothe a tearful toddler with quiet talking in the middle of the night, you are modelling self-help skills. When your child is ready to cope with these challenges on his own, he will call up images of the good feelings he had while falling asleep in your presence. And bingo, he'll fall asleep.

easing your toddler off to dreamland – fifteen tips

We'll begin with fifteen tips that apply to nearly all toddlers. These are practical strategies aimed at 1) getting little ones off to dreamland and 2) teaching them a healthy attitude toward sleep. The second half of this chapter turns the spotlight (or a very dim nightlight – don't want to wake the kids) on common toddler sleep concerns – and solutions – that tired parents have shared with us.

One night my daughter called out "Mummy, I need you!" I went straight away to her room, fed her, and she sleepily said, "Thank you, Mummy" and drifted off to sleep. I thank God that she knows we are here for her and that she uses us when she needs us. I hope that this will be a life-long pattern, not just in sleep, but with her everyday life.

1. Tire out your toddler

Encourage your child to be active during the day. The more physical activity that children – and adults – get during the day, the better they sleep at night. Babies who are not yet walking can be encouraged to play on the floor, cruise and crawl. Take your toddler to the park and run, jump, and bounce on the playground equipment. Toddlers get their exercise in bursts of activity. They don't take long walks or set out to jog three miles as adults do. They take frequent rest stops during active play, but they don't mind being active much of the day. Toddlers should not be plugged in for more than a half-hour a day playing video games or watching television.

Sears' Sleep Tip: Kids who are couch potatoes by day tend to sleep less at night.

2. Set consistent bedtimes

Infants and toddlers generally go to bed "too late". Or they go to bed at different times every night. Modern families' busy daytime lifestyles encourage this "whenever" approach to bedtime. Unless your family's lifestyle allows for your toddler to sleep later in the morning, try to set an early and consistent bedtime for your little one. Even if a later bedtime is what works best in your family, try to be consistent about when your child goes to bed. By putting kids to bed at the same time night after night you are programming their internal sleep clock to fall asleep easily at this set time.

3. Set the stage

Toddlers and preschoolers are not going to go to bed willingly if there is a lot of activity going on in your household. They don't like to miss out. When it's time for your toddler to go to bed, turn down the lights all over the house, turn off the television (you can record what you're missing), and channel older children's energy into quiet activities. As you turn down the household activity level, let your child know that bedtime is coming. Set the kitchen timer for 10 or 15 minutes and tell your child that when the timer

nighttime props for tots

While a mother's breast, a father's arms, and a familiar voice singing a lullaby will always be your child's favourite sleep inducers, there are times when parents need some reinforcement. Try these:

- *An aquarium.* The bubbles, the graceful fish, the hum of the heater, the lights and shadows – the slowly changing patterns all built into this cute container are mesmerizing. They will calm toddlers and eventually bore them to sleep.
- *White noise machines.* A favourite of adults, these bedside sound machines allow you to choose various monotonous sounds, such as a bubbling brook, ocean waves, rainfall, and melodious chants, that soothe young and old into sleep. (See "More Sounds to Sleep By", page 22).
- *An air filter.* A HEPA air filter not only rids the bedroom air of dust, allergens, and other nose stuffing and night waking irritants, but also produces white noise that blocks out other sounds that may awaken a light sleeper.
- *A dimmer switch.* Gradually dimming the lights will help ease your toddler into sleep. See if you can find a dimmer that can be operated with a remote control. Or put a dimmer on the reading lamp next to the bed.

goes off, it's bedtime. Or use an egg timer and say, "When all the sand hits the bottom, it's time to start getting ready for bed". Kids are less likely to argue with a timer than with a parent.

4. Enjoy a variety of bedtime rituals

Bedtime rituals are all the things you do consistently, every night, starting a half hour to an hour *before* tired time. Bedtime rituals help the busy toddler wind down and make the transition from an exciting and active evening to the quietness and relative boredom of sleep.

You can't force a child to sleep, but you can create a quiet, soothing environment that allows sleep to overcome the child. Avoid stimulating activities, such as wrestling or running around the house for a while before bedtime. Save exciting activities that rev up a child's mind and body for late afternoon. Children need a buffer zone between a busy day and bedtime. Quiet activities and a regular bedtime routine can help kids make the transition from awake time to sleepy time.

Bedtime routines don't have to be exactly the same from night to night. Toddlers enjoy novelty. Bedtime with Mum may be different from bedtime with Dad, but that's good.

Even children who are very tired may not be willing to give up and go to bed. They don't want to be separated from you or miss anything interesting. This is why bedtime rituals need to be creative and include quality time with parents. Bedtime routines should be interesting and special, even as they wind children down from an active day.

Ritual tips. Different babies enjoy different rituals at different ages. Be flexible. What works one month may not necessarily work the next. Here are some tried and true favourites:

- The Bedtime B's: bath, bottle or breastfeeding, backrub, book, and clean bottom (if bath time revs up your child, bathe her during the day).
- Strolling through the house with baby in a sling (see "wearing down", page 19).
- Reading a poem or singing "Twinkle, Twinkle Little Star".
- Saying goodnight to everyone: toddlers love long goodnight lists: "Good night, toys, good night, pets, good night, Mummy, good night, Granddaddy", etc.
- The bath and favourite, calming book combination.
- Back rubs. Give your child a massage and gradually lighten your touch as your child drifts off to sleep. Or "plant a garden" on your child's back using different touches for the different kinds of seeds your child asks to plant. Gradually lighten your strokes as you smooth out the soil.
- Listen to music and hum or sing along. Choose quiet, gentle songs, not get-up-and-dance-along music. You may find that playing or singing one *special song* becomes part of your settling-down-to-sleep routine.

- Your child may fall asleep more easily if there is quiet background activity in the household instead of complete quiet. A little bit of noise reassures her that you are close by.
- Feeding to sleep – a perennial favourite.

I'd save all my phone calls and return them when I knew my toddler was ready for sleep. Toddlers always want to feed when you're on the phone, so take advantage of that and let the quiet ebb and flow of your voice lull baby right to sleep.

Signing off. The bedtime ritual that worked best for us with our toddler, Matthew, who had a hard time winding down and leaving the excitement of daytime activities, was one we called "signing off". When it was near his bedtime, we made the rounds: "Say night-night to the toys, night-night to Mummy, night-night to Princess (the cat), night-night to Honey Bee (the dog)." As we walked upstairs, we said night-night to the relatives in the photos on the wall, and night-night to whatever else we encountered between the family room and the bedroom. When we finally arrived in the bedroom, we completed the wind-down ritual by saying night-night to the toys and pictures on the wall. This slow signing off seems to help children who are so engrossed in their play that they have a hard time transitioning into bedtime.

The fish story. When Matthew was three, an evening of exciting activity often meant that he would have a hard time falling asleep. So after he had climbed in bed, I would tell him a "fish story". It was not an exciting tale about the one that got away. Instead, it went like this: "When I was a young boy, I used to go fishing … and I would catch one fish, two fish, three fish …" With each fish my voice got lower and slower. Some nights it was a ten-fish story, other nights I caught twenty fish before Matthew was peacefully asleep. Basically, I was boring him to sleep.

Before bed prayers. Nighttime prayers are a way to share your faith with your child. We have always felt that the words children hear as they drift off to sleep are imprinted more deeply in their minds than words spoken during the day. You can say the same prayer every night, either a traditional child's prayer or one you make up in your family, or use a basic prayer with variations based on the child's day ("Thank you, God, for …") This prayer is likely to stay in your child's memory for the rest of his life.

5. Respond to sleepy signs

Throughout this book, we have urged you to respond to signs that your baby is tired. Toddlers, like babies, go to sleep more easily when they are feeling sleepy. Watch for signs that your child is tired and ready to wind down and go to sleep:

- Activity slows, lies on floor, rubs eyes, yawns (younger toddler)
- Activity picks up – to fend off the send off (older, wiser toddler)
- Picks up cuddly and ambles toward bedroom (fairy tale toddler)

If you wait to start your ritual until after tired signs begin, you'll miss this window of opportunity. For some toddlers, preparations for going to sleep can wind them up. If you wait until he's tired to start getting ready for bed, he may be all charged up again by the time he's clean, dry, and in pyjamas. Bathe him, brush his teeth, put his pyjamas on and get him all ready for bed *before* the usual time the drowsy signs occur. Let your child become drowsy while you do the quiet part of your ritual like stories, massages, and snuggling.

Rather than do the whole ritual thing, we simply did quiet things until our toddler gave off tired signals. If she wasn't in pyjamas, no big deal. I'd feed her to sleep and that was it. As long as clothes are clean and comfortable anything can be "pyjamas". Tooth brushing can be whenever, too. And if you get caught by tired time and the clothes are dirty, change them once baby is out. Do the main thing, feed off to sleep when the window opens or it will close while you're fiddling around with toothbrushes and outfits.

6. Enjoy bedtime stories

A story tops off the day, like dessert at the end of a meal. Reading to your child is an important part of nighttime parenting, one that most parents enjoy most of the time. (There may be one or two stories that your child absolutely *loves* that you might get a *little* tired of.) If you treasure the time you spend reading bedtime stories, you will radiate patience and relaxation as you read them. If your child senses you are tense and just trying to get to the last page (or trying to actually *skip* pages), she won't fall asleep as quickly. Here's how to get the most out of books for babies:

- *Love your books.* Since you're going to spend a lot of time reading, pick stories that *you enjoy too,* so that when your little one pleads, "Read it again", you won't mind. Martha and I have been reading bedtime stories for 38 years now. Our last child, Lauren, was no longer breastfeeding as a toddler (she's ours by adoption), so it took a large stack of books, and she loved every one. It was a great way to get our biggest night owl to lie still long enough to get relaxed and drift off. Some of our favourites that are appropriate for children ranging from two to five years are listed in Appendix B, page 259.
- *Use your sleepy-soothing voice.* Speak gently, quietly, and in a monotonous voice. Avoid exaggerated facial expressions or sudden change in volume, which can startle a child awake. Gradually pause longer between sentences and read more slowly and softly toward the end of the story.
- *Keep it simple.* Read age-appropriate stories with simple pictures. Try to keep to *one* book. Otherwise, your child may awaken during the pause while you search for another book.
- *Position for sleep.* Have your child lie in her most common sleeping position while you read to her.
- *Don't stop too soon.* Even though their eyes are closing, children's ears are very keen to follow a story. We once heard a child instruct his mother to "Keep reading – I can still hear you even when I'm sleeping."

I read to my three-year-old daughter at bedtime, and then she tells me "good night, love you, sweet dreams" and then rolls over and goes to sleep on her own.

7. Put a "cuddly" to bed, too

As you tuck in your toddler, put a favourite stuffed toy, doll, or other "cuddly" to bed next to her. Help her tuck her little friend under the covers and give her cuddly a hug or a kiss goodnight. Watch her parent her doll or toy off to sleep the same way you help her sleep – this will help her wind down. On nights when your child is reluctant to go to bed, tell her, "Let's go put dolly to bed". As she shares in dolly's bedtime ritual, she will get ready for sleep herself.

I stumbled upon a way to get Ashton to fall asleep once when she was just resisting. I went cheek to cheek with her as if I was giving her a hug and I nibbled her earlobe with my lips. I immediately felt her body relax and her eyelids start to droop. The rhythmic nibbling combined with the warmth of my breath and our closeness to each other sent her quickly into dreamland. It was also very soothing for me and a good tool for my partner to try.

8. Offer sleep cues

Find a few favourite phrases that relax your child. Say these over and over in a singsong voice as your child is falling asleep or when he needs assistance in getting back to sleep. The child hears your soothing voice, but doesn't have to think about what you are saying. Dr Bob used to repeat, "Rest your eyes" to his son over and over again. Try:

- "Nighty-night"
- "Go night-night"
- "Sleepy-sleepy"
- "Time for sleep"
- "Sleep now"

Find a phrase that is reassuring to your child during the day and use it consistently to help him recover from a meltdown, something like, "It's okay!" Soon your child will learn to associate "It's okay" with settling. When he awakens from a scary dream or some other reason, hearing the familiar "It's okay" may quickly resettle him back to sleep.

Our two-year-old loves trains. Sometimes he wakes up during the night fussy and upset and we say, "Can you hear the train?" and we make train noises. He listens, nods, and stops crying. He knows we can't hear the real train, but at least he will stop crying to listen carefully.

9. Enlist help from a sibling

At age six, our daughter Hayden could easily "mother" her two-year-old sister, Erin, to sleep (because she had plenty of it when she was little). We would occasionally encourage Hayden to lie down with Erin and sing to her or look at a picture book and get her to sleep "just like Mummy and Daddy did with you". Erin fell asleep, and sometimes Hayden did too. We got a lot of mileage from sibling co-sleeping. When we had two close-in-age children that we wanted to go to bed at the same time, we would announce, "Whoever is in bed first, picks the story."

Sears' Parenting Tip: Your future grandchildren will value the parenting-to-bed skills you taught their mother or father.

10. Make peace before bedtime

Children, like adults, have difficulty sleeping when they are angry or upset. If children have been arguing or fighting during the day, help them make up before bedtime and go to bed friends. If you and your child have been at odds all day, or if it has been an upsetting day for other reasons, take time to talk it out briefly, then do something pleasant with your child before bedtime. Maybe this is a night for an extra bedtime story, or for a tale from your adventures as a child. Cuddle your child off to sleep and help him clear his mind of upsetting thoughts. This can even be a part of your sign-off prayer to help it happen in a neutral way.

11. Try a reward chart

If bedtime is not going well at your house, try a reward chart. Set the timer to announce bedtime, and tell your child that if he goes to bed without complaining, he will get a gold star on his chart. After three good nights in a row, take him out for a fun reward (fun as in play, not as in a junky treat). When you've had a success or two, change the reward schedule to once every 7 days. Soon he'll forget all about the chart.

12. Water your child

"I need a drink of water" is a classic stall tactic. Head this off by giving your child a drink of water in the bathroom before bed. Call it the "last drink" so she knows she can't keep asking for water. Or, put a trainer cup or water bottle next to the child's bed to quench the thirst that invariably hits as soon as the child is under the covers. He'll enjoy the independent feel of having it on hand for himself, especially if he feels he's had a good dose of hands-on nighttime parenting.

13. Use a nightlight

Sleep researchers have shown that the brain is able to sleep better at night with no light on, but some children are afraid of complete darkness. Try using a dim night light in your child's room. An older child may feel more secure with his own flashlight or a reading light next to his bed that he can turn on if he wakes up. With our daughter Lauren we found that when she was older and in her own room she was happier when we let her keep the light on. We then turned it off when we went to bed.

14. Try the "fade away" strategies

Getting your baby to sleep independently implies helping your baby get used to needing less of you and comfortably relying on his own self-settling abilities. "Fading away", means gradually weaning your child from breast, bottle, arms, voice, and eventually your presence at his bedside as he falls asleep. (See pages 160–1 for examples of this getting-baby-to-sleep-alone strategy.)

15. Just go to bed!

You know your child is tired, you've been through the whole wind-down ritual, but he will not go to sleep. In this case, tell your child to go to his bedroom, lie in his bed, and either look at books or play quietly. If he still needs you close by, read your own book or magazine in his room. If he has to entertain himself, he will probably soon be ready to sleep.

The rule is he doesn't have to go to sleep. He just needs to stay in bed. He is allowed to read as long as he wants. He seems to get to sleep earlier and easier when he feels he has some control of his sleep time.

teaching your young child to fall asleep alone and happy

Putting your child to bed while you are there snuggling with her is easy. The challenge that most parents face is getting a child to learn to fall asleep without Mum or Dad there. All the steps so far in this chapter are designed to help your child feel comfortable and happy at bedtime, but how do you move towards sleep independence in a way your child will accept?

A better question is this: is it realistic for parents to expect all young kids to fall asleep alone? In our experience the answer is no. Around age two or three a child's imagination kicks in and they develop a fear of being alone in the dark at night. They can imagine monsters in the closet or under the bed. Or they may simply want you there for no particular reason. This is normal behaviour for a child. But because these fears are irrational, most parents don't take them seriously and simply expect their child to get over them. Even kids who slept alone as babies can begin to fear sleeping alone later on.

So how can parents get their kids to be happy going to bed alone? Slowly, gradually, and as peacefully as possible. Getting your child to sleep independently implies helping her get used to needing less of you and comfortably relying on her own self-settling abilities. It means gradually weaning your child from your arms, voice, and eventually your presence at her bedside as she falls asleep.

If you have been staying with your child while she falls asleep up to this point, then there is probably very little stress to overcome. If your child used to fall asleep alone but has stopped, and you now realize that there may have been some months of stress while you've tried to accomplish sleep independence again, then you will probably need to take a step backwards in the weaning process, reconnect with your child, spend a few weeks or months letting your child fall asleep worry-free with you right there next to her, then begin what we call the "fading away" process.

On pages 160–1 we go into detail on how to slowly fade out of your child's bedroom. Skip ahead now and read those pages if you are currently trying to achieve this goal.

We would like to summarize the fading away idea here for the purposes of this chapter:

- *Snuggle to sleep.* Lie in bed with your child while he falls asleep.
- *Camp out next to bed.* Sit on the floor next to your child while she goes to sleep.
- *Move in and out.* Leave the room for brief intervals, but come back frequently.
- *Check on your child.* Hang around in the hallway or next room, but peek your head in to let your child know you're there.
- *Infrequent checks.* Come back to your child's room every 5 or 10 minutes until he's asleep.

Realistically, this is not a welcome idea for parents who used to enjoy the evenings alone when their baby was a good sleeper. No parent wants to go *backward* in this weaning process. But if you don't re-create a stress-free bedtime, your child will likely continue to have nighttime fears, anxiety, and stress for many years. Put in a little time now. View this as a short season in your parenting career. In the long run, your child will be better for it.

In chapter 7 we will go into more detail about how to transition a toddler from needing your presence to fall asleep. We will also discuss how to move a child out of your room and into his own.

food for sleep

Toddlers have tiny tummies. They usually need a snack before going to bed. Just remember that what children eat affects how they sleep. Some foods contribute to restful sleep – we call them "sleepers". Other foods – "wakers" – get in the way of a good night's sleep. "Wakers" are caffeine- and sugar-containing foods that stimulate neurochemicals that perk up the brain. "Sleepers" are foods that contain *tryptophan*. Tryptophan is an amino acid that the body uses to make serotonin and melatonin, neurochemicals that slow down nerve traffic and relax the busy brain.

It's a good idea to eat tryptophan-containing foods with complex carbohydrates. The carbohydrates help usher more tryptophan into the brain so it can manufacture more sleep-inducing neurotransmitters. Without carbohydrates to help, other amino acids that ride along with tryptophan, such as tyrosine, can perk up the brain and keep the child awake. High-protein, low-carbohydrate menus are best saved for breakfast, when it's time for the sleeping brain to wake up and be busy.

Carbohydrates all by themselves are not good sleeper foods. There's no tryptophan in these foods, and sugary, junk-food carbohydrates eaten all by themselves can set you up for a blood-sugar roller coaster ride. First, you get a jolt of energy from the sugar. A couple hours later, when your blood sugar falls, causing your body to release stress hormones, you feel restless. If you're sleeping, you may wake up.

Calcium is another "sleeper" nutrient. It helps the brain use tryptophan to manufacture melatonin. Magnesium, another sleep-inducing mineral, is found especially in whole-grain cereal, sunflower seeds, spinach, tofu, and nuts.

So what makes a good bedtime snack? The best sleepy snacks contain protein, healthy carbohydrates, and some calcium and magnesium. So how about grandma's classic bedtime snack of homemade biscuits and milk? The glass of milk contains tryptophan, healthy carbohydrates (lactose), and calcium. Homemade oatmeal biscuits contain healthy carbohydrates to partner with the proteins in the milk.

Best snooze foods

Here are foods that contain significant amounts of the sleep-inducing amino acid tryptophan. Try these for dinner and bedtime snacks.

- dairy products: cottage cheese, cheese, milk
- soy products: soy milk, tofu
- seafood
- meats
- poultry

- whole grains
- beans
- hummus
- lentils
- hazelnuts, peanuts (Nuts and seeds are not safe for children under three; try nut butters, or grind up nuts into a fine meal and sprinkle them on other foods)
- eggs

Don't worry, be sleepy!

Stress stimulates the body to release cortisol, which can deplete the brain of tryptophan. This is one of many biochemical ways in which stress keeps you awake. So enjoy those bedtime snacks in a stress-free, peaceful environment, to get the maximum benefit from tryptophan.

Best sleepy snacks

For good snacks to sleep by, try these protein-carbohydrate-calcium combinations:

- milk and whole-grain biscuit (e.g. raisin-oatmeal)
- milk and whole-grain cereal
- a hard-boiled egg and a slice of whole-grain toast
- a half peanut butter sandwich on whole-grain bread (see age advice above)
- homemade apple pie and ice cream (our favourite)
- tofu and fruit

The above snacks contain just enough carbohydrates, calcium, and protein to relax rather than perk up the brain. It takes about an hour for all these sleep-inducers to reach the brain.

Best dinners for sleep

The foods you serve your child at dinner can help him get to sleep, too. Here are some dinners to help wind down your family. (These foods, in small portions, make great bedtime snacks too, even if they're a bit unconventional.)

- chilli with beans, not spicy
- sesame seeds (rich in tryptophan) ground and sprinkled on salad with tuna chunks, and whole-wheat crackers
- tuna salad on whole wheat sandwich
- tofu stir-fry with hazelnuts
- scrambled eggs and cheese
- meats or poultry with veggies
- hummus with whole-wheat pita bread
- seafood, pasta, and cottage cheese
- whole grain pasta with parmesan cheese

faqs about toddler sleep

You'll run into many detours on the road to getting your toddler to sleep. Some of them can exhaust your patience. If you can manage to hang on to your sense of humour, some are actually pretty funny. Here are the most common questions we get asked in our medical practice and on our website:

Bedtime procrastinator

We begin putting our 2½-year-old to bed at 8pm, but he has a load of excuses that prolong the routine: he needs a drink of water, he has to go to the toilet, he asks us to 'read again (and again)' … Sometimes it takes me an hour to an hour and a half to get him to sleep. We're tired after a day's work, and we often could fall asleep before he does. Where should we draw the line?

The main reason kids procrastinate at bedtime is stress. They aren't worried about the actual getting-ready-for-bed routine. They are anxious about the very end of the routine – when you leave them alone to fall asleep. Fear of going to bed alone will make the whole routine stressful and your child is much more likely to act out in any way he can to delay the impending alone-in-bed time. This makes the whole bedtime hour less enjoyable for you too.

Get behind the eyes of your child and understand bedtime procrastination from his viewpoint. Ask yourself, "If I were my child, what would I need from my parents at bedtime?" Answer: my parents! Instead of regarding bedtime as a chore, think of this prolonged going-to-bed ritual as *quality* time you spend with your child. This may be the only time during the whole day when he has your focused attention, so of course, he wants to make the most of it and reconnect with you. If you can relax and enjoy this time, you will both be happier.

Parents in this situation will usually need to take a step backwards and spend a few weeks or months sitting by their child's bedside using the fade away technique introduced above.

This can be difficult, since you are tired and your tired child is being very demanding. You may be wanting some time with your partner or time just for yourself. Take it as a compliment that your child enjoys this special time with you. We worry more about babies who are not so "demanding" of their parents at night. And keep it in perspective – those early years fly by quickly.

Sears' Sleep Tip: It's all about attitude. Instead of dreading prolonged bedtime rituals, view them as *treasure times* that you are storing up so that you can all sleep better later on.

Develop a consistent bedtime ritual using the tips from earlier in this chapter. On nights when you know you don't have enough patience for the whole routine, call in a crutch. Listen to an audiotape of your child's favourite story, or watch a calm video together. You can snuggle up on the couch with your child, enjoying bedtime closeness without expending a lot of energy. Many nights when Matthew was three to four years old he and I snuggled together in a beanbag and he dozed off to *Lady and the*

tuck me in, dad

Little minds are in a receptive state at bedtime. Bedtime stories can help a child reflect on her life, and you can tuck a little teaching into the stories you tell. Events from your growing-up years are a great source of bedtime tales.

You can also use bedtimes as *teachable moments* to implant into your child pleasant thoughts and admirable values as she drifts off to sleep. Do this night after night and these bits of wisdom will be filed away in her library of experiences. Years later these bedtime lessons will be an important influence in her life.

Bedtime prayers are a time-honoured tradition for smoothing out the wrinkles of life and for passing on parental values and beliefs. Teach your child a familiar prayer, or make up your own prayers of gratitude and concern for others.

Dr Bob remembers toddler Andrew used to ask while snuggling to sleep, "Tell me good things, Daddy." Bob would create peaceful scenes for Andrew to imagine. "We are sitting next to a quiet river in the warm sunshine with little fish swimming by." Four or five little images would help Andrew settle into sleep peacefully.

Tramp. Meanwhile, Martha was free to be with baby Stephen.

After one or two stories, if she wanted more I said something like, "Mummy needs to go put on her pyjamas now, and I'll be back to check on you in a few minutes." I encouraged her to look at the books we had just read together. She was okay with that and would often be asleep by the time I got back.

Wants to stay up late

Our two-year-old fights going to bed until 10 or 11pm. I know he's tired, certainly we are. How can I get him to sleep earlier?

The most important aspect of helping a toddler go to bed early, especially when you know he is tired and is just fighting it, is to learn what his tired time is (review page 5), anticipate it, get into the bedtime routine early, set the stage for sleep (review page 9), and do this consistently night after night. You may also need to eliminate any afternoon naps (see "Getting Baby to Nap at Predictable Times", page 189). (See related situations, "Establish a Set Nap Schedule", page 190.)

Also, take inventory of what else is going on in your family. Does your child miss you during the day and want to make up for it at night? Are changes in your routine, such as a move, a change in childcare providers, or the arrival of a new baby, upsetting your child? Some children don't want to go to bed because they are afraid of going to sleep. Others resist bedtime because they don't want to be separated from their parents or because they want more "quality time" with their parents. In our family we noticed that the busier and more preoccupied we were during the day, the more our children lobbied for quality time at night.

You know that your son needs to get to bed earlier so that he can get enough sleep. And you and your partner may need some couple time in the evening. So how do you take what you have figured out about why your child is resisting bedtime and use this insight to get him to sleep earlier?

If there are stressful situations that make it hard for your child to sleep, try to remedy them. Make an effort to spend quality time with your child at times other than bedtime. Encourage lots of active play, so your child really is tired at night. Turn off the television.

Plan ahead for an earlier bedtime. Start your winding-down-for-bed routine earlier. Have your child take a bath and get his pyjamas on earlier in the evening. Then at least he is ready for bed, and you don't have to hurry through the whole routine when you are both tired and cranky. Then use the time between bath and bed for quiet games and other activities that you do together.

It may be that your child is just not ready to go to sleep before 10pm. Throughout this book we have stressed the importance of earlier bedtimes, especially for infants and children. Yet, an early bedtime may not work well in your family. With today's busy schedules, parents may not have much time with their children during the day. As a result, children demand more attention from their parents in the evening and balk at bedtime. If your child is, on the whole, well rested (maybe he's taking a long afternoon nap that helps him stay awake at night), a later bedtime may be more realistic. When your child goes to bed is not as important as going to bed at the same time from one night to the next.

Wakes up too early

Our almost three-year-old wakes up at 5am to play. He's bright-eyed and bushy-tailed and ready to go, but I'm not.

Some children are like roosters. They wake up and are ready to go with the first ray of sunlight on their little faces. This doesn't necessarily mean you have to get up at the crack of dawn.

Put blackout curtains on the windows in your child's room. This should keep the little rooster asleep for an extra hour or two. But you will probably have to let him stay up an hour later at night. To do that he may need a slightly later nap. In other words, everything gets pushed forward clockwise – later rising, later nap, and later bedtime. You have to decide if you want more time for yourself in the morning or in the evening. You won't get both.

If Dad gets up early, your toddler can tag along with him while he does all the guy things – shower, shave, dress, fix breakfast – while you get longer to sleep. It's a good father/son "alone together" time.

If that's not going to happen, you can get up and lie with your toddler on the couch – while he plays quietly, you can snooze or at least be horizontal long enough to feel more rested once the clock says it's a more reasonable hour. By modelling that it's still sleepy time for you, your toddler will get the message that it's a good idea to play quietly. Of course this assumes that your house is thoroughly childproofed, the doors to outside are locked, and any off-limit areas are gated off. Even though most youngsters won't wander all over the house when they could be by you, you'll rest easier knowing he won't get in trouble if you really doze off. Dr Bob's partner positioned her toddler on the couch in a way that he'd have to crawl over her to get down, which meant she'd know if he was on the move.

Place a child safety gate in your child's doorway. Set up a water bottle and small snack (something non-chokable) on your child's nightstand before you go to bed. Teach your child to play and eat quietly and safely in his room when he wakes. You can even set an alarm clock and tell him he can call for you when the alarm goes ding. Even better is a music player with a timer that you can set to come on with your child's favourite music (a regular alarm buzzer may be too scary).

Wakes up to play

Our eighteen-month-old baby sleeps in a cot next to us and sometimes she wakes up in the middle of the night eager to play. It's cute, but we're not in the mood to play at 3am. How can we stop this habit?

First, you can be encouraged that this is usually just a phase as baby discovers new milestones. It often passes within a few weeks. Despite this, your toddler needs to learn that nighttime is for sleeping, not for playing. Here's how we discouraged middle-of-the-night playmates.

When our toddler was sleeping close to us and woke us up, we acknowledged her presence but then told her "time to sleep". Then we pretended to go back to sleep. If we "played dead" long enough, she would decide that it wasn't very interesting to be awake in the dark, and she would go back to sleep. If baby protests this silent treatment, you can cuddle her close to you (use a firm hand) and repeat the sleep cue: "time to sleep" or "sleepy-sleepy". Or roll over and lie with your back to baby. Most babies eventually give up and after a few nights, go back to sleep easily.

If this phase lasts too long, and is obviously not going away, in the interest of letting one of you actually get to stay asleep, the one who is feeling generous can get up and walk or rock baby back to sleep. Don't turn on any lights (there will be enough "night light" coming in to find your way around). After she gets bored she'll be ready to go back to sleep. Then you can both make your way back to her cot, or your bed.

Discouraging the midnight visitor

Our two-year-old comes into our room, where he used to sleep, at all hours of the night. How can I get him to stay in his room short of locking him in, which I obviously don't want to do?

Like salmon returning to their birthplace to spawn, children often naturally gravitate back to their preferred sleeping place. Those middle-of-the-night visits, though disrupting, are a usual developmental stage, especially if your child is making the transition from sleeping in your room to sleeping solo in his own. Here's how to give your child extra nighttime security without disrupting your sleep:

- Have an open-door policy, but with rules. Put a futon, mattress, or a cute sleeping bag at the foot of your bed and market this as his "special bed". Then show and tell him this rule: "You can come into Mummy and Daddy's room at night if you need to and sleep in your special bed, but you must tip-toe in as quietly as a mouse and not wake up Mummy and Daddy. Mummy and Daddy need their sleep, otherwise we will be cranky the next day. And a cranky Mummy and Daddy are no fun to be with …"
- Try not to view this nighttime visit as bad behaviour. It is natural and normal. It will diminish in time without you even needing to discourage it.
- To reinforce both your availability and the message that nighttime is when everyone sleeps, go on to tell him, "If you wake Mummy and Daddy up, you have to go back into your room." Try another show and tell game. During the day walk with him from his room into yours and show him how to slip quietly into his special bed without waking you up.

Here's how some parents in our practice negotiated with their midnight visitor:

After we moved, our four-year-old, Josh, wanted to sleep with us all the time. Even after he fell asleep in his own bed, he'd creep in with us at about three o'clock in the morning. Even though we enjoy cuddling with him, especially as we all fall asleep, he's an after-midnight kicker, and we'd spend most of the nights he was with us crossing our arms over our sensitive body parts. So we made a deal. We told Josh that we loved sleeping with him, but now that he was bigger, we didn't sleep well when he was in our bed all the time, and this made us tired and grumpy parents. We further explained that we could probably handle feeling that way once a week. So we made up a chart and told Josh that if he stayed in his own bed all night Monday through Saturday, he could sleep with us all night on Sunday. Now Josh is eager to sleep "well" on his own so that we can all enjoy our Sunday night snuggles.

Weaning off nighttime bottles

Our two-year-old still insists on a bottle at bedtime and if he wakes during the night. I know this isn't good for his teeth, but he really seems to need the comfort. I also wish he'd stop needing the bottle during the night. What can I do?

This is a common dilemma. A toddler who is used to the comfort of sucking on a bottle to get to sleep won't give this up easily, but it's true that milk or juice sugar that stay on the teeth at night can cause cavities. In chapter 6 we'll discuss this situation in detail, but here's the basic approach we recommend:

- *Go sugar free.* Slowly dilute the milk or juice with water over a couple weeks until it is all water. If your child clues in to this trick, back off for a few days then continue again. This at least eliminates the risk of cavities.
- *Have a bye-bye bottle party.* Have a ceremony where you toss the bottles into the outside dustbin, watch the rubbish trucks take it away

if possible, celebrate with songs, dancing, cake and presents. Encourage your child that he is all grown up now and tonight will "go night-night as a big boy". Have a hidden spare bottle handy in case your child decides he doesn't like this idea come bedtime and his hysterics are beyond what you feel is ok. Some of his presents can be other bedtime props, like a musical stuffed toy, new pillow, or blanket.

- *Substitute yourself.* You may find that once you've taken the bottle away you need to find something to take its place. Your child may declare that that something is *you*. You may need to spend a few weeks helping your child go to sleep if you feel he needs you.

If you're using other substitute props, make sure your child knows how to find them during the night when he wakes up and asks for the bottle.

If you feel your child really needs the comfort of a bottle with water, that's okay. You know best when to be rid of the bottle once and for all.

Becoming a bed hog

Our thirteen-month-old has been sharing our bed, and up until now it has been great. Lately he has started moving around while he sleeps. It's like he thinks he owns the bed. My partner and I are starting to feel the effects of a third person in our bed. Help!

Funny – and not so funny – things happen when baby shares your bed. Three familiar, though sometimes annoying, sleep positions that family-bed babies seem to enjoy are the heat-seeking missile, the starfish, and the H-sleeper.

The "heat-seeking missile" snuggles comfortably into a parental armpit or a breast and refuses to back off. Like a mother hen, you instinctively put your wing (your arm) over the top of your baby's head. He may want to stay in touch with, or actually attached to, your warm body all night long. Baby sleeps great, but you may not. No worries, though, about this baby falling out of bed.

With the "starfish", baby sprawls his arms and legs out as far as they can go, sometimes stretching out so much they seem to force you right off the bed. Starfish sometimes become *thrashers*.

The H-sleeper enjoys physical contact with both parents. He falls asleep between the parents, parallel with their bodies, and then strategically rotates himself until he is perpendicular to the parents, resting his head on

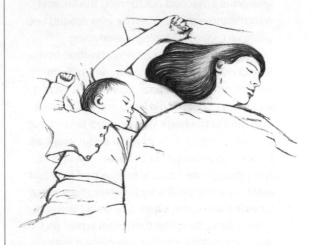

Baby's head in mother's armpit.

one parent and his feet on the other. Isn't that nice? He loves you both! Again, baby sleeps comfortably that way all night – but you may not, especially if you're the one getting kicked in the ribs.

Usually when an infant or toddler starts taking over the bed in these positions, dads announce, "It's time for a big boy bed!" Is Dad right?

Here are your options. If everybody is sleeping reasonably well, you may be able to laugh this off and hope it's passing phase. Yet if baby's nighttime frolicking means baby is the only one who is sleeping well, you need to take some action:

- "Draw the line." Put a line of pillows between you and your toddler. He gets one-third of the bed space; Mum and Dad get the rest.
- Try Dr Jim Sears' trick he calls "staying in your own lane": Jonathon sprawled across the bed with arms stretched out forming the letter H with the three of us. When he was around two years old, I was watching a swimming competition and I was paying attention to the lane dividers that kept the swimmers from swimming on top of each other and it gave me an idea. What if I could keep Jonathon in his own lane in the bed? We had tried pillows but they just took up a lot of room and it was hard to have an entire pillow between him and us. Even though we had a king-size bed they just didn't seem to do the trick. When I saw these lane dividers in the swimming pool I thought, "hmm, something like that might work" so I went downstairs into our garage and noticed that we had some of those water woggles, long

thin cylinders made of firm foam. Using ones that had hollow centres, I slid broom handles in to add some rigidity. After Jonathon fell asleep I placed one on each side of him, each one running the length of the bed, and this worked beautifully. If he started to roll over or rotate sideways the foam was firm enough to keep him from going over it. These were perfectly safe because they were rigid enough so that he didn't become entangled and light enough that he wouldn't be hurt if he somehow slipped under. They were also easy to store under the bed when not in use. One point: I don't suggest using old woggles that have been sitting in the pool in the sun for months because the foam tends to break down and be quite flaky and makes a mess. Go out and get some new ones.
- To give everyone more space, put a twin bed next to your queen- or king-size bed.
- Take bed sprawling as a sign that it's time to start transitioning baby to his own bed. Dad may be right! (See chapter 7, "Moving Out!")

Fear of monsters

Our three-year-old wakes up yelling about the "monsters" in his room. I try to tell him there really aren't any monsters and that Daddy has chased the monsters away. Is this the best way to deal with this? I don't want him to believe that there really are monsters in his room.

Children's dreams distort reality, and young children have difficulty knowing what's real and what's pretend. Therefore, if they see a monster in their dream, they may believe that the monster is real. There are two schools of thought on monsters and other imaginary creatures. The usual suggestion is to play along and just get rid of the monsters. Or, try to teach your child that monsters are fun and friendly. When your child wakes up frightened about them, you search the bedroom and say things like "no monsters anymore", "monsters went bye-bye", "Daddy scared the monsters away". If he worries at bedtime, you can make a show of ordering the monsters out of the bedroom and reassure your child that they're not coming back. While we are sceptical of this approach, for some children it does work. The problem is, *it's not true*. When you chase monsters away, you're reinforcing the child's concern about monsters, and since you say those monsters are indeed real, they can come back.

Here's a better alternative: tell your child the truth. Monsters don't exist. They are pretend. If your child is going through a "seeing-monsters-in-his-sleep" stage, avoid scary TV or cartoons that could be distorted into monsters in his dreams. Your child trusts you. If you say there are no monsters, he will believe you. You might also talk about other things besides monsters that are only pretend, to help your child learn to tell the difference between what's real (a family pet, elephants at the zoo) and what's not (characters in cartoons, such as Monsters Inc., animals in story books who talk).

Nighttime anxiety

Our three-year-old had been sleeping well on his own for a few months, but now he's waking up and coming into our room at night. He seems really upset. How can I help him get back to sleeping through the night in his own room?

Realize your child has a need. He is growing and developing, and new fears and worries are going to come along. Sometimes they will disturb his sleep, and you are right in thinking that he needs your help to cope with his nighttime anxiety.

Why is your child suddenly feeling insecure about nighttime? There are many possible reasons. Here are just a few:

- *Imagination.* As kids get older they develop the mental ability to imagine that there is a monster in the closet, a giant hand under the bed (that was Dr Bob's fear as a child), or something looming in the darkness outside. They don't necessarily have to see these things first on TV or hear about them in stories. Kids can create these fears all on their own.
- *Separation anxiety.* This occurs not only around nine months of age, it can also show up again between age 2 and 3. Your happy sleeper becomes anxious because you are not there. Your child needs your physical presence as reassurance that he is safe because you aren't going anywhere.
- *Life changes.* Changes in a child's life, such as starting preschool nursery or childcare, moving, or having a younger sibling can trigger some temporary nighttime anxiety. Changes in the family's life, such as in a parent's work schedule, can also affect how well a child sleeps.

Here are some ideas you can try to help your child learn to sleep through the night again:

what's on your child's mind?

Do you think that your awake-at-night child is purposefully trying to manipulate you? Do you think he is lying in bed thinking, "Hmmm. I know Mum and Dad are having a relaxing evening. How can I disrupt them? I know, I'll get up and go ask for a drink of water. I know they hate that!" If your child is really thinking like that at the age of three, then good luck. But we really don't think kids are that devious (well, not until they are older).

When your child gets out of bed at night to come find you, you may be tempted to send him back to his own bed with firm orders to stay there. Instead, put yourself into the mind of your child as he crawls back into his own bed, wide awake, and lies there, staring at the wall. "I'm afraid, and my Mummy won't help me", he thinks. Or, "I wish my Daddy was here with me." Remember that a child's needs are not always rational from an adult's point of view.

I don't want her nighttime memories filled with her screaming from her cot. I don't want my memories filled with hearing her scream from her cot.

- *Talk it out during the day.* Sit your child down in the afternoon and tell him that you want to help him with his nighttime worries. Decide on a plan together. Perhaps you will go back to his bed with him when he wakes up, and lie down with him until he falls asleep again. Maybe you will decide to put a mattress or a comforter on the floor in your room, where he can sleep if he gets scared during the night. Maybe you and your child will come up with another idea.
- *Act quickly at night.* When your child wakes up in the night and comes into your room, don't get into a debate with him about going back to his own bed. Just do what you planned to do. Take him back to his room and fall asleep together in his bed. Or, get him settled in his little bed in your room. Or let him climb in bed with you. The object here is to get everyone back to sleep without feeding your child's nighttime fears.
- *Enjoy a peaceful day with active play.* As we have said before, minimizing the stress in your child's daytime life will minimize nighttime problems. If the daytime stress is unavoidable, be prepared to live with a few sleep problems until things settle down. Encourage your child to run, jump, and be active during the day. This tires him out, and it also alleviates tension and anxiety.
- *Wean him back to sleeping alone.* As your child starts to feel more secure at night, you can begin to work on getting him back to sleeping alone. He may decide that if he wakes up he will join you in his special bed in your room without waking you. Or you can take him back to his bed, staying with him just until he's nearly asleep. Tell him "I'll be back in a minute to check on you", and then be sure to come back.

- *Dim the lighting.* Too much light may keep your child awake, but a nightlight may keep him from being afraid when he wakes up alone in the dark. Keeping the hall light on with the door open is another good option.

why nighttime parenting matters

Long-term nighttime stress can lead to long-term sleep insecurities that can create daytime insecurities and problems with self-confidence. That's a mouthful, but we want you to understand it. Picture the following two scenarios:

Alex is four years old and had been sleeping well in his own room. Bedtime was a relaxing routine of stories, hugs and kisses, and sweet dreams. Until tonight. When his Dad tries to put him to bed, he protests that he wants his Dad to stay with him. When Dad says no, Alex asks for an extra hug and kiss, a longer story, tucking in the covers better, or whatever else he can think of to keep Dad around for an extra minute or two. Dad leaves his room, and Alex starts getting out of bed every five minutes to ask for a drink of water, to find out what his parents are watching on TV, to ask what he's doing tomorrow, or to complain that he's hungry. His parents send him directly back to bed, alone. On subsequent nights, Alex's tactics escalate into complaints of tummy aches and headaches. He takes a long time to

fall asleep and doesn't seem quite as happy and secure in the daytime anymore. He even starts wetting the bed (something he'd never done before). This goes on for years, and as he grows through childhood he feels that bedtime is a time of loss and separation.

Now let's meet the same child, but with different parental responses.

Alex is four years old and had been sleeping well in his own room. Bedtime was a fun routine of stories, hugs and kisses, and sweet dreams. Until tonight. When his Dad tries to put him to bed, he protests that he wants his Dad to stay with him. His Dad gives him an extra long hug, stays in the room for a few minutes pretending like he's putting some clothes away, lingers in the hallway busily, then tells Alex goodnight (kiss, hug, and tuck again), and leaves. Alex is asleep in two minutes. He just needed a little extra something that particular night, and his Dad gave it to him.

Dad discusses this situation with Mum. While they want to keep their early bedtime routine with Alex (they like their evenings uninterrupted, and don't want to have to waste an extra hour every night trying to cater to their child's bedtime fears), they also have been sensitive to his changing needs over the years. They didn't push it when he needed some time getting used to starting preschool. They didn't leave him crying with a babysitter, but took the time to help him feel comfortable and playful. They've yet to go on a holiday without him. Now they realize that their child is trying to tell them he is feeling anxious about being away from them at night. They understand that if they fulfil his needs now for the short term, they won't turn into long-term unfulfilled needs that will leave him feeling insecure over the years. They also know that if they meet those needs without Alex continuously having to ask (or protest), his needs should diminish faster. Plus, everyone will be happier.

So the next night when Alex protests when Dad turns to leave the room, Dad sits on Alex's bed and says "I don't mind staying with you for a little while. You rest your eyes, and I'll sit by the bed here for a few minutes." Dad winds up spending the next three weeks lingering in Alex's room or the nearby hallway at bedtime. Sometimes he folds laundry while waiting for Alex to fall asleep. He sits in the chair and uses a tiny clamp-on book light to read without turning on the overhead light. He doesn't interact much with Alex, he's just there. Sometimes he tells Alex that he needs to go in the other room, but he will be back to check on him in a few minutes. He putters around, making just enough noise for Alex to know he is close by. It is a very slow weaning process that, while time-consuming, really pays off in the long run. Eventually Alex returns to his former easy-to-sleep routine, and his parents get their evenings back.

Bedtime was always a drawn-out affair in our family. The routine took forty-five minutes to an hour, especially with my oldest son, who has always been very tuned in to what's going on around him. Now, many years later, everybody goes to bed on their own. My three children are expert sleepers who rarely have trouble falling asleep at night. I'm the one who needs to stop at my kids' bedroom doors to chat for a few minutes and connect with them before I can fall asleep.

chapter 3

the facts about infant sleep
and what they mean for parents

The steps and tips on how to get your infant and toddler to sleep that we shared with you in the first two chapters of this book are based on general principles about how babies and toddlers sleep. When you know why babies do the things they do, it is easier to work out how to respond.

Learning more about how babies sleep and why they wake up during the night will help you understand the nighttime parenting strategies we suggest in this book. It will also help you bring a helpful attitude to caring for your baby's nighttime needs.

learn the facts of infant sleep

Read all about it! We want you to understand why babies sleep the way they do – or don't. First, here are some general facts about sleep.

How adults sleep. There are two main states of sleep – REM (rapid-eye-movement sleep) and non-REM. The term "falling" asleep is biologically correct. As you drift off to sleep, you enter non-REM sleep, and over the next hour and a half you descend through the levels of this sleep state until you are at level four, the deepest level of sleep. You may even sleep through a phone ringing, or here in California, through earthquakes. If you are awakened from this deepest level of non-REM sleep – say, by a persistently crying baby, you are more likely to be disoriented and grouchy than when you are awakened from lighter levels of sleep.

After the first 90 minutes of gradually descending into non-REM sleep, your brain begins to arouse and move into a lighter and more active kind of sleep, the state of REM sleep. During REM sleep the brain is quite active (it's when you dream), although the rest of your body is usually relaxed and relatively quiet. You experience rapid eye movement even though your eyes are closed (hence the term REM sleep), and men can get erections. During REM sleep, facial muscles may twitch, producing "sleep grins". It's fun to watch for this in babies. Since this is the lightest stage of sleep, it is easiest to waken out of REM sleep.

Adults cycle through REM and non-REM sleep approximately every 90 minutes. Early in the night the periods of non-REM sleep may last as long as 60 minutes, and REM periods may last from 10 to 30 minutes. Toward morning the proportions of non-REM and REM reverse, so that much of early-morning sleep is REM. The length and pattern of these sleep cycles varies greatly between individuals and at different ages. However, during an average eight-hour sleep adults may spend two hours in REM, or active (light) sleep, and six hours in non-REM, or quiet (deep) sleep.

Both of these states of sleep are important for a person's overall well-being. Non-REM, or deep sleep, is necessary to help the body rest and recuperate. It is known as the restorative state of sleep. REM sleep is necessary for brain development. Understanding these sleep cycles explains why human babies awaken so easily and why it may not be wise to fiddle around too much with babies' natural sleep cycles.

How babies sleep. Why do babies wake up so much? This is probably the question new parents ask most. The simple answer: because they're babies. Babies sleep differently from adults.

Babies go to sleep differently. Infants take longer (at least 20 minutes) to drift off and enter deep sleep. On the other hand, adults and older children "crash" into deep sleep, drifting into non-REM sleep in just a few minutes. The younger the infant, the longer it takes him to drift into deep sleep.

What does this sleep fact mean to parents? Babies awaken easily during this drifting off period. Parents don't have to be sleep scientists to figure this out. Many parents describe their baby as "difficult-to-settle", or they say "she has to be fully asleep before I can put her down". Many parents have had the experience where they think their baby is asleep, so they gently carry her to her cot and lay her down – but she wakes up as soon as Mum or Dad turns to tiptoe out of the room. Baby is not truly asleep until he arrives in the state of deep sleep, 20 to 30 minutes after closing his eyes. Trying to hasten the bedtime routine can leave parents very frustrated.

You can see why the advice from sleep trainers to "put babies down in their cots awake" doesn't work, especially for babies less than three months old. Babies need to be gentled through this first period of REM sleep, so that they can stay asleep until deeper sleep overtakes them. Between three and six months babies begin to drift more quickly into non-REM sleep. They can be put down awake, or partially awake, and they will enter deep sleep fairly quickly.

Bottom line: babies need to be patiently parented to sleep, not just put to sleep.

Babies stay asleep differently. While adults cycle from deep to light sleep approximately every hour and a half, infants move through these states every hour. The younger the infant, the shorter the sleep cycle. What does this mean for parents? When passing from one state of sleep to another, the brain is more likely to awaken than at other times. We call this the "vulnerable period". If by chance an *arousal stimulus* (teething pain, loud noise, hunger, separation anxiety, and so on) bothers baby during this vulnerable period, baby is likely to awaken. Because babies have shorter sleep cycles, they have more vulnerable periods – more times during the night when they are likely to wake up. In addition, babies spend more time in REM (light) sleep in the second half of the night. This explains why babies often wake up more during that time.

Bottom line: minimize arousal stimuli during vulnerable periods for night waking.

As babies grow, their sleep cycles lengthen and the percentage of deep sleep increases. There are fewer vulnerable periods during the night when they can awaken easily. They also sleep more deeply and they stay asleep longer – a sleep maturity milestone called *settling*. The age at which babies settle varies greatly according to the sleep temperament of the baby. The good news is that all babies eventually settle.

Babies' developing sleep patterns are much like their changing feeding patterns. In the early months babies take small, frequent feedings and short, frequent naps. About fifty per cent of the total sleep of a newborn is REM sleep. This percentage is even higher in premature infants. As you can see from the graph below, as babies grow, they learn to sleep and feed more like adults. These five things happen:

- REM (active) sleep decreases
- Non-REM (deep) sleep increases
- Sleep cycles lengthen
- Vulnerable periods for night waking occur less frequently
- The total number of hours of daily sleep lessens.

This is called *sleep maturity*.

Babies are designed this way. Why are babies' sleep patterns so different from adults'? Answer: because babies need to sleep this way. How babies sleep is one of many things throughout infancy and childhood that parents can't control, and it may even be unsafe and unwise to try to change. Keep in mind that babies sleep the way they do – or don't – because they are designed that way for both developmental and survival benefits.

Babies sleep smarter. REM sleep is more than an annoying nuisance that keeps parents as well as babies from sleeping more deeply. The fact that babies' developing brains don't turn themselves off as well during sleep as adult brains has developmental benefits. Sleep researchers believe that REM sleep stimulates the infant brain at a time when it is growing very rapidly. Blood flow to the brain increases during REM sleep. The lower brain centres fire off electrical stimuli toward higher brain centres. This stimulation works like mental exercise to help the brain centres develop. The mental activity of dreaming helps the brain grow more neurons. This theory that REM sleep stimulates brain growth is supported by the fact that the young of highly intelligent animal species spend more time in REM sleep than the young of less intelligent species. One day as I was explaining the light sleep/better brain correlation to a tired mother of a wakeful infant, she chuckled, "In that case, my baby is going to be very clever."

Babies sleep healthier and safer. Not only do these immature sleep patterns help babies grow smarter, they help them grow healthier and sleep safer. Suppose your baby slept like an adult. Suppose baby slept so deeply that he couldn't signal when he was hungry, cold, had a stuffy nose and was having difficulty breathing, or was just plain scared? Baby's well-being would be threatened. Babies come wired to awaken so that they can let nearby caregivers know what they need to thrive and survive. What does this mean to parents? These arousals are thought to be *protective arousals*, and they are beneficial. Training babies to sleep too deeply, for too long, too young is not in the best interest of the baby's development and well-being.

Sears' Sleep Tip: Now that you understand infant sleep, when people ask, "How does your baby sleep?" you can answer, "Like a baby".

There are sleep trainers who ignore these basic biological facts and insist that babies should be able to put themselves to sleep and sleep through the night. As you can see from the information in the previous pages, putting a baby down to sleep alone in a cot and leaving the baby to cry himself to sleep, and back to sleep when he awakens, is biologically and developmentally wrong. We are passionate about helping parents understand their babies' basic sleep needs and giving them tools to cope until their babies reach sleep maturity, so we

hope you'll keep these biological facts in mind when making all decisions about your baby's sleep.

how babies sleep at various ages

As with all developmental milestones, the age at which babies wake up less and start "sleeping through the night" varies from baby to baby. Here are the general sleep patterns that most babies follow at various stages along the way to sleep maturity:

- *Newborn period.* In the first month, babies tend to sleep a total of sixteen to seventeen hours a day. They sleep in three to four hour stretches with an equal amount of sleep during the daytime and nighttime hours. At this age babies wake up mainly from hunger (which they don't experience until they're born, so it's very scary for them at first).
- *One to three months.* Between six and eight weeks of age, babies begin to "consolidate" their sleep into shorter periods during the day and slightly longer periods at night. They sleep from 15 to 16 hours a day. At this age, most babies wake up at least once a night and need a feeding and help to resettle (many will wake up two or three times). Babies start waking up not only from hunger, but also from a need for closeness (being alone is also very scary).
- *Three to six months.* Babies sleep a total of around fifteen hours a day, taking two or three

babies sleep differently

Notice how babies sleep differently than do adults and imagine what could go wrong if they didn't.

Infant Sleep

- Designed to easily awaken
- Designed to sleep less deeply
- Need night feedings
- Short sleep cycles, 60 minutes
- Mostly REM (active) sleep

Adult Sleep

- Designed to stay asleep
- Designed to sleep more deeply
- Don't need night feedings
- Long sleep cycles, 90 minutes
- Most non-REM (quiet) sleep

two-hour naps during the day and doing the rest of their sleeping at night. By six months, most babies will begin to sleep four- to five-hour stretches at night. At this age babies also begin having shorter REM periods of sleep and longer non-REM.

- *Six to nine months.* Babies sleep around 14 hours a day and may drop one of their naps. Most babies between six and nine months take one morning and one afternoon nap. They may start sleeping seven-hour stretches at night. Most continue to wake up several times a night, and some can self-soothe back to sleep. Developmental changes start triggering night waking at this stage. They practise their motor development, such as sitting up, while still half-asleep. Add teething pain to this list and you have a recipe for night waking even in babies who were previously "good" sleepers.
- *Nine to twelve months.* Babies sleep between thirteen and fourteen hours a day, still with two naps. Some babies may sleep ten hours at

night, occasionally maybe even twelve hours (often interspersed with one or two feedings). While babies still need a morning and afternoon nap, the morning nap will usually be shorter.

- *One to two years.* Babies sleep from twelve to thirteen hours a day, with ten to twelve hours at night, and two shorter naps. Around (or even before) eighteen months of age, some infants will begin to relinquish the morning nap, but need the afternoon nap. Some need two naps one day and one nap the next. Between 12 and 18 months babies often start waking up because of *separation anxiety.* From 18 months to two years, the concept of *person permanence* clicks in, enabling babies to fall asleep on their own more easily because they can understand that their parents are nearby in another room even though they can't see them.
- *Two to three years.* Toddlers sleep between eleven and thirteen hours in 24 hours, and often give up the morning nap. Nightmares and sleep terrors may begin, as well as sleep fears and

sleep needs

Age	Total Hours Sleep	Number of naps	Total Naptime Hours
Newborn	16–17	3	6
1–3 months	15–16	3	4–5
3–6 months	14–15	2	3–4
6–9 months	14–14½	2	3
9–12 months	13–14	2	3
12–24 months	12–13	1–2	2
2–3 years	11–13	1	1–1½
3–4 years	11–12	0–1	½–1

fear of the dark. Previously "good sleepers" may become fretful sleepers at this age. Most toddlers graduate from cot to bed between ages two and three.

- *Three to four years.* Finally by this stage most children's sleep patterns become like those of adults. By four years, many children no longer nap during the day, yet still need eleven to twelve hours of sleep at night.

why babies wake up

Understanding all the things that can go on in that little body and mind when you put her down to sleep at night may help you understand why babies wake up so often, develop some creative tips to help her sleep, and above all sympathize with your baby. Here are the main reasons why babies awaken frequently.

1. They're babies! As discussed in detail on page 53 babies have shorter sleep cycles. Every hour or so as they pass from the state of deep sleep into light sleep, they go through a vulnerable period for night waking. If they sense any upset or discomfort during this vulnerable period, they cry for assistance. For safety's sake, babies' sleep patterns have *easy arousability*, which means that if anything threatens their well-being (such as SIDS) they wake up more easily than do adults. Exhausting as it may be to their caregivers, these are survival and developmental reasons why babies are prone to night waking.

2. They're hungry. Tiny babies have tiny tummies and fast metabolisms. They can't go as long without food as adults can. And breastmilk moves through baby's stomach faster than formula. Many infants don't start clustering their day feedings and dropping night feedings for at least six months, and most breastfeeding babies continue to need a night feeding for sometime thereafter. While some books may say infants don't need night feedings after a certain age, try telling that to a baby with an empty tummy.

3. They're thirsty. If your baby was used to feeding several times at night, or getting a bottle or two, but has now learned to sleep without this (thankfully!), he may start to feel the lack of fluids at night. This becomes truer during the toddler and preschool years. If you find your child is waking up and feeling thirsty, have a handy trainer cup or water bottle nearby that your child can drink from before he fully wakes up. Also be sure to provide a good size drink of water before bedtime (unless, of course, you are potty training at night).

Doctor Bob's third child used to wake up between 18 months and 2 years asking for water (even though he was still breastfeeding). He wouldn't even open his eyes. He'd just lie there asking for water, and when we gave him a drink, he'd fall right back to sleep.

4. They're growing. Growth hormone levels are much higher during sleep. Thus, the saying, "he seemed to outgrow his baby clothes overnight". Growth hormone also stimulates hunger. Waking to feed frequently is the baby's way of making sure he has enough fuel to do the growing. Babies typically will experience growth spurts around three weeks, six weeks, three

months, and six months. During these stretches your baby will go on feeding marathons day and night. Don't worry. If your baby is generally a good sleeper, things should go back to normal within a few days. If your baby has been a night waker all along, then you probably won't even notice the difference. Growth spurts are just another way that Mother Nature robs us of sleep (when we say "us", what we really mean is you mums out there, and you dads who are noble enough to share the nighttime duty.)

This is not the age to discourage night feeding. Don't fall into the trap of thinking that you don't have enough milk. Your body responds to baby's increased feeding by producing more milk. Your baby is feeding more at night during this growth spurt because he needs more "grow milk" at night. These normal, but tiring, phases of breastfeeding and infant growth are dubbed "frequency nights" or "marathon feeding".

When younger babies increase their night feedings, mothers need to decrease their daytime commitments so they can accommodate. Temporarily shelve all energy-draining activities that can be put on hold for a while, so you can conserve your energy for extra feedings. Enjoy nap feeding so that you can sleep when the baby sleeps. (See strategies for easier nap feeding, page 187). Housework can be put off or delegated. Realize no one's growth is going to be affected if the housework doesn't get done for a few days. Go to sleep when baby does in the evening. Explain these growth spurts to your partner and enlist his help for more "father nursing" during non-feeding times.

5. They're developing. During major motor achievements, baby may start waking up at night to practise what he's learned. Typical times for this are four months for rolling over, six months for sitting up, between seven and nine months for crawling, and between nine and 15 months for walking. These milestones are adorable during the day, but not your idea of a good time at night. Night "practices" usually only go on for several nights, then baby may go back to his normal sleep patterns.

6. They're teething. Baby's first four months are often termed "the honeymoon" when it comes to sleep. Baby may wake up once, twice, or not at all, and life is good. Enter the fifth month, and your worst nighttime opponent enters the game – teeth. Babies begin to feel teething pain as early as three months of age, even though the teeth may not break through for another two months or more. Teething phases sometimes last for only a week, and just when you begin to get really frustrated, baby starts to sleep well again. You'll usually get a couple months' break between teething cycles. However, some teeth will seem to take forever to come in, and you may be in (or up) for a rough month or two. This is also a common problem for toddlers. The infamous two-year molars can surprise you, and your toddler may need more of you during this month or two. Fortunately, that's the last of the teeth until age six.

7. They hurt. Many irritating things go on in those growing little bodies that can wake baby up. (See chapter 11, "Medical and Physical Causes of Night Waking".)

8. They're lonely. Let's step into your baby's mind for a moment. Your baby just spent the last nine months being carried around inside your body, and as baby grew, so did her awareness of your warmth, heartbeat, body sounds, and your motion as you walked. Now that baby is born, where does she spend much of her day? She is cuddled in your arms to feed, carried in a soft carrier, lovingly caressed during baths and while being dressed, passed back and forth between caring friends and relatives, and rocked to sleep. If baby is experiencing so much of you during the day, why wouldn't she want some of you at night? Some babies wake simply because they miss you and want a bit of Mum or Dad (once again, usually Mum) to get back to sleep.

I think he wakes up to check that I'm still there.

9. They're anxious. Closeness, not separateness, is a normal psychological and emotional state for a baby, especially during the first year or two. Just as babies feel incomplete if separated from mother during the day, they may feel the same at night. To a baby, separateness doesn't start just because the sun goes down. Many infant development specialists believe, and we agree, that separation anxiety (during the day and night) is a built-in survival mechanism for babies, since naturally it is safer for them to be closer than distant from a caregiver. So, when baby wakes up alone, he feels out of touch. Separateness and aloneness is not a normal state for a baby. When a baby wakes up alone in a dark, quiet room – behind bars – a sort of "what's wrong with this picture?" anxious thought process goes on. More mild-tempered babies will sometimes simply accept nighttime aloneness and go back to sleep. Those with more persistent personalities will cry out in the night, as if summoning their caregivers, "Something is not right here. Please make it right!"

10. They're afraid. You will find that your toddler and preschooler may begin to develop some nighttime fears as their imagination sets in and they begin to fear what may be lurking in the dark. Your two-year-old may be dreaming about a giant dummy chasing him through the sandbox. We will discuss sleep fears in chapter 12.

11. They're conditioned to. In our medical practice we have noticed a phenomenon we call *conditioned night waking,* which is most frequent in babies who are privileged to breastfeed and co-sleep Baby awakens, mother presents breast, baby feels comforted and goes back to sleep. He gets to like this immediate gratification. And, of course, any smart baby is literally going to "milk" this nighttime perk for all he can get. "Ah, nightlife is good!" he imagines. And, since babies instinctively do what brings them pleasure and helps them thrive, they are reluctant to give up the very relationship that they not only want, but also believe they need. A good habit can become a need. Once babies realize that they thrive on night feeding (even at the expense of Mum), they are unlikely to give it up without a protest. That's why we believe this becomes a need rather than a habit. Habits are easy to break, needs are not.

normal night noises sleeping babies make

Babies are not sound-less sleepers. They sigh, snort, gurgle, coo, snore, sputter, squeak, squeal, hoot, toot, cough, even whimper and mumble a bit. Your baby's night noises are as unique as her personality, and most of them are not signs of distress. These normal sleep sounds, which often occur as babies are transitioning from one state of sleep to another, may be lovingly misinterpreted as, "Oh, he's about to wake up. I better get to him before he does." Sometimes, if you wait out these sounds, you realize that these are not cries for attention. They're just normal sounds, and you don't need to rush in to pick up and comfort baby. He may not even wake up. He may put himself back to sleep without your help if he does wake. If baby's noises escalate into cries, this indicates that something is "not right here" and that he needs something from you to make it right. It might be food, it might be holding, it might be a few soothing words, but you can't go wrong by paying attention to these more insistent nighttime noises.

Joshua (Dr Bob's son) will sometimes cry out for one second, and then go right back to sleep. We don't go to him unless it's obvious he's awake.

adopt a nighttime parenting attitude

Helping a baby learn healthy sleep habits is not like housetraining a puppy, and it's more than simply following a list of methods. There's an important relationship involved. It's a little human being who needs to be taught how to fall asleep comfortably and fearlessly and how to go back to sleep after awakening at night. Teaching these lessons in a nurturing way will also teach your baby to trust you.

You'll notice throughout this book that we use the term "nighttime parenting" rather than simply "getting your baby to sleep" or worse, "sleep-training". Calling what you do with your baby at night "nighttime parenting" reminds you that this is part of the whole parenting package. You want your baby to feel that she can rely on you and trust you to help her feel good during the

helping others sleep!

Share your wisdom and nighttime experience with others. In our pediatric practice we encourage experienced mothers and fathers who have survived and thrived while helping their own children sleep better to share their experience with new parents. As a perk, you get a "helper's high" – that warm, fuzzy feeling of knowing that some parents and babies are sleeping better because of the advice you gave them. Truthfully, that's what keeps us writing books.

night as well as during the day. Your attachment to her is something that she can always count on. You show this attachment differently at night, because you need to sleep, but the relationship you have with your baby continues. Once you approach baby's sleep time with this nighttime parenting attitude, you will naturally view the time you spend helping your baby sleep as an opportunity to build your relationship. You will rely more on yourself and your own intuition to get your baby to sleep better rather than using a bunch of gadgets and insensitive techniques to "break" baby of night waking.

Having said that you are going to be parenting your baby at night as well as during the day, we have to add that *it's important not to neglect your own nighttime needs*. Many first-time mother, in her zeal to be a good mother, ends up becoming a martyr mother at night: "My baby needs me so much at night, that I don't get the sleep I need. But that's okay. Baby comes first." While some sleep disruption inevitably goes with the territory of being a parent (with children of all ages), neglecting your own need for sleep is *not* okay. Sleep deprivation can compromise your emotional and physical health, and it is neither a necessary nor normal part of nighttime parenting. Your baby needs parents who are well rested enough to be responsive and fun during the day. Babies need sleep to thrive, and so do mothers and fathers. It helps to have the attitude: "I'm going to keep working at getting *all* of us the best sleep possible."

Some say easy sleepers are born, not made. There is some truth to this. Sleep is not a state you can force a baby into, but some babies have temperaments that allow them to fall asleep easily and to go back to sleep without much help. How you parent your baby also affects how well your baby sleeps. Some parents are more careful to create an environment that allows sleep to overtake baby. Some are more persistent about sensitively teaching their babies how to put themselves back to sleep. How well your baby sleeps will depend on both baby's individual temperament and on how you parent at night.

A realistic long-term goal is to help your baby develop a healthy attitude about sleep: that sleep is a pleasant state to enter and a secure state to remain in. Many sleep problems in older children and adults stem from children growing up with fears and anxiety about falling asleep. Just as daytime parenting is a long-term investment, so is nighttime parenting. Your short-term goal may be to teach your baby sleep habits that help you get more sleep yourself, but you want to do this in a way that will also accomplish your long-term goal. Teach your baby to have a healthy attitude toward sleep in the first year, and both you and your baby will sleep better in the years that follow.

I've noticed that some of the parents in our area have adopted the cry it out method of getting their children to sleep. In the first couple years they used to boast about how their children would "sleep through the night", while I would often doze off to sleep for a catnap during the neighbourhood meeting because I was up feeding at night. Yet, when their kids got older, they would wake up with nightmares, see monsters in their room, and seem to be afraid of sleep. Now these mothers are the ones nodding off during the day and losing sleep while my child sleeps happily through the night, as do I.

unclutter the daytime life of a nighttime parent

It's hard to cultivate a positive attitude towards nighttime parenting at 4am. At that hour, you do what you have to do to survive and get back to sleep. The real work of helping the whole family sleep better begins in the daytime, as you adjust your lifestyle to accommodate the changes a baby brings to your family's life.

New mothers often fail to anticipate the toll a baby takes on their energy, especially at night. They believe they'll continue their previous busy lifestyle and baby will somehow fit in. Not so! Tired mothers of new babies often ask, "When will my life get back to normal?" I respond, "This is a new kind of normal. Life won't ever again be the way it was before."

Evaluate your lifestyle. Take inventory of all the things that drain away your energy, but that don't necessarily have to be done by you. You want to spend your energy where it matters – on your baby and on your own well-being. Consider the following:

- What jobs can you delegate?
- What commitments can you get out of or put off?

sleepy mums advise ...

Mothers who have survived, and thrived, through many years of nighttime parenting offer these attitude helpers:

- I look at this like an investment that will pay off. It's what I signed up for.
- Our daytime and general life is so hectic that I actually look forward to those special times of night feeding.
- We have good nights and bad nights, but we make a point of celebrating the good ones rather than bemoaning the bad.
- We tried everything to get our baby to sleep through the night and nothing was working. So I tried changing my attitude. I found expecting my baby to sleep through the night when this wasn't happening was making me angry, which only kept me awake more. Once I changed my attitude and reminded myself that a baby waking up at night was normal, natural, and expected, I slept better. It's much more difficult to get angry about something you expect and perceive as usual.
- When my baby woke during the night, I was careful not to look at the clock, not to count the feedings. Keeping track of how much sleep I was missing made it much harder to get back to sleep and harder to function the next day.
- How good a parent you are is not demonstrated by how long your child sleeps. I mention this because someone is bound to ask you the magic question, "Is he/she sleeping through the night?" or "Is he/she a good baby?" You will dread those questions and learn to ignore them.
- Don't make sleep a control issue. You'll both probably lose.
- Every mother goes through a period where they are sleep-deprived. We just cope by saying: "This is only for a short time." Before you know it you'll be sleep-deprived because you're waiting for your teenager to get home after a date.
- Sometimes the best way to get over sleep problems is to redefine "good" sleeping. Often there really isn't a problem, except that people have been told that kids should sleep a certain way.

- How can you change your daytime schedule to sneak in extra naps? (See "Creating Healthy Nap Habits", page 185.)
- What can you do during the day to help yourself sleep better?

I just had to redefine my daytime priorities. I had to realize that I couldn't be "Supermum" and do everything! Once I discontinued almost all outside commitments and gave myself the freedom to have a not-so-perfect house, I felt less resentment about getting up at night and was able to be more accepting. And, after a while, I think I just got used to it.

Have a restful day. Babies – and adults – sleep better at night if they have enjoyed a restful day. Think about especially stressful days in your past and the restless nights that followed. When you go to sleep with a bloodstream full of stress hormones, you set yourself up for a restless night. Daytime stress is one of the reasons why infants have difficulty settling at night after a move, mother returning to work, or an illness. When daytime stress can't be avoided, at least have a restful evening, as a prelude to better sleep.

Have a peaceful house. Computer screens, TV, loud music, noisy guests, and loud conversations make the atmosphere in your home super-charged. Turn off the TV, the radio, and the bright lights, and make your home a quiet, peaceful place. Your baby will sleep better and so will you.

Strive for a daily pattern. Newborns come disorganized. All of their physiological functions are irregular. They don't follow a predictable pattern. If Mum and Dad's life is also unpredictable, baby will have a much harder time settling into regular routines for sleeping and eating. Notice we use the term "pattern" rather than "schedule". Your Palm Pilot may have run your pre-baby life, but babies need some flexibility. They change from week to week. Don't expect to have a "day planner baby". You will get more joy out of parenting if you create a routine that fits your baby, rather than trying to make

your baby fit the routine. Yet, babies are creatures of habit, and the more predictable their day, the more restful the night is likely to be.

Get some exercise. You will sleep better at night if you are active during the day. Put your baby in the baby sling or stroller and go out for a walk. Run and play with your toddler at the park. Stretch the kinks out of your back and shoulders with yoga or other forms of exercise.

Take naps. Adult lifestyles don't often allow for the luxury of napping, but parents of babies who are awake at night are entitled to sleep during the day. Don't use naptime to get the housework done. Use this downtime to rest, or to do things that rejuvenate your tired spirit.

Don't compare, don't complain. When parents of babies get together, they inevitably talk about sleep. Sometimes this is helpful, sometimes it's not. It all depends on who you're with. Don't be discouraged by parents who brag about their own babies sleeping through the night at an early age. Seek out experienced parents who share your parenting values and who have helpful, positive ideas to share.

Have reasonable expectations. If you expect your baby to sleep for twelve hours straight, or even half that amount, every single night, you are bound to end up frustrated. This is not the way babies are made. If you understand why your baby wakes up at night and expect this, it will be easier to live with.

get connected

The concept of nighttime parenting that we have described above is part of *attachment parenting*, a style of parenting that we advocate. We'll summarize this style of parenting briefly in this chapter. Other chapters in this book apply the ideas of attachment parenting to various nighttime challenges. If you want to learn more about attachment parenting in the daytime, read some of our other books, including *The Baby Book, The Fussy Baby Book* and *The Good Behaviour Book*.

Even though we started using this term in 1980, attachment parenting (AP) is not a new-fangled way of raising children that we and others have dreamed up. It's what mothers and fathers would do instinctively if they were raising their baby on a desert island without the advice of sleep books, in-laws, and psychologists. It is a high-touch, highly responsive style of infant care. Parents invest a lot of time and energy in their relationship with their baby, yet they get a high return on this investment. They learn to know and understand their child, and children respond with trust and respect. Attachment parenting (AP) is what many parents naturally do without realizing it has a name.

AP helps parent and child get to know and trust each other by using the connecting tools we call the eight Baby B's:

- *Birth bonding.* Start the connection as soon as possible after birth.

- *Breastfeeding.* When you breastfeed, you learn to read your baby's cues – both day and night. The physical closeness of breastfeeding rewards both mother and baby with good feelings.
- *Babywearing.* Wear your baby in a carrier several hours a day. Babies who are held are calmer and more fun to be with. A baby who is happy and peaceful during the day will sleep better at night.
- *Bedding close to baby.* Sleeping within an easy distance for touching and feeding lessens nighttime separation anxiety, both in baby and in mother.
- *Belief in the language value of baby's cry.* Babies cry to communicate, not to manipulate. When parents respond to babies' cries, babies learn to trust Mum and Dad and their own ability to communicate.
- *Beware of baby trainers.* Rigid advice that says you must put your baby on a schedule or let your baby "cry it out" to sleep puts a distance between you and your baby. (See chapter 10 for an exposé on how rigid baby-training can sabotage your parent-child relationship.)
- *Balance.* Use your knowledge of your baby to decide when to say "yes" and when to say "no" to your baby. Also, have the wisdom to say, "yes" to caring for your own needs.
- *Both.* Babies need both parents to share in their care, day and night.

AP is flexible. The Baby B's are not a set of rules for parents to follow. They are tools that you use to accomplish your goals of knowing and enjoying your baby. These tools are based on biology – how your baby and you are "wired" to respond to one another. There may be medical or family circumstances that prevent you from being able to practice all of these Baby B's all of the time, and some will work better for you than others. Do the best you can with the resources you have. The most important thing is to get connected to your baby. As you and your baby learn to fit together, you can adapt and modify the Baby B's to suit your circumstances.

AP is not indulgent or permissive parenting. A frequent criticism of attachment parenting is that it puts baby in control, rather than parents. But can parents control babies? Actually, parenting your baby at night forces you to come to terms with the realistic fact that you *can't* control your child's behaviour. Parenting, by day and by night, should not become a control issue. Parenting depends on trust. Because AP allows mutual trust to develop between you and your child, you learn to respond to your child's needs *appropriately*, knowing when to say "yes", when to say "no", when to intervene, and when to back off and let children work through a problem on their own.

Instead of controlling their children, AP parents *shape* their children's behaviour, like gardeners tending their plants and flowers. While there are plenty of things in a garden that you can't control, such as how many buds are on the plant or when those buds open up into flowers, there are also plenty of things that you can do: you pull the weeds and water and prune the plant so that the plant blooms more beautifully. Over our many years of experience as parents and as pediatricians, we have noticed that the Baby B's of infancy often lead to the childhood C's. These children are more likely to become: cuddly, caring, compassionate, considerate, and confident.

AP shines at night. Using the Baby B's to help you get connected to your child during the day will give you an important advantage in working out the best plan for nighttime parenting. When you know your child so well and are confident in your parenting, you can work out a sleeping plan that is custom-made for your baby. You don't have to flounder around in the dark, following a book or someone else's ideas about how your baby should sleep. You'll think about your baby and the problem you are trying to solve, and a light bulb will go on. AP helps turn on those switches.

AP parents do not buy into the cry it out approach for getting babies to sleep and feed according to a rigid schedule. Nor are they big fans of sleep-inducing gadgets that fill in for parents on night duty. The sensitivity AP parents develop toward their babies tells them that what babies need most is a parent's presence. Leaving a baby to cry feels wrong to these parents, because they know that baby trusts them to respond to crying.

AP offers high-touch parenting in a high-tech world. This style of parenting encourages you to take time out and smell the roses. Busy lifestyles have made this a sleepless nation, and less responsive styles of parenting may only make it worse. Could there be any correlation over the last decade between the flurry of sleep-training books and the fact that sleep disorder clinics for children have sprung up in nearly every major town? The current epidemic of

connected kids sleep better

In our practice, we have noticed that parents who use the Baby B's have babies and children with fewer sleep problems, especially as they get older. Investing in this style of nighttime parenting when your baby is small will bring dividends of restful nights in the years to come. Connected kids tend to be less afraid of the dark and have fewer nightmares and episodes of sleep terrors. They tend to sleep better as older children. One reason for this is that these children have lower levels of stress hormones, by day and by night, so that they *sleep less anxiously* than less connected children.

AP allows you to be so intimately in touch with your baby and young child's needs that when you are faced with parenting challenges at night, you are able to create an action plan that works for you and your child. If AP parents reach a point where they feel that the family would be better off if baby learned to sleep more independently, they find sensitive ways to help baby learn to do this, ways that do not violate the trusting relationship between child and parents.

Children who are products of insensitive cry it out sleep-training methods do appear to "sleep through the night" at an earlier age. But they are sleeping more anxiously (see supporting research, page 23), and the result of this is that they tend to have more sleep problems as toddlers and preschoolers.

sleeplessness could be compared with the epidemic of childhood obesity. When children grow up with junk food, they become fat. When children begin life with junk sleep, they grow up anxious. Connected kids sleep better as older children because they slept less anxiously as infants.

Keep working at it. No single approach to nighttime parenting will work with all babies all the time, or even all the time with the same baby. Babies have different nighttime temperaments and families have varied lifestyles. Develop a style of nighttime parenting that fits the temperament of your baby and your own lifestyle. If it's working, stick with it. But if your sleep programme isn't working for your family, don't persist with a bad experiment. Be open to trying other nighttime parenting styles, especially as your child enters new developmental stages. Follow your heart rather than some stranger's sleep-training advice, and you and your baby will eventually work out the right nighttime parenting style for your family.

get to know your baby's sleep personality

You probably entered parenthood with some definite ideas about what type of parent you wanted to be and with some plans for how your new baby would fit into your life. Some of your plans probably are working out just fine, but some other things – say, nighttime – might not be going so well, because your baby seems to have plans of her own. She has a personality, which may not have figured into your original plans.

Your baby's sleep habits are in large part determined by your baby's temperament, which is not something you can change. Temperament is the part of a person's personality that is inborn and genetically determined. For example, some people are naturally calm, or sociable, or high-strung. This is true even of tiny babies. When your baby is born, you spend the first few months just getting to know your newborn. You are finding out what kind of baby you have been blessed with. Your baby's temperament will be an important influence on how you parent baby at night.

Easy babies. Of course, easy babies aren't "easy" – no baby is. But some babies are easier to care for than others. They need less of your time and energy to be content. Sure, they love to be held and played with, but they will also be happy to sit in an infant seat or lie in the cot and entertain themselves for a while. These babies also tend to need less of you at night. They fall asleep more easily and stay asleep longer. If your friend's baby is "sleeping through the night" at three weeks, she probably has this type of baby. (Or she's not giving you the whole story.)

Even though parents may report that their infants "sleep through the night", videotape studies show that most infants wake up at least once at night during the first year. Yet some infants (called "settlers") are able to put themselves back to sleep, so parents don't ever know they woke up. The main issue is not night waking, but *self-settling*. The goal of most sleep books is for an infant to learn to be a self-settler. To some extent our book has that goal also, but with the caveat that different children attain this goal at different ages and that the parents' job is to sensitively help babies learn to sleep, not just stand back and let them teach themselves.

High-need babies. Babies who ask more of their parents can be just as pleasant and just as much fun as easy babies, but they *need more* input from you to stay that way. (In chapter 5 you will meet "Miss More", our first high-need baby, daughter Hayden.) Some will term these babies "fussy babies". We find that they are more outgoing, energetic, and anxious than easy babies. A high-need baby likes to be held much of the day. In fact, high-need babies *need* to be held much of the day. They just aren't content to be put down for more than a few minutes. Tiringly, the high-need label holds true for nighttime as well. These babies need more attention from Mum and Dad when they fall asleep, and they wake up more often because they need a "dose" of Mum or Dad (okay, usually Mum) to stay asleep.

I feel that our one-year-old is a very good sleeper. I usually get a full eight hours of sleep each night. I think I was able to achieve this because I followed my instincts and cared about what my son wanted rather than go with the socially-acceptable "Let him cry it out" method. I feel good as a parent that I met my son's needs rather than forced him into the misery of lonely nights for my convenience. Besides, when I cuddle him to sleep at night, I remember that these are moments that

*last a relatively short time. In my son's entire life,
how many years will he want to be at Mummy's
side? I feel that by working with my son's
temperament, I am making the most of my
mother-son relationship, teaching him trust, and
ultimately self-reliance; he will realize that he is a
person of worth because I've shown him that he
is.*

**How does your baby's personality type predict
her nighttime needs?** If you are reading this
book because your baby is having sleep
problems, you have probably just now decided
that you have a needier baby. Some high-strung
babies are just not fans of sleep in general. And if
you are parents just getting to know your
newborn, you are probably thinking, "Oh please
be the easy kind of baby, please please
pleeeeeease!"

The truth is all babies have nighttime needs.
Easy babies will make these needs known less
often, and parents may find it easier to teach
easy babies to sleep longer at night. High need
babies are a different story. Here's why:

- *Need to touch.* High need babies thrive on
touch. They've been inside Mum for the past
nine months and they aren't ready to give up
that feeling of being enclosed and held. They've
grown used to Mum's movements and heart
sounds. Now that they are out in the world, they
can experience this closeness just as intensely,
but in different ways. They hear you, smell you,
see you, feel you and even taste you (during
breastfeeding). When Mum isn't near, high need
babies feel unsettled and incomplete. They can
sense that something is missing even if they are
sound asleep. They may sleep for hours on end
when sleeping next to someone, but wake up
every half hour if sleeping solo.

- *Need to suck.* High need babies usually have a
great need to suck for comfort. Whether it's your
breast or finger, or a bottle or dummy, comfort
sucking is almost as important as food for these
babies. They won't easily fall asleep without it,
and when they stir during the night their "suck
alarm" goes off and they start looking for
whatever they can get their mouth on. If you're
not there, your baby will let you know loud and
clear that she needs you.

- *Need to move.* You probably know by now if
your baby is one of those "always needs to be
rocked or bounced" babies. High need babies
are not content to simply be put down to fall
asleep in a cot or bed that doesn't move. There
is something soothing about the gentle rocking
of a parent's arms, a baby swing, or a cradle,
and your baby knows it. It's almost as if your
baby needs to be "coached" into falling asleep –
as long as you keep moving, baby won't notice
that sleep is sneaking up on him.

- *Balancing baby's nighttime needs with yours.*
Are your baby's needs unreasonable? Is your
baby really hungry every 2 hours at night? Does
your baby really *need* to sleep near you or does
she just *want* to sleep near you? Do you sleep
close to baby because baby wakes up
frequently? Or is baby waking up at night
because you are close? And where does your
need for sleep fit into the picture?

The art of nighttime parenting is about making
choices that get everyone's needs met most, if
not all, of the time. The choices you make for

your family will depend on both your baby's sleep temperament and your own sleep needs. Keep in mind that how you parent your baby at night may change as your baby matures. A two-month-old high-need baby may *need* to feed every two hours at night, but a fourteen-month-old high-need toddler may be ready to cut back on nighttime feeding, with some firm but loving guidance from parents. Some babies need more help than others in learning to fall asleep and stay asleep. There are different ways to provide this help, and in this book, we try to give you lots of options. We won't tell you exactly what to do with your baby in every situation, but we will help you understand your baby, so that you can sensitively meet his needs and get enough sleep yourself. You don't have to be a sleepwalking zombie during the day just because you are meeting your baby's needs at night.

matching you, your baby, and your sleep plan

Now that you have more insight into your baby's temperament, how does this affect your baby's sleep habits, and how will it affect your nighttime parenting approach? Here are some ideas to keep in mind as you continue to work through our sleep plan:

Easy babies and independent sleep. Babies with mild, easy-going temperaments are often the best sleepers. They have a low level of need at night. They will therefore easily learn self-soothing techniques, accept independent sleep associations (see page 12), and probably learn to sleep through the night relatively soon. For parents who are hoping that baby will go to sleep fairly easily, sleep well in his own bed, and not wake too often during the night, this is the baby for you! Sounds like a mattress commercial. Unfortunately (or rather, fortunately!) we don't choose what our baby's temperament will be. Easy babies are born, not made.

Easy babies and attachment-based nighttime parenting. Easy babies also thrive when parents choose a closer nighttime arrangement, such as feeding to sleep and co-sleeping. Because such babies are mild mannered, they may not demand such closeness at night, but they will certainly welcome it!

High-need babies and independent sleep. Parents who are hoping that baby will learn to sleep well in a cot in the other room with minimal night waking, and are blessed with a high-need baby, are in for a big surprise. Such a baby is very unlikely to learn to fall asleep unassisted, in a cot, in their own room, and sleep through the night. When a high-need baby is subjected to the cry it out method of sleep training, a very long and unfortunate battle of wills ensues. We feel that it is important for parents to understand what their baby's nighttime needs are in this type of situation and listen to their own instincts. A high-need baby will thrive and blossom into a self-confident and independent child if his needs are met in the early months and years. Read chapter 5 for more insights.

High-need babies and attachment-based nighttime parenting. This is a wonderful mix of a baby with many needs, and parents who are open to meeting those intense nighttime needs by breastfeeding at night and co-sleeping. However, *both* parents must team up and share night duty (and day duty) because a high-need baby can be really demanding. In chapter 5 we detail how parents can team up to thrive as a family unit with a high-need baby and avoid mother burnout.

As you work through your sleep plan, keep in mind what your baby's needs and temperament are. Always run any advice you get from us or anyone else through your own parenting instinct filter. Go with your gut feelings. You will be right 99.9% of the time.

sleep safety

Here are practical ways to help your baby sleep comfortably and safely during naptime and nighttime.

Sleepwear – how to dress your baby safely and comfortably for sleep

The more comfortably you dress your baby at night, the better she is likely to sleep. Try these suggestions:

Sleep cool. Get used to feeling your baby's forehead for clues that she's too hot. A hot, sweaty head may indicate a need for a cooler room or less clothing. Other signs of overheating include damp hair, rapid breathing, a prickly heat rash, and restlessness. If you are worried that your baby is too cold, check her hands and feet. While it is normal for the extremities to be slightly cooler than the body, if your baby's toes and fingers are truly cold she may need an extra layer of clothing. If your baby was born premature, your doctor may advise you to cover your baby's head with a cap for the first month or two, since babies lose a lot of heat through their heads. Term babies should not wear a cap or hood while sleeping, after the first night or two, since this may lead to overheating. Babies who co-sleep should not be dressed as warmly at night as babies who sleep solo. (See "Create a Comfortable Bedroom Temperature", page 11.)

Sears' Sleep Tip: As a general guide, babies sleep most comfortably covered like mother, *plus* one more layer.

After an entire winter of being completely sleep deprived, I decided one night to take my nine-month-old out of her long-sleeve outfit and dress her in a short-sleeve one piece at bedtime. It worked like magic! She is now sleeping much better, only waking up once. When she sleeps with only her nappies on, she sleeps even better.

Cotton is cool. Cotton absorbs body moisture and allows air to circulate more freely. Also, the occasional infant may be sensitive to synthetic sleepwear, and the itching may keep her awake. Flame-retardant cotton sleepwear is now available.

Sleep loose. Most babies prefer to sleep loose. Buy your baby's sleepwear to fit loosely enough to allow free and comfortable movements. There are two types of sleepwear for tiny infants: loose, baby sleeping bags, and footed sleep suits. Warm sleepwear is more practical than blankets, since babies often kick off blankets. Sleeping bags tend to be more loose-fitting, fit better for longer, and are easier for changing nappies. It's harder to get a good fit in footed sleep suits for the rapidly growing baby. Some babies sleep well in sleep suits that cover the feet. Others prefer to have their feet uncovered or covered with booties instead. Remove labels if they are rough, scratchy, or irritating to baby's skin.

I found that when my now toddler was able to choose his own number of blankets, he chose none and slept better. I wonder if I had just kept him too warm earlier.

Sleep safe. Sleepwear for babies should not have dangling ribbons, strings, or ties longer than eighteen centimetres to avoid danger of baby strangling. If baby co-sleeps, she will need less clothing than if solo sleeping, since she gets extra heat from the warm body next to her. Babies who are too warm at night may be at greater risk of SIDS, since overheating diminishes the protective arousals from sleep. If you choose to swaddle your baby to help her sleep longer, avoid overheating from other covers. Arms-free swaddling is the least restrictive and allows baby more freedom of movement. Use a single cotton blanket and avoid heavy comforters. To keep the cot-sleeping baby from sliding under the covers, tuck the bottom portion of the blankets snugly beneath the end and each side of the cot mattress, yet don't fit the blanket so tightly as to restrict baby's freedom of movement. (See more information about safe co-sleeping and safe cot sleeping, pages 74–7.)

Prefers Tummy Sleeping

I have a four-month-old who used to sleep fine on her back. But now that she can turn over, she often flips in the middle of the night. I know that sleeping on the back is important to prevent SIDS. What should I do?

"Back-to-Sleep" campaigns have been the biggest breakthrough in lowering the risk of SIDS. In most countries, back sleeping has lowered the risk of SIDS by around fifty per cent. So, always put your baby to sleep on her back, at least for the first six to nine months.

There are several reasons why back sleeping lowers the SIDS risk. We believe that the main reason is that back sleepers rouse from sleep more easily and sleep less deeply than tummy sleepers. As we discussed on page 58, easy arousability from sleep is an important protective mechanism. Another reason why back-sleeping is safer is that babies lying on their backs are less likely to become overheated because back-sleeping leaves the internal organs more exposed so they can radiate heat more easily than when on the tummy. Another possibility is that when sleeping facedown, a baby may press her head into a soft surface and suffocate.

To alleviate your worry, consider the numbers. The tummy-sleeping/SIDS risk is a statistical correlation only. It does not mean that if your baby sleeps on her tummy she is going to die of SIDS. Current SIDS rates are around 1 in 2,000 babies, meaning that there is a much greater than 99.9 per cent chance that your child will do just fine, regardless of her sleep position.

Here is another consideration. Many SIDS researchers believe that babies will naturally assume the sleep position that allows them to breathe more comfortably during the night. If your baby habitually flips over to sleep on her tummy after you've put her down to sleep on her back, this may be the right sleeping position for her. If you want to be completely safe, however, you might want to turn her onto her back when she is in a deep sleep on her tummy.

If she still flips over onto her tummy, try encouraging side sleeping. To lessen the chances of a side-sleeping baby rolling onto her tummy, stretch her underneath arm forward as shown in the illustration below. This arm can act as a stabilizer to keep baby from rolling onto her tummy. If the baby's arm stays closely tucked into her side, it will be easier for her to roll onto her tummy. Wedges to keep babies positioned on their back have never been proven to be either safe or effective and are generally discouraged.

Because of medical conditions, there are some babies who sleep more safely on their tummies, such as babies who suffer from gastroesophageal reflux (see page 214) or infants with small jawbones or other structural abnormalities of the airway. For babies with GER, an alternative to tummy sleeping is to place your baby to sleep on her left side as shown in the above illustration. Using the outstretched-arm technique, a side-sleeping baby is then more likely to flip over onto her back than her tummy.

Safe co-sleeping

Co-sleeping is safe, if you follow some simple, sensible precautions. Here's what you need to know to safely share sleep with your baby.

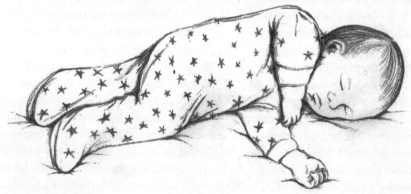

Side-sleeping with arm extended.

- Place baby to sleep on his back. Back sleeping is associated with a lowered risk of Sudden Infant Death Syndrome.
- Take precautions to prevent baby from rolling out of bed. It's unlikely that a small baby sleeping next to mother will roll out of bed, since, like heat-seeking missiles, they automatically gravitate toward mother's warm body. But to be safe, use a guardrail when baby sleeps between mother and the edge of the bed. Guard rails made of plastic mesh are safer than those with slats, which can entrap baby's limbs or head. Be sure there are no *crevices* that baby could sink into between the mattress and guard rail, the mattress and the head board, or the mattress and the wall. Push the mattress as *flush* as possible against these structures and fill in any gaps with folded towels or blankets.
- Trust your mother radar. Baby will be okay in bed with you.
- Place baby adjacent to mother, rather than between mother and father. Mothers we have interviewed on the subject of sharing sleep feel they are so physically and mentally aware of their baby's presence, even while sleeping, that they would be extremely unlikely to roll over onto their baby. Some fathers, on the other hand, may not enjoy this same sensitivity to baby's presence while asleep, so it is possible they may roll over or throw out an arm onto baby. After a few months of sleep sharing, most dads seem to develop a keen awareness of their baby's presence.
- Use a large bed, preferably a king-size.
- Do not sleep with your baby if you are under the influence of any drug (such as alcohol or tranquillizing medications) that diminishes your sensitivity to your baby's presence.
- Do not allow older siblings to sleep with a baby under one year of age. Sleeping children do not have the same awareness of tiny babies as do parents. Ditto this precaution for substitute caregivers.
- Avoid overheating from over bundling. Because baby is sleeping next to a warm body, a co-sleeping infant may need to be dressed less warmly than a baby who is solo sleeping. If you bring your baby from cot to bed, you may need to remove a layer of clothing. (Overheating can diminish baby's natural arousability from sleep.)
- Don't fall asleep with baby on a couch, beanbag, or any other soft surface that could cause baby to suffocate. One of the dangers of sleeping on a couch is that baby may get wedged between the back of the couch and the larger person's body, or baby's head could become buried in cushion crevices or soft cushions.
- It's safest not to lie down and breastfeed your baby on a cushiony surface, such as a couch, as a tired mother could fall asleep breastfeeding and roll over onto the baby.
- Recliners or adjustable armchairs are a favourite for dads falling asleep with babies, since some dads are used to these anyway. Be cautious about this practice. Baby can slip sideways from your chest and become wedged between you and the sides or arms of the chair.
- Do not sleep with baby on a free-floating, wavy waterbed (those without internal baffles), as a sleeping infant's face can be trapped in the depression formed by the weight of the head and the body. "Waveless" waterbeds are safer for sharing sleep. As an added safety measure, baby could sleep on a firm sleep mat rolled out on top of the firm waterbed.

- Don't wear dangling jewellery or lingerie with string ties longer than eighteen centimetres. Baby may get caught in these.
- Avoid pungent hairsprays, deodorants, and perfumes. Not only may these camouflage the natural maternal smells that baby is used to and attracted to, but also foreign odours may irritate and clog baby's tiny nasal passages. Reserve these enticements for sleeping alone with your partner.
- No smoking in baby's bedroom. Smoking greatly increases baby's risk of SIDS. Even the odour of smoke in your hair, clothing, or breath is a risk.
- Place your mattress and base directly on the floor. Put your bed frame away for a couple years. Assume that baby will crawl or roll out of bed at some point, and this will shorten the fall and avoid injury.
- If your bed is on a hard floor, you can soften baby's landing by placing rugs, futons, or pillows on the floor around your bed.
- Do not use extra soft padding on your mattress. This can make baby's sleeping surface too soft and may block baby's breathing if baby's face sinks into the soft padding. A pillow top mattress may also be too soft. If you feel your mattress surface is too soft, you can place a waterproof bedwetting protector pad under the sheet. This will provide a firmer surface for baby. It will also protect your mattress when baby's wet nappy leaks during the night.
- Remove pictures or any other hanging decorations from the wall near the bed. Such objects can come loose and fall onto baby. An active older baby may pull them down. Blinds and curtain cords near the bed are also potentially dangerous.

- If you are extremely obese, your infant could be at greater risk of smothering when snuggled close to you. Consider an alternative to co-sleeping such as an Arm's Reach Co-sleeper.
- It's safest and easiest for breastfeeding to place baby's head at the level of your breast. Your blanket will then end up around your rib cage. Choose sleepwear that keeps your neck and shoulders warm, so that you don't need to pull the covers up and over baby's head.
- For an in-depth analysis of the science of safe co-sleeping, see page 106.

When baby sleeps alone on an adult bed:

- Follow the same precautions as above.
- Use a baby monitor so you can hear when baby stirs. Immediately check on baby when you hear rustling to make sure baby isn't crawling or rolling off the bed.
- Cover baby with a small baby blanket only. Pull the bed sheets and blankets down to the foot of the bed.
- Teach your mobile baby (once baby starts scooting on tummy or crawling) how to safely crawl backwards down off the bed. Practise this over and over during daytime play. Since your bed is close to the floor (off the bed frame) baby can safely climb down. A futon on the floor will provide a soft landing pad.
- Place bed rails on both sides of the bed.

Safe cot sleeping

To keep your cot-sleeper safe, go through this checklist:

- Place baby to sleep on his back. Back sleeping is associated with a lowered risk of Sudden Infant Death Syndrome.
- Use a cot labelled BS EN 716 which shows that the cot conforms to British safety standards.
- Be sure the mattress fits the cot perfectly. An undersized mattress will leave a gap along the side or end of the cot where an infant's head can get caught. There should be no more than a four centimetre gap between the mattress and the side or end of the cot. If you can fit more than two fingers between the mattress and the cot, the mattress is too small.
- The firmer the mattress, the safer.
- Make sure the cot bumper fits snugly around the entire perimeter of the cot and is secured by at least six ties or snaps. To prevent your baby from chewing on the ties and becoming entangled in them, trim off excess length.
- Remove bumpers and toys from the cot as soon as the infant begins to pull up on the cot rails, because they can be used as steps for climbing over the rail.
- Place the cot in a safe area in the room, preferably near your bed. Don't place a cot near a heater, against a window, near any dangling cords from blinds or curtains, or close to any furniture that the infant could use to climb out of the cot.
- Don't attach cot toys between side rails or hang them over the cot after baby is old enough to push up on hands and knees (usually about five months). Be sure pacifiers and mobiles do not have strings longer than eighteen centimetres.
- Don't place breathing blockers in baby's cot or wherever baby sleeps. Breathing hazards include pillows, fuzzy stuffed animals and toys, string toys, and tiny chokable toys.
- Spread sheets and under sheets smoothly and tuck them in tightly beneath the mattress. This lessens the chance of wrinkles on the bedding that could obstruct baby's breathing.
- Check cot railing and hardware for splinters, sharp joints, or cracks where baby's fingers could get pinched or stuck. Frequently check the mattress support system to be sure it is secure.
- Be particularly vigilant when travelling, since baby will be sleeping in an unfamiliar and potentially unsafe environment. Bring along a firm, roll-out, safe-sleeping mat, since the beds and cots in hotels may not be up to the same safety standards you have at home.
- No smoking in baby's bedroom. Smoking greatly increases baby's risk of SIDS. Even the odour of smoke in your hair, clothing, or breath is a risk.
- Best to avoid pillows until an infant is around two years of age. As a general guide, when a child is ready to graduate from cot to toddler bed, he's old enough to use a pillow. Be sure the pillow is not too squishy. Foam pillows are safer than feather pillows.
- To check updates on cot safety, consult www.dti.gov.uk/ccp/topics1/safety.htm

chapter 4

meet different families
with different sleep plans

In the first two chapters you learned general tools to help your infant and toddler sleep happier and stay asleep longer. In chapter 3 you learned some general facts of sleep, which were necessary to help you understand why babies sleep the way they do.

Now we're going to put the information you learned into practice by relating the most common night-life situations that we encounter in our pediatric practice and helping you put your baby's individual sleep plan (ISP) into practice. We will take you on a step-by-step roadmap on how to bring together the many sleep tools listed throughout this book to help you formulate your baby's own individual sleep plan. As we journey through these real situations we will refer you to the appropriate pages in the book that deal with this situation in detail.

Working out your baby's ISP will take time. The longer baby has had tiring sleep habits, the longer it's going to take to reshape them. Your baby may be unwilling (or unable if there is a medical problem causing the night waking) to "get with the plan", but be patient and persistent, and keep modifying the plan. It is not an overnight cure, nor an every night cure. There are no quick fixes in daytime or nighttime parenting situations. Any sleep plan that will last and is sensitive to your baby's nighttime needs and your individual lifestyle will take time. Hopefully, you can identify with some of the following nighttime challenges and apply the advice to your family.

newly-born or soon to be

We're expecting our first baby. How can we help her learn to sleep well right from the start?

Meet the Newborners. Neil and Natalie were first-time, dual-career parents. They both had PhDs and worked in the field of scientific research. In fact, when we saw them for prenatal counselling, they opened the discussion with,

"Doctor, this is a well-researched baby." Neil went on to tell me, "We have done a lot of reading and we've decided that the attachment style of parenting is best for our baby." Natalie added, "It's amazing how much research there is out there showing that babies of responsive parents grow up to be happier, healthier, and smarter."

We frequently see parents like this in our pediatric practice. We dub them "high investors". They realize that investing early in a high-touch attachment style of parenting will bring great rewards down the road. Here's how we worked with their family through the early years with their baby.

When Neil and Natalie brought baby Naomi in for her one-week check-up, they told us how glad they were to have studied up on sleep tools before their baby was born, since they don't have much time to read now. They didn't regard sleep as a problem. Natalie said, "We're sleeping with our baby, since naturally breastfeeding and co-sleeping go together."

At little Naomi's one-month check-up, Natalie told us that co-sleeping was working well for her. "It just makes sense to have her sleep next to me and breastfeed. It would disturb my sleep a lot more if I had to get out of bed in the middle of the night, pick up a crying baby out of a cot, and sit up and feed her. It would take both of us a long time to resettle. With her next to me at night, I don't even wake up completely. I just instinctively feed her, and we both quickly drift back to sleep. Sometimes in the morning I don't even know how often she fed during the night." She added, "I am going to be working part-time out of our home, so I'm glad that co-sleeping is helping me to get a reasonably good night's sleep."

This mother and baby had discovered nighttime harmony. Their sleep cycles were in sync, and both got their nighttime needs met. Natalie got enough sleep, and Naomi got enough milk, along with the closeness she needed. She was growing well and was alert and calm during her check-up.

Neil agreed that co-sleeping was working well for the family. "Frankly", he joked, "I like it because I don't have to get up and feed the baby in the middle of the night." He continued more seriously. "I may not be able to breastfeed Naomi, but I try to be involved in every other part of her care. I do baths and nappies. The other night, Natalie handed her to me after she had fed her, and I walked her around the house until she fell asleep on my shoulder. While breastfeeding is Naomi's favourite thing in the whole world, it's nice to know that she feels safe and trusts me to take care of her too. Natalie's been trying to get out and take a walk every day when I get home from work, and usually, Naomi is content with me during that time, as long as I focus on her and not the match."

As the months went by, Natalie and Neil encountered some challenges. Naomi went through a couple high-need periods when she fed several times during the night, but Natalie was prepared for these growth spurts, and Neil stepped in to comfort Naomi when he could, and to take care of Natalie when he couldn't do much with Naomi. Neil spent a lot of time with Naomi on weekend mornings, allowing Natalie to escape to the university library and concentrate on her work.

When Naomi became a toddler, night feeding became more challenging for Natalie. Naomi sometimes wanted to feed all night long, as she slept, and Natalie often found this tiring. She wanted to continue to meet her baby's needs at night, and she realized that continuing to have positive feelings about feeding was also important. So when she fed Naomi during the night, she was careful to ease her baby off the breast as she drifted off into sleep and to button up her pyjama top to discourage Naomi from latching on every time she stirred. If Naomi fussed a bit, Neil or Natalie gently rubbed her back and soothed her. This didn't work all the time, but it worked often. When Naomi turned two, Neil and Natalie got her a "big girl" bed, and over the course of the next year, Naomi learned to sleep by herself, although Natalie continued to feed her to sleep in her own bed. If Naomi woke up during the night, one or the other parent went in to comfort her. Sometimes Dad ended up sleeping in Naomi's bed.

When her parents brought Naomi into our office for a two-year check-up, Natalie and Neil reflected on how far they had come since Naomi's baby days. Naomi still fed to sleep at bedtime, but some nights she fell asleep during her bedtime story or while her mother rubbed her back. Natalie said, "I never thought I'd see the day when Naomi would fall asleep without feeding. But she's getting there. Someday I know she won't need me at all at bedtime, and I will miss snuggling with her."

As we follow families like this over the years, we find that one word describes them best, "Thriving!" These babies and children not only get bigger; they thrive, which means growing optimally – physically, emotionally, and intellectually. The parents thrive too. They become astute and sensitive disciplinarians, and they truly enjoy being with their children. A deep trust and mutual respect between parents and child grow out of this early investment in nighttime parenting.

If you have a newborn or you are expecting a baby soon and would like to give your baby a healthy sleep start by studying up on baby sleep like the Newborners did, try these steps:

1. Choose your parenting style. Read about the attachment-parenting style of baby care on page 66 and see how many of the Baby B's you want to practise. Since your baby is not yet born, you will not be able to decide fully. Begin your parenting career with as many of these eight attachment tools as you can, and modify them to fit your baby's individual temperament and your lifestyle. Once you "get connected" you will naturally use all the other sleep strategies in ways that best fit *your* baby.

2. Get Dad involved early. Read "Twenty-three Nighttime Fathering Tips", page 166. The high-touch style of attachment parenting can lead to mother burnout unless Dad shares some of the nighttime parenting.

3. Make the bed and bedroom safe and sleep-friendly for you and baby:

- Start your nighttime parenting career off in the right bed. A king-size bed is a must since whether you expect it or not, nearly all infants, even toddlers, will need to spend some time in your bed during their journey toward nighttime independence.

- Turn on sounds to sleep by (see page 22)
- Darken the bedroom (see page 9)
- Dress baby safely and comfortably for sleep (see page 72)
- Create a comfortable bedroom temperature (see page 11)

4. Try a variety of bedtime rituals. It's important to get baby used to a variety of ways of going to sleep – and back to sleep – early on so mother doesn't get burned out. Study the bedtime rituals listed on pages 12 and 33.

5. Teach baby how to sleep longer stretches. Early on your baby will need you to parent him to sleep. As he grows into sleep maturity, teach him self-help tools to peacefully go to sleep – and back to sleep – without always needing your help. Especially in the early months, don't expect to put an awake baby down in a cot, pat her "night-night" and expect her to go to sleep. If your baby could talk, she would say, "No one has yet taught me how to go to sleep on my own. I'm just a baby." Study the sleep-longer tools listed on page 28.

6. Make night feedings easier. For tips to both meet your baby's nighttime nutritional needs and get enough sleep yourself, study the night-feeding suggestions on page 134.

doing it differently with the next baby!

We're expecting our second baby. Now that we have an active toddler in the house, I want to find ways to sleep with our baby, but not have to feed so much at night.

Let's meet the Doitdifferentlys. David and Debbie are expecting their second baby. Their first child, Daniel, is now three years old. The three have enjoyed the family bed from day one. Daniel is now weaned and sleeps in his "big boy" toddler bed on the floor next to Mum and Dad's bed. David snuggles Daniel down to sleep every night.

As these parents sought counselling on sleeping better with the next baby, Debbie confided, "Sleeping close to Daniel, and even the frequent night feeding, was a wonderful bonding experience. I wouldn't change it for the world. We are so close and he is such a secure child. However, I do remember his frequent night waking sometimes made me sleep deprived, so I was cranky and resentful the next day. I don't want to be one of those mums who fall asleep at the wheel driving kids to school. I need help figuring out a way to get more sleep with our next baby than I did with Daniel."

With the next baby, can she breastfeed, co-sleep, *and* get a better night's sleep herself? Yes she can, yet right from the start she will need to teach her new baby other ways of falling asleep, in addition to breastfeeding. Here's the plan we worked out for her.

Be realistic. We praised Debbie on having the wisdom to know her limitations and on planning ahead to prevent resentful problems before they occurred. She realized that she had to work out a way to get more sleep at night in order to care for two children during the day.

Start early. During the first month David and Debbie got to know their new baby. Debbie naturally fed Daisy whenever she wanted to be fed. Toward the end of the first month with Daisy's first growth spurt and consequent marathon day and night feeding, Debbie started thinking, "I'm going down the same road I did before. It wasn't a bad road, but it was a tiring one with Daniel." To avoid going down the same tiring road, they started using the following list of ways of helping baby thrive, yet also getting baby used to other "nursings" to sleep. Here's what we advised:

Sears' Sleep Tip: We cautioned these parents not to tinker too much with the supply and demand recipe for successful breastfeeding. Being too forceful at scheduling too soon runs the risk of baby not getting enough milk.

Get Dad involved early. See "Twenty-three Nighttime Fathering Tips", page 166. After reading these tips, David learned not only how to "father nurse" his baby, he learned ways to help Debbie get more rest so she could night feed more easily. In the first few months David's role was mainly to free Debbie from many of the non-baby care chores that would drain her energy away from the children. As Daisy got more used to accepting father's "nursings" at night, she would step up her daytime feedings yet not demand to be breastfed so often at night.

Make feeding easier. Read the section "Fifteen Ways to Make Night Feeding Easier", page 134; and "Twelve Tips for Getting Baby to Feed Less at Night", page 147. By teaching baby how to cluster her feedings more during the day, baby's need to feed at night lessened, yet she still got enough nourishment to thrive.

When Debbie fed Daisy down to sleep and back to sleep when she awakened, she didn't feed her *completely* to sleep. As Daisy was just about to fall asleep after feeding, she would do the "hand off" to Dad who added the finishing touch by walking baby down in the neck nestle position and experimenting with a variety of "finishing touches", as listed on page 179. David also took his nighttime fathering role seriously, and found creative and effective ways to put Daisy to sleep so she wouldn't get hooked on just breastfeeding to sleep.

Over the next few months when we saw the family for Daisy's regular checkups, they were happy to report the above tips were working. Debbie confided, "It's really not that we're giving Daisy less quality care than we gave Daniel, it's just now we've learned some strategies to both meet his needs and get enough rest for ourselves."

baby training

We went to a class that listed ways of getting baby on a predictable feeding schedule so she would sleep through the night. I'm tired and this method sounded very convincing. Is it okay to put our baby on a set feeding schedule so she doesn't need to be fed so often, especially at night?

Be discerning about baby training. Observe these precautions:

- Insensitive baby training *forces* baby to sleep rather than *teaches* baby to sleep, just the opposite of our sleep-training philosophies.
- Neither a book nor a class should tell *you* when *your* baby needs to be fed. Only the hungry baby knows when he needs to be fed. Only the one who shared the umbilical cord with baby – Mum – knows when baby needs a response from her. Baby training teaches you to follow a book rather than learn how to read your baby.
- Do your homework. Read "Ages and Stages of Feeding at Night" (page 131) to understand why babies, especially those who are breastfed, need to be fed more frequently.
- Most baby-training methods are variations of the tired old cry it out theme. Be aware of the possible health consequences of scheduling a baby's feedings by the cry it out method (see below). Scheduling feedings too rigidly, too young is risky. One of the most common causes of the "failure to thrive" syndrome is failure to listen to and respond to baby's feeding cues. When babies are not listened to, they stop cueing their needs. As a result, baby gets less milk and Mum therefore produces less milk, and neither mother nor baby thrives.
- Let's now meet the Baby trainers, well meaning, yet vulnerable, new parents who let themselves be convinced that scheduling was convenient and suitable.

One day new parents, Bob and Belinda, brought in their three-month-old baby, Billy, for his routine check-up. When I had talked with this family during previous exams, parents and baby seemed to be thriving, though the parents had occasionally voiced their desire that he would sleep longer. At this visit I noticed several differences in the way the parents cared for baby Billy. First, they carried him in a plastic infant seat rather than wearing him in the baby sling as they had done at previous examinations (cry it out clue 1). Second, they put their baby down a few feet away from them and started talking to me without looking at the baby (CIO clue 2). Then father proudly piped up, "We've got him trained to sleep through the night, and he's such a good baby. He rarely cries" (CIO clue 3).

As I began examining this "good baby", I became concerned. There was no sparkle in his eyes. He didn't connect with me. His muscle tone was weak, and when I weighed him I found that he had gained only a few ounces during the past month. I asked the parents what they were doing differently. They mentioned they had gone to a baby-training class where, as the father reported, "We learned how to get him to sleep through the night by letting him cry it out, and how to get him on a feeding schedule during the day so that he wouldn't control us." Mum added, "It was initially hard on me, but now I get more rest." Alarm bells went off in my head. This baby probably was not getting enough to eat. In addition, the baby had developed what I call *shutdown syndrome,* or failure to thrive. His basic biological cues were not being listened to, and his needs were not being met. So he had given up on trying to connect with his caregivers.

These were caring, yet tired, parents. When I explained to them what was going on, they were wise enough to realize that their baby-training plan was not working for baby Billy. I asked them to go back to feeding their infant more frequently and wearing him in a baby sling like they used to. I advised them that "sleeping through the night" was not a reasonable expectation for a three-month-old. Basically, I asked them to soften and follow their hearts like they had done before the CIO crowd sabotaged them. We worked out a more sensitive way to help their baby sleep longer at night using the tips mentioned in chapter 1. When they returned a couple weeks later for a re-check, Billy's muscle tone had improved, he had gained weight, there was sparkle in his eyes, and the family seemed reconnected, though the father half-jokingly admitted, "He's no longer such a good baby."

baby fights sleep

Our baby fights going to sleep. By 10pm we're exhausted, but he's still awake. Help!

Meet the Sleepfighters. Steve and Sylvia came to our office for help with three-month-old Sammy. Steve and Sylvia reported their main struggle with Sammy was that he wouldn't settle down easily at bedtime. They spent hours trying to get him down, but he fussed, squirmed, and just wouldn't give in to sleep. Here is how we helped them make bedtime easier.

Step 1: Learn baby's tired time

As you learned on page 5, taking advantage of baby's natural tired time to put baby to sleep makes the whole routine much easier. Sylvia wrote down Sammy's tired times every night for one week (the times he actually showed signs of being tired, not the time he ended up falling asleep). Sylvia wasn't surprised to find that these tired times varied from as early as 7:30pm to as late as 10pm. There was no predictability to Sammy's evening tired times. We shared with Sylvia our ideas in chapter 9 about scheduling baby's naptimes to create a predictable bedtime. Sylvia wasn't sure about this idea:

I never really wanted to schedule Sammy's naps. I'm more of a play-it-by-ear kind of parent. I'm used to letting him nap whenever he wants. Nap scheduling sounds like a lot of work.

Step 2: Focus on the timing of naps

She logged baby's naps for a week and found an obvious pattern. On the days that Sammy had a late afternoon nap, he wasn't tired until 10pm that night. When an early afternoon nap occurred, he was tired earlier in the evening. We asked Sylvia to take the next two weeks and do whatever it took to make sure Sammy napped around 2:30pm each afternoon. Sylvia put her afternoon activities on hold for these two weeks as she got that nap done consistently. This also necessitated making sure the morning nap was consistent.

Some days when Sammy didn't seem likely to go down for a nap, Sylvia "tricked" him into napping using our ideas on page 187, especially co-napping. Baby Sammy couldn't resist snuggling next to Mum for some special high-touch time in the early afternoon. She tried her best to make sure he napped for at least an hour in the afternoon so that he was happy through the evening. Sylvia happily reported to us at the end of two weeks that Sammy started showing tired signs around 8pm almost every night. We explained to her that once she learned what his tired time was, she could begin the bedtime routine about a half hour before this time so that when tired time hit, he would more easily fall asleep.

Step 3: Create an environment conducive to sleep

This was another key step for Steve and Sylvia to focus on. They set the stage for sleep very thoroughly by using many of our ideas on page 9. They began to get Sammy used to this soothing environment as a prelude to sleep. When tired signs came, Sammy would already be relaxed and ready for sleep before he could begin to fight it.

Step 4: Try a variety of sleep routines

Steve and Sylvia used to take turns rocking, walking and bouncing baby while he fought his way to sleep. They wished Sammy would learn to fall asleep on his own (an independent primary sleep association), but they were willing to use attachment associations if necessary (see page 66). We suggested they spend the next week or two trying a number of different ways to lull baby to sleep (page 18). They would never know what works best until they tried it all. They borrowed a friend's baby swing to try. They rocked him in a cradle. They laid him in the cot and shushed him down. They carried him around. They snuggled with him in bed. They made sure he was well fed, burped and changed before they began the ritual. These were all the same things they had always done, but now they were doing it at his natural tired time. Sylvia was thrilled to tell us:

Some of these rituals get him to sleep fairly quickly, especially when we use motion. He will even settle down and go to sleep in his cot, although it takes a bit longer.

They decided to take advantage of Sammy's love of motion and try a swinging hammock bed. It worked like a charm. He now went to sleep fairly quickly and consistently every night around the same time. He usually awoke once each night, but Sylvia accepted this as a normal part of parenting.

high-need sleepless baby

Our baby is wired, day and night. He's calm as long as we hold him during the day and sleep close to him at night. We're exhausted! How can we get him to sleep longer stretches?

Meet the Highneeders. This family has been blessed with what we call a high need baby (see page 68 for a discussion on baby personalities and sleep temperaments). Hugh and Harriet shared with us in the first month how much work their baby is both day and night. Now at two months of age, they are looking to make nighttime easier. Here is how we worked through our plan with them:

Step 1: Be realistic about baby's nighttime needs

We helped Hugh and Harriet understand baby Hannah's high-need level. We suggested that she would be unlikely to sleep through the night in a cot in the next room at an early age. She would need more daytime and nighttime touch.

Step 2: Find out where you and baby sleep best

Hugh and Harriet had Hannah's nursery all painted and furnished weeks before her birth, but baby wanted nothing to do with it. She wouldn't sleep more than 15 minutes in her cot. They bought a Moses basket and let baby sleep right next to their bed, but she still woke just as often. We suggested they try the one thing they've been reluctant to do; let Hannah sleep with them in their bed. They didn't like this idea. They envisioned an easy baby who would easily learn to sleep alone, but our explanation of what a high need baby is makes sense to them, so they were willing to give it a try.

Hannah slept better in their bed, but still awoke every 1½ to 2 hours, and the only way she would go back to sleep was to feed. What's more, she often kicked and squirmed in her sleep, which kept both parents awake. Hugh and Harriet weren't happy, so they tried cot sleeping again with the mattress slightly upright at our suggestion (in case it's reflux heartburn, as illustrated in our next story). Hannah didn't buy it. She demanded to sleep snuggled close, so Harriet resigned herself to this arrangement. Like many dads, Hugh couldn't sleep in a bed with a baby that tosses and turns all night, so he set up a mattress on the floor of baby's nursery (ironic, isn't it?), where he got a full night's sleep.

Step 3: Learn baby's tired times

Hugh and Harriet knew that Hannah routinely got tired and would feed to sleep around 10pm. They tried changing the naps so that she'd go to sleep earlier, but she seemed innately wired to stay awake through the evening. They decided just to go with what works, and not try to force an earlier bedtime.

Step 4: Get baby to accept more than one way to fall asleep

When Hannah was three months old, Harriet gave us an update:

Honestly, the baby sleeps very well. As long as she is in my arms or baby sling for naps, or snuggled up in bed next to me at night, she's happy. She wakes every hour or two to feed, and as long as I respond quickly, she feeds right back to sleep.

Harriet looked tired, but happily adjusted to her role as a very involved mother. She seemed willing to give whatever it takes to help Hannah thrive through her high need personality. She admitted to us what the drawbacks were:

It would be nice to sleep in the same bed as my partner. It would be nice to have twenty minutes to myself once a day. It would be nice to sleep more than 2 hours straight without having her attached to my breast.

We encouraged her that her investment will pay off. She's helping a very energetic and intelligent baby thrive into a self-confident, outgoing, head-of-the-class type of child.

Yet, we shared with her two very important cautions for parents of a high-need baby:

- Avoid mother burnout.
- Share the daytime and nighttime parenting with Dad.

Because high-need babies turn into high-need toddlers, who turn into high-need preschoolers, who finally mature into confident, outgoing older children, it is critical that Hannah learn to be equally bonded to both parents. Baby needs to feel comfortable being parented by Hugh so Harriet can take a break. Harriet may feel like she can do it all now, but

she may eventually get burned out. We made a few suggestions that have worked with many high-need families:

- Try to get Hannah comfortable with falling asleep in Hugh's arms or in the baby sling with Dad. (See "Twenty-three Nighttime Fathering Tips", page 166.)
- See if Hannah can learn to fall asleep without always feeding, but with rocking and walking instead. (See "Fifteen Ways to Make Night Feeding Easier", page 134.)
- Have Hugh hold Hannah as much as possible when he's home, and especially get Hannah used to being worn in the Baby-sling.

Hugh confided in us that he was tempted to urge Harriet to just let the baby cry it out. We shared with him the many ideas we discuss in chapter 10, and the simple fact that cry it out is not for high-need babies. A baby as persistent as Hannah will just keep crying harder.

Hugh and Hannah spent a few weeks focusing on the nighttime (and daytime) fathering techniques we present in chapter 8. Instead of feeling shut out of the parenting relationship, Hugh decided to jump right in and take on a more sensitive and supportive role. Hugh tried to give Hannah bottles of pumped milk at night, but she didn't buy it. He took more naptime and nighttime duty on the weekend, often wearing Hannah in the sling so Harriet doesn't need to. Some fathering techniques worked well and kept Hannah happy, and sometimes she demanded Mum, no matter what. At least Harriet did get a break from time to time.

The one thing that they couldn't change, however, was Hannah's need to snuggle close to a parent during sleep and to feed several times during the night. Hugh still often sleeps in the next room, and continues to take some nighttime fathering duty when Harriet burns out. When friends jokingly ask, "So when are you having a second baby?" Hugh and Harriet always laugh the loudest.

Step 5: Help baby stay asleep longer

Harriet used every technique we suggested, and still Hannah would only go to sleep, and back to sleep at night, by feeding.

By three years of age Hannah learned to fall asleep and stay asleep without feeding, and all family members finally slept through the night. Years later after hearing glowing reports about Hannah's school progress, both parents told us: "It was a long, hard road, but we're seeing the rewards of our investment!"

painful night waking

Our baby wakes up a lot shrieking, not just crying. He cries a lot during the day, too. I just know something is wrong with him. Help!

We met this family when their baby was two months old. Let's call them the Refluxers. He had been waking up every hour since three weeks of age, and he wouldn't nap more than 30 minutes when lying down. Ryan is a thriving breastfed baby who is easy-going and happy during the day. He just won't sleep long without waking up crying, unless Mum or Dad is holding him. Then he'll sleep for hours.

First, instead of immediately pigeonholing this baby into the category of "bad sleep habits" or "conditioned night waker", we listened carefully to the clues the astute parents provided.

This story immediately rang a bell inside our head that said GastroEsophageal Reflux. GER occurs when milk and stomach acid move up into the oesophagus and throat and cause painful burning, and therefore night waking. Baby Ryan has some classic clues:

- He wakes up frequently when lying down, but sleeps well when upright in parent's arms (in the upright position, gravity keeps food and acid in the stomach).
- He cries when laid down flat, but sits happily for long periods of time when upright in an infant seat.
- Parents instinctively knew their baby awoke because he hurt somewhere.

Rob and Rhona share with us that their friends told them to let Ryan cry it out, to stop tending to him at night, and that they were spoiling him. Their previous doctor called the problem "colic" and didn't think of GER. Ryan didn't have some of the other classic signs of GER (discussed thoroughly in chapter 11 on page 214). This hidden type of GER is called *silent* GER, and is often missed. Thankfully, Rob and Rhona listen to their intuition and come looking for answers. As listed on page 215, we took them through the steps of finding out hidden medical causes of night waking, such as GER and intolerances to some foods in a breastfeeding mother's diet (often these two causes are both present). After a few weeks of trying all the treatments listed on page 216 (see related story, page 217), they found that Ryan slept best in a swinging hammock bed. It's upright position and gentle rocking motion helped to minimize the reflux and easily soothed baby back to sleep.

won't sleep well in cot

Our two-month-old is still waking up every few hours and we're tired of stumbling down the hallway to get him back to sleep. How do we get more sleep?

Welcome the Sleepaloners. Sam and Susan have been trying to get a good night sleep ever since baby Sean was born two months ago, and it's just not happening. He has been sleeping in his cot in the nursery and Sam and Susan were hoping he would be just like all the other babies in the playgroup – sleeping through the night by now. Two months of stumbling down the hallway to put him back to sleep several times each night has left Susan tired and cranky during the day. She wanted him to stop waking up so much. We shared with them the idea that each baby has unique nighttime needs, and Sean needed something different than the easy sleepers that their neighbours have. We also reminded them of the many normal reasons why babies wake up at night (page 58). We suggested they start over

at square one with baby and take our sleep plan step by step. Here's how we helped them get more sleep.

Step 1: Rule out a medical cause of night waking

We asked Susan several questions to make sure Sean doesn't have a hidden medical cause of night waking (page 213). We determined he probably does not.

Step 2: Create an environment conducive to sleep

Sam really wanted Sean to stay in his own room and cot, so Susan and he followed all our recommendations on page 9 and made sure the room temperature, bedding, and clothing were all comfortable for Sean. Susan had been breastfeeding Sean every time he woke up because he seemed hungry and she found it much easier to give him the breast than to mix a bottle during the night. Sam surprised Susan by volunteering to give Sean a middle-of-the-night bottle.

We give him one or two bottles of formula each day. Why not give one at night too? His tummy will stay full and he might sleep longer.

We explained to Sam that in theory this sounds logical. We have seen it work with some babies and not with others. We offered a word of caution: "Feeding at night helps maintain Mum's milk supply. The more formula you give, the less breast milk Mum will make." We suggested that if they want to try this they should lessen the amount of formula during the day. Sean needed to breastfeed more during the day to make up for less feeding at night. We also offered the option of pumping breast milk for Sam to give in a bottle at night, but Susan said pumping just isn't for her.

Step 3: Open your box of sleep tools

At three months Susan reported that Sean was still waking up every 2 to 3 hours, except for a four-hour stretch when Sam gave him a bottle. We went through the many secondary sleep association tools that they could use to help Sean stay asleep longer (pages 28). Susan and Sam tried them all and found that using white noise and leaving a used breast pad in the cot helped some.

Then teething pain began at four months and Sean began waking up even more (we explain this phase on page 60). We offered ways to treat teething pain (page 226) which helped, but not enough. Susan told us she is burning out and was worried that Sean wasn't learning to be a good sleeper.

Step 4: Determine where baby sleeps best

We offered advice that seemed drastic to Sam, but made good sense to Susan. We suggested that it was likely their baby was stressed by sleeping alone. We explained how long-term sleep stress is very unhealthy for babies (page 23). Would Sean sleep longer and happier if he

were closer to his favourite people in the world? Susan confided:

"I've always wondered if he'd sleep better in our room, and maybe in our bed. Sam has resisted this suggestion because he doesn't want to get stuck with the baby in our bed for years. But I'm the one who usually gets up with Sean during the night. I need more sleep!"

We asked Sam if he'd rather have a baby who sleeps very well in their room or bed for the next few years, or a baby who keeps waking up stressed. We shared with him the many advantages of sleep sharing from chapter 5. He saw our point but worried letting Sean sleep near them would create a long-term bad habit. We agreed that if this didn't work, it would create a long-term "habit", but a good one. We reassured Sam that many babies sleep close to their parents, and all these babies eventually do move out of their parents' beds. After Sean, Susan, and Sam enjoyed months or years of happy, stress free sleep, we showed them how to wean Sean from their bed and room (as we discuss in chapter 7).

We explained the various co-sleeping options (page 4) and Susan decided to bring Sean right into their bed. We advised them how to do this safely (page 74). After a few nights in bed with Mum and Dad, they found Sean still woke up just as often, but fell back to sleep more easily because Mum tended to him more quickly. More importantly, Mum's sleep was less disrupted because she didn't have to get up.

Sam, however, wasn't happy. Sean's squirming, grunting, and breathing kept him awake much of the night. He hung in there for a week because he saw Susan was getting more rest, but then he had enough. He needed sleep to function well at work so he ended up sleeping on a futon in Sean's room for a few nights. He was not happy about that. Susan was torn between her need for sleep and both their need for a close marriage. She decided to try another sleep option with Sean nearby.

They tried a co-sleeper (which we have seen work very well for many families – see it on page 123). Sam sleeps a little better now (back in bed with Susan), since he didn't feel Sean's squirming.

At six months Susan reports to us that in the co-sleeper Sean still woke up twice each night. She breastfed him at one waking, Sam gave him a bottle feeding at the other, and things were overall much better than before. They thought this might be because there's more space between them during sleep. They still wished that Sean would only wake up once, or even better, not at all, because that's what their neighbour's baby did. And surely, by the time he's in college, he will!

feeding all night

I love feeding our baby to sleep but she still wakes up every 2 to 3 hours at night and won't go back to sleep without feeding. I'm burning out! What I don't know is just how long this night waking pattern is going to last. I don't mind a couple more months of this, but I'll go crazy if she's still doing this at nine months or fifteen months.

Meet the Night feeders. Six-month-old Nicole has been sleeping with Nigel and Natalie since birth. They found this arrangement natural for them, and Natalie knew there would be some night feeding involved. Natalie knows sometimes Nicole is hungry and needs to be fed, yet now she sees baby Nicole has developed a habit of waking more often than Natalie can cope with.

Babies who night feed seem to follow one of two courses: they either naturally begin to sleep longer stretches and only wake once or twice to feed (and Mum gets enough sleep), or they develop a habit of waking up more frequently because they know they get to, and love to, feed (yet Mum *may* get burned out). The dilemma is, in the early months of breastfeeding when babies need to feed at night, we don't know which babies will gradually feed less as they get older and which ones will continue to wake up because they are conditioned to expect the comfort of feeding.

So what can Nigel and Natalie do right now with their six-month-old that will insure less night waking down the road? The main thing they are going to try to change is to help baby Nicole learn to fall asleep and back to sleep without breastfeeding. By changing her association between sleep and feeding, they hope she will wake less at night because she knows she won't always get to feed. Here's how we helped them work through their individual sleep plan:

Step 1: Decide if night feeding is a problem for you

We counselled Nigel and Natalie that many breastfed babies need one or two night feedings during the first six months of life. Baby Nicole has been demanding three or four feeds, and shows no signs of letting up. We knew that some day she would sleep longer, but Natalie confided in us that she isn't one of those mums who can just hang in there and wait it out. She needed a change now!

Step 2: Evaluate where baby is sleeping

It helped to try various arrangements if baby isn't sleeping well in your current setting. Some families in this situation find putting baby to sleep a short distance away, such as in a co-sleeper or Moses basket next to the bed, will help baby wake less often. Other babies will sleep more soundly in a different room altogether.

Nigel and Natalie were happy having baby in their bed. They wanted to work through the rest of the plan without changing this.

Step 3: Create an environment conducive to sleep

Nigel and Natalie knew that if Nicole is going to fall back to sleep at night easily, she'll need a soothing setting to fall asleep in. By reading through the options on pages 8–12 they gained several new ideas they could use to make Nicole's nighttime environment more sleepy.

Step 4: Evaluate the bedtime ritual

Natalie shared with us that she always fed Nicole to sleep. We shared our thoughts about primary sleep associations on page 14 and encouraged her that this was a very natural choice for a breastfeeding pair. Yet, if she now wanted to decrease night feedings, she needed to change Nicole's association between breastfeeding and sleeping. She could gradually and sensitively help her learn other ways to fall asleep. Natalie and Nigel both felt they wanted Nicole to learn attachment-based sleep associations, but wanted to see if this could occur without always breastfeeding.

They spent two weeks trying many of our sleep association rituals from page 28, writing down what works best in their sleep log, and finding Nicole falls asleep the fastest when being carried around or rocked (no surprise!). Natalie told us that this routine actually took more work than simply sitting down and breastfeeding to sleep, and we advised that she could choose to go back to doing this. Natalie, however, really wanted to help Nicole learn other sleep associations and was willing to keep trying. Nigel and Natalie hoped that once she got used to falling asleep without feeding, this would translate into less night waking to feed.

We made sure they were equipped with ways to "lay baby down" once she was asleep, as outlined on page 18.

Step 5: Learn baby's tired time

Since Nigel and Natalie chose to get baby Nicole to sleep at bedtime without breastfeeding, they took some time to learn her consistent tired times (page 5) and used this to their advantage.

Step 6: Take measures to lessen night feeding

Now that Nigel and Natalie had thought out some changes to their bedtime ritual, we now focused on their main concern – frequent night waking to breastfeed. We knew that when mums get burned out on night feeding, they are tempted to "let baby cry it out". Instead, we offered Natalie twelve tips to lessen night feeding (page 147) that don't involve excessive crying. She and Nigel worked on these methods for a month and came back to discuss their progress.

She's still waking up every few hours and won't go back to sleep unless I breastfeed her. I tried a dummy, rocking, walking, a water bottle – everything! She fusses until I give her the breast. I followed your suggestions on nap feeding to catch up on my sleep and tanking her up with more frequent feedings during the day, but she's still waking up to feed.

We noticed she said "I" did all this, and asked how Nigel was involved in the nighttime parenting.

"What can I do?" he says. "I don't have breasts, and that's all the baby wants at night."

It was time to get Dad involved. We discussed with Nigel our ideas on nighttime fathering in chapter 8. Nigel spent the next few weekends following many of our ideas to get baby Nicole to accept him as a substitute for falling asleep for daytime naps. He sometimes got up at night and "father nursed" Nicole back to sleep. As expected, she took longer to get back to sleep without feeding, and often spent several minutes fussing in Mum or Dad's arms. This understandably led to frustration on Nigel's part.

At 3am in the morning I hand her back to Natalie and say, "Just feed her back to sleep, please!"

We encouraged Nigel to hang in there. Nicole learned that she had two parents, and came to accept either one to comfort her back to sleep.

Nigel found that he could successfully get Nicole back to sleep about half the time. Natalie found that at least once a night Nicole truly seemed hungry, and she couldn't imagine withholding food in the name of better sleep. Natalie decided to get out of bed with baby and fed in a chair (so baby learned that feeding didn't occur in bed) once each night. She also started baby food (Nicole was seven months old) and hoped this would help keep her tummy full through the night. Nigel also kept a trainer cup with water or pumped breast milk handy to see if this would get her back to sleep without waking Mum.

Step 7: Help baby stay asleep longer

Natalie shared with us that Nicole, at eight months, was only waking up twice each night. Because she learned that breastfeeding no longer happened while lying in bed, she would often go back to sleep using our "back to sleep" ideas on page 25, such as gentle shushing, laying on of hands, or using a dummy on occasion. Natalie was able to cope with the one long breastfeeding each night in the rocking chair. As expected, Nicole gradually woke up less often to feed once Nigel and Natalie taught her other ways to go to sleep and back to sleep.

family burned out from frequent night feeding

Our whole family is falling apart because of sleep deprivation. I'm depressed, and our marriage is suffering. We have tried everything we can think of to get our night-feeding baby to sleep more. Is it okay to use the cry it out approach as a last resort? Is there a sensitive way to do this?

I realized how serious the family's sleep deprivation was when mother revealed that she almost fell asleep at the wheel the other day. They needed a solution to their infant's night waking, and they needed it NOW!

Many kids ago we learned an important survival principle: IF YOU RESENT IT, CHANGE IT! When the whole family is falling apart, it's time to take some action. Here's an example.

Meet the Burnouters. I recently saw tired parents Ben and Beth and their son, Barney, for sleep counselling. Ben is an obstetrician, and Beth is a full-time mother, and they had driven an hour and a half to talk with me about Barney's frequent night feeding. At fifteen months he was still waking up every two hours during the night to feed, and this kept Beth from getting the sleep

she needed. When the family came into my office, I observed that the baby was thriving, but the parents looked absolutely wiped out. I was happy that Ben had come along for this consultation. In my experience, mothers tend to downplay the serious impact of baby's sleep patterns on the family's health. Dads are more honest about the situation.

I observed the family dynamics. Beth was a very nurturing, yet supersensitive mother. If Barney made so much as a peep, she would scoop him up in a millisecond and feed him. She told me, "It's just easier for me to comfort him before he gets so worked up. I refuse to let him cry. I just can't." Ben told me that Beth was so tired that she was becoming depressed and was considering taking anti-depressant medication. He, too, was tired at work, and their marriage was suffering. Basically, the whole family was falling apart because of lack of sleep.

Ben was proposing that they just let the baby cry. Beth didn't want to do this. I found myself in a dilemma. On the one hand, I couldn't agree with Dad's remedy of putting the baby in his cot, closing the door, and letting him cry. (The first day in medical school you learn, "First, do no harm!") On the other hand, things couldn't continue the way they were. I had already seen Ben and Beth once before and given them our usual sleep plan, but apparently this approach had not helped. The situation had reached a point where Mum's need for sleep had to take priority. So, these were the steps we went through:

1. Explain the problem. I explained to the parents that Barney had become a conditioned night-feeder. He was so accustomed to feeding to sleep and feeding back to sleep when he awoke in the middle of the night, that he didn't know any other way to relax and go to sleep. So he stayed attached to Mum's breast for much of the night. (In reviewing baby's early history, I suspect that Barney had GER in the early months and that this had taught him that sleep is a painful state. He had outgrown the GER, but the anxiety about falling asleep remained. See page 161 for explanation of post-GER conditioning).

2. Realize that a change needs to be made. It took a while to gently convince Beth that what her baby needed most was a happy and rested mother and that she couldn't be the good mother she wanted to be if she didn't get some sleep. Beth and Ben were aware of the saying, "If Mum isn't happy, nobody's happy!" but Beth had been willing to sacrifice her own need for sleep to keep her baby content at night. With her partner's support, she finally agreed that Mum's need to sleep was the priority here. I reassured her that turning over nighttime parenting responsibilities to Dad doesn't mean that she is an uncaring or insensitive mother. On the contrary, she's ultimately doing what's best for baby.

3. Present the plan. I first reassured Beth that this plan was not the standard cry it out programme of nighttime neglect. We would like to call this "the no-fuss sleep plan", but let's be honest. Of course a high-need baby with a persistent personality is going to protest when his favourite all-night café shortens its hours and his favourite waiter is on holiday. The critical difference was Barney would not be left to cry *alone*. I was also careful not to offer these tired parents a quick fix. I explained to them that this problem could not be solved overnight, and that it might take a month or two before Barney learned to sleep in five or six-hour stretches. Here is what I suggested Ben and Beth do to help Barney learn to sleep better.

Beth would continue feeding Barney frequently during the day. She would continue wearing him in the baby sling and doing all the other things she had been doing that have built their close attachment.

Ben would put Barney to sleep at night. At first, Beth and Ben would use the *add the finishing touch* technique as described on page 179. Beth would feed Barney until he was almost asleep, and then hand him off to Dad to complete the process with rocking, shushing, and whatever else it took. When Dad was home, he would also take care of getting Barney down for naps.

When Barney woke and cried at night, Ben would be in charge of helping him go back to sleep. He would be the "father nurser". Fortunately, Ben was ready and willing to do this. He planned to take a week off from work in order that he wouldn't have to worry about getting enough sleep. Beth would sleep in a room as far away from baby as possible. I could see that this part of the plan made Beth uneasy. She did not want Barney to cry at night. I explained to her, "Allowing a baby to cry in someone else's arms is vastly different from leaving a baby alone to cry in a cot. Crying in the arms of someone he knows and trusts is not the same as crying it out alone." It could be called CIDA – crying in Dad's arms. (If there is no dad in the house, it would be someone baby is close to.) I told her because she had been so sensitively responsive it would be very hard for her to hear Barney crying, even though she'd know he was with Dad. But we (Ben and I) reassured her that if he saw that Barney was "over the edge", Ben would come get her.

In a follow-up conversation a month later, the parents happily reported that Barney was sleeping longer and that Beth was getting more rest. The whole family was now thriving. Beth reported that allowing Ben to struggle with comforting Barney at night was one of the hardest things she had ever done, yet she had come to see that there was more than one way to comfort Barney at night. She had moved beyond the unrealistic ideal she had tried to live up to as a mother and had found a practical solution to Barney's sleep problem.

Ben confided that it had been hard for him, too. "It was so hard to hold a crying, arching baby when I knew that if Beth just fed him he would go right to sleep. But now Barney and I are closer than we ever have been, and I have a lot more confidence in my ability to calm him."

Depending on your baby, your family situation, and your own gut feeling as a parent, you might choose to try letting your baby fuss – but in a way that respects his need to communicate. Here are some guidelines:

Try other approaches first, and give them time to work. Go through the step-by-step approach in chapters 1 and 2. Realize that teaching your child to sleep better by any method will take time and dedication on your part.

Check the list of causes of night waking on page 229 before trying the crying in Dad's arms approach. You want to be sure that your baby's night waking is not caused by a medical problem.

Don't try this approach unless you believe that in your particular family situation it is necessary for you and your baby. The older your baby can be when you do this, the better. We feel that a baby under 15 to 18 months will have more trouble handling this kind of frustration. So, if you do it with a baby younger than that, be very careful to watch for the "warning signs" we have on page 211. Don't persist with a failing experiment. Be alert for changes in your baby's behaviour during the day. If your observations and your "parent gut" tell you this is too hard on your baby (and only you can tell), try something else. Experiment with other alternatives. If these don't work, try this approach again when baby is more mature and accepting.

Baby is not left to cry alone in a room. Instead, baby cries in the arms of a nurturing caregiver. Even if baby can't have Mum, he should have *someone*.

Increase your nurturing and attachment during the daytime.

Remember, it takes time. Do not follow anyone else's pre-set schedule. Your baby has unique needs and you have a unique sensitivity to those needs. One top-selling sleep-training book answers the question "How long can I let my baby cry?" with "One hour!" The book doesn't know the effects of an hour of crying on a particular baby. An hour, even five minutes for a younger baby, is like a hopeless eternity. If, when, and how long to let your baby cry in Dad's arms is a cry-by-cry decision. Again, only the people who know the baby very well can make the right decision.

Focus on night-to-night progress, not the achievement of a fixed goal such as "sleeping through the night within a week". Expect to take two steps forward and one step back. If baby gets a cold or a tummy ache, is teething hard or being weaned from the breast, or even if you take a trip or have visitors, expect that her nighttime needs will increase for a time.

Remember, parenting is a long-term investment. Listen to your babies when they are young, and they will listen to you when they are older.

chapter 5

the joys of sleeping
with your baby

"Ah, the simple pleasures of nestling next to Mummy!" If babies could talk, this is what they would say about the oldest sleeping arrangement in the world – co-sleeping. When we are asked "Where should baby sleep?" our usual reply is "Baby should sleep where all family members sleep the best." But where would babies themselves prefer sleeping?

Suppose you were a baby. Would you rather sleep alone in a dark room, behind bars, or snuggled close to your favourite person in the whole wide world? The choice is obvious.

Sears' Sleep Tip: If babies could vote, do you think they would choose to sleep alone in a dark room, behind bars, or nestled next to their favourite people in the whole wide world?

Not only do babies give the family bed the thumbs-up, so do mothers. Most mothers cherish the special closeness of sharing sleep with baby. At international parenting meetings we have asked mothers from other countries what they thought about sleeping with their baby. They found this question as odd as, "Should I breastfeed my baby?" Mothers whose opinions are not skewed by Western sleep books and "sleep experts" do not regard co-sleeping (or breastfeeding) as optional. They believe it's the only natural thing to do. Even in Western cultures, many mothers we have interviewed feel the same way. As one mother volunteered, "Just because it's nighttime, that doesn't mean my baby needs me any less."

Not only do mothers instinctively feel that their babies belong near them at night, many fathers feel likewise:

When my partner entered our bedroom and saw our newborn lying alone in the Moses basket next to our bed, he said, "Our son is sleeping in THAT? He will get cold, and how will we know that he's breathing?" My partner took our son out of the Moses basket and brought him into our bed.

Even sleep experts believe this is where babies belong. In a conversation with Dr James McKenna, Director of the Mother-Baby Sleep Laboratory at the University of Notre Dame, and a leading expert on mother-infant co-sleeping, I voiced my amazement that in some circles co-sleeping is considered weird, even unsafe. Dr McKenna replied that, on the contrary, cot sleeping is what should be considered abnormal and unsafe. We believe he is right, and later in this chapter we will tell you why.

Sleeping with your baby is a natural part of the whole parenting package, and it fits in well with modern lifestyles. Co-sleeping is becoming more popular in today's society, partly because more mothers are breastfeeding and co-sleeping makes nighttime breastfeeding much easier. Employed mothers who are away from their babies for long hours during the day have also popularized co-sleeping.

You may choose not to sleep with your baby, but no Sears' book would be complete without the message of this chapter. If you want to know how we have parented our babies at night, this chapter will tell you. We practise what we preach in these pages.

Though we are known for being advocates of parent-infant co-sleeping, we haven't been so "preachy" about co-sleeping in the other chapters of this book. We have written *The Baby Sleep Book* to help all kinds of parents with sleep problems, no matter what parenting style they use. We understand that where your baby sleeps is a very personal choice. We want to help everybody be more sensitive to their baby's nighttime needs (and we want you all to get a good night's sleep, too).

Honestly, there is nothing better than having my baby in bed with me in the morning and waking

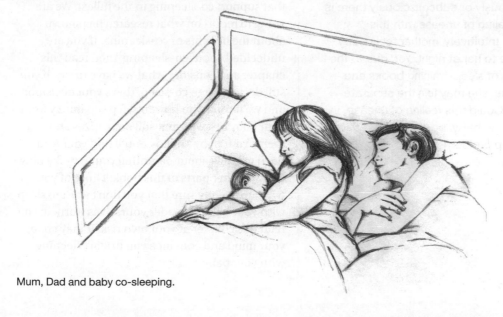

Mum, Dad and baby co-sleeping.

sleep anxiety

The deeper we get into our sleep counselling, the more we see a condition we call "sleep anxiety" – in baby, and in mother. Recent studies have shown that sleeping alone may not be in the best physiologic or emotional interest of a baby, especially in the early months. Experiments have shown that infant animals separated from their mothers have a higher level of stress hormones (see explanation, page 106). Could a baby sleeping alone become an anxious sleeper? Dr James McKenna has videotaped infants and mothers sleeping in various arrangements. Research has shown that solo sleepers are often fitful sleepers, even though they may not always completely awaken.

Sleeping apart from her baby could cause mother to become an anxious sleeper because either consciously or subconsciously there is an internal feeling of unease with this arrangement. Intuitively, mother feels baby belongs close to her at night. Yet, due to the dire warnings of sleep-training books and societal norms, she may join the separate-sleeping set. Could this feeling of unease, in both mother and baby, be one of the reasons for many sleep problems?

up with slobbery "raspberries" (his favourite thing to do in the whole world), or hearing him babble "da da da" over and over. I know it won't last, so I'm trying to soak up as much "touch time" as I can.

We know that some of you *love* sleeping with your babies and wouldn't trade it for the world. If you have read other books we've written, you have found encouragement and support for this style of nighttime parenting, yet *this* book is also written for parents who may not share sleep with their baby. We would ask you to notice, however, that nowhere have we encouraged parents to try the cry it out-alone method of getting babies to sleep. While we feel that there are many ways to meet babies' needs at night, our hearts (*and* our brains) tell us that this is not one of them.

We are going to say things in this chapter that support co-sleeping to the fullest. We are going to report on what research has shown about the benefits of co-sleeping. If you are undecided about co-sleeping, then read this chapter and consider what we have to say. If you still decide not to co-sleep, that's your decision; and we'll show you how to sleep separately from your baby in a way that still recognizes and meets your baby's needs. You'll find what you need to know about parenting your cot-sleeping baby in other parts of this book. Those of you who are already sure that you don't want to sleep with your baby, consider yourselves warned: you read this chapter at your own risk. It may change your mind and convince you to start sleeping with your baby.

our co-sleeping experiences

Dr Bill and Martha: our first three babies were easy sleepers – there was really no demand for them to share our bed, except for the occasional early morning snuggle when they were awake before we were ready to get up. Then along came our fourth child, Hayden, in 1978. Right from the start, we knew she had a different temperament. She slept fine for six months in her cradle right next to Martha, waking two (now and then three) times a night to feed. Then she graduated to a cot across the room. Hayden hated her cot and woke more and more often. Finally one night, out of sheer exhaustion from being up every hour, Martha brought Hayden into our bed, and they both slept. All Hayden needed was to be close to Martha, and from that night on we all slept much better – together. We slept so happily together that we did it for four years, until the next baby was born.

Even as we ventured into this "daring" sleeping arrangement, we were aware of what the baby books said. They all preached the same old tired theme: don't take your baby into your bed. Martha said, "I don't care what the books say, I'm tired and I need some sleep!" We had to get past all those worries and warnings about our baby manipulating us and about terminal nighttime dependency. You're probably familiar with the long litany of "you'll-be-sorry" reasons. Well, we were not sorry; we were happy. As we write this book, Hayden and her partner, Jason,

are sharing sleep with our one-year-old granddaughter, Ashton.

Here's what Hayden wrote just after the birth of her daughter, Ashton:

Our first night together outside my womb was very tender. She slept so peacefully nestled up against me in our bed. She was only inches or so away from where she had spent the last nine months. Maybe her peaceful demeanour came from the familiarity of my body movements, breathing, heartbeat, smell, voice, and touch.

Sleeping with Hayden opened our hearts and minds to a nighttime parenting style that is as old as the human race but that was new to us. We learned that there is more than one way to care for babies at night and that tired parents need to be flexible and use whatever arrangement gets all family members the best night's sleep. Over the next fifteen years we slept with four more of our babies (one at a time). While it's nice now to have the bed to ourselves, our minds are full of beautiful nighttime memories of sharing that bed with our children.

We must have made sleeping with our young ones look not only normal but also pleasant because our other grandchildren's parents, Dr Bob and Dr Jim and their wives, Cheryl and Diane, have also enjoyed sleep sharing in their families. Here is Bob's story:

When Cheryl and I first got married, she thought my parents were crazy. "I'm not going to have a baby in our bed", she stated firmly. I didn't co-sleep with my parents when I was a baby, but I'd seen them do this with my younger brothers and sisters. I wasn't sure what I wanted to do with my own kids. I just figured we'd wait and see.

When child number one came along, he spent the first night in his cradle next to our bed. Well, at least that was the plan. After Andrew woke up six times in the first five hours I finally said, "Why don't you just keep him next to you and let me sleep?" (Yes, I was a compassionate, sacrificing, I'm-right-there-with-you-babe type of husband even back then.) She kept Andrew in bed next to her, and I slept the rest of the night. So did she. So did baby Andrew. The two of them slept until 10 o'clock the next morning. And we all slept wonderfully for the next two years, though we were a little squished in our queen-sized bed. (Note – get a king! It's worth it!) Oh, and Cheryl doesn't say that my parents are crazy anymore, at least not in regards to co-sleeping.

The cot ended up being used as a nice laundry basket in "Andrew's room". I put "Andrew's room" in quotes because I don't think he ever went in there. It ended up being the extra room where we folded laundry, stacked books and boxes, and stashed anything else we didn't know what to do with. We ended up selling the cot when we moved.

the truth about co-sleeping

At least once a year we are guests on some TV show about "Should baby sleep with parents?" or some such "controversial" title. First, let's take the confusion and controversy out of this normal and healthy sleeping arrangement.

It's not an unusual custom. At first we (Bill and Martha) thought we were doing something very unusual when we slept with our babies, but we soon discovered that other parents slept with their babies, too. They just weren't telling their doctors or in-laws about it. In social settings, when the subject of sleep came up, we would admit that we slept with our babies, and then other parents would confess that they did, too. We wondered why parents thought they had to be so hush-hush about this nighttime parenting practice. Why did they feel as if they were doing something strange? Most of the world's parents sleep with their young ones. Why is this natural human parenting behaviour still taboo in our society? How could a culture have made so much progress in other areas, yet be so misguided about parenting styles?

In 1989 a renowned anthropologist, Dr Melvin Connor, reported on a study of sleeping practices in 173 developing societies around the world. In 76 of these societies (44 per cent), mother and infant shared a bed. In another 44 per cent of the societies, mother and infant at least shared a room. Dr Connor also found that parents in "primitive" societies consider solo sleeping as barbaric and abusive. After listening to Dr Connor read a "spoiling" passage in a famous baby book, one African mother replied, "Doesn't he understand it's only a baby? That's why it cries. You pick it up. Later, when it's older, it will have the sense and it won't cry anymore."

What to call it. Sleeping with babies has various names: the earthy term "family bed", while appealing to many, is a turn-off to parents who imagine Mum and several kids squeezing into one bed, along with Dad and the family dog. "Bed-sharing" is a term frequently used in medical writings. We prefer to say "sleep-sharing" because, as you will learn, parents and babies share more than just bed space. Infants and mothers sleeping side by side share lots of interactions even when they are sound asleep. Co-sleeping seems to be the newest term. The prefix "co-" means "together", so that one word, co-sleeping, sums it up pretty well. It's the word we will use most often in this book.

With Ashton asleep next to me, I feel like I am mothering her in my sleep.

Co-sleeping* is a mindset. Sharing sleep involves more than a decision about where your baby sleeps. It is a mindset, an attitude of acceptance which acknowledges that your baby is a little person with big needs. You understand that your infant trusts you, his parents, to be continually available during the night just as you are during the day. In our culture, co-sleeping also means that parents trust their own intuition

---

* Co-sleeping does not imply that baby must sleep immediately next to mother in an adult bed, although for physiological reasons mentioned on page 107, this is the ideal. "Co-sleeping" really has a broad array of options, such as baby in a co-sleeper or in a hammock, cot, cradle, or Moses basket next to parent's bed. Sleep researchers broadly define co-sleeping as any arrangement in which the child is in seeing distance of a caregiver. Ideally, one would add all the senses: hearing, smelling, seeing, and touching. We define co-sleeping as a sleeping arrangement in which baby and mother are close enough to one another to be mutually influenced by each other's nighttime physiology and sleep cycles, and close enough so that the infant is able to effectively cue the mother of his nighttime needs, and the mother is in close enough sleeping distance to easily respond with a minimum disruption of sleep.

co-sleeping – everyone's doing it!

A National Centre for Health Statistics survey from 1991 to 1999 showed that 25 per cent of American families always (or most always) slept with their baby in their bed, 42 per cent slept with their baby sometimes, and only 32 per cent of families said they never co-slept with their baby. Research carried out in NE England found that 65 per cent of parents do share their bed with their babies at some point, even if they had no intention of so doing before the birth. For those of you who co-sleep, or are thinking about co-sleeping, you're in good company.

about parenting their baby, instead of unquestionably accepting the norms of your peer group. When you accept and respect your baby's needs, you don't worry about spoiling your baby or letting him "manipulate" you when you welcome him into your bed. Co-sleeping parents are flexible and adapt their nighttime parenting style to their baby's changing needs.

Healthy things happen. In the early years of sleeping with our babies, I turned it into an informal research project. I would observe Martha and the baby cuddled up next to her. I began to see that there was a special connection between them. Was it brain waves, motion, or just something mysterious in the air that made them seem to be so closely in touch? Specifically, I noticed these special connections:

cute quotes from co-sleepers

Some memorable moments from co-sleeping families:

- At 20 months, when I try to put my daughter back in her cot after she wakes at night, she just looks up at me very pitifully and says, "Bed, Mummy" wanting to come into our bed. How can I resist?
- One of the joys is the way our child wakes up, and we do, too. He wakes up smiling, and we wake up to this precious bundle next to us.
- My daughter would ask me to sing the Barney "I love you " song when she woke in the middle of the night between her Dad and me. I sang it, though these were not exactly the sentiments foremost in my mind at the time.
- One morning I woke up to find my two-year-old kneeling over me trying to pull my eyelids open.
- When I feed her off to sleep her sleep grins fill me with such joy that all the worries of the day just melt away and I can rest knowing my daughter is happy.

- Martha and baby naturally slept alongside each other. Even if they started out not touching, the baby, like a heat-seeking missile, would naturally gravitate toward Martha. Sometimes, they faced each other, a breath away. Most of the sleep-sharing mothers I have interviewed tell me that they spend most of their night naturally sleeping on their backs or sides, as do their babies. Not only is back-sleeping the safest for baby, this position gives mother and baby easy access to each other for breastfeeding.
- Martha and baby seemed to share even the air as they slept face-to-face, almost nose-to-nose. I wondered if the carbon dioxide that mother was exhaling might influence baby's breathing? See "Science Says: Co-sleeping Is Healthy" on page 106 for detailed research on this fascinating breathing connection.)

- As I watched the sleeping pair, I was intrigued by the harmony in their breathing. Sometimes when Martha took a deep breath, baby would take a deep breath. I also noticed that when I carried a baby on my chest, she or he would take a deep breath when I directed my exhalations onto baby's scalp. It was as if my breath was a sort of "magic breath" that shaped the baby's breath.
- The sleep-sharing pair often seemed to be tuned in to each other. Martha and baby would often enter a state of light sleep together. They would move around a bit, gravitating toward one another. Martha would turn toward baby and feed or touch her, and the pair would peacefully drift back to sleep, often without either one awakening. Also, they seemed to stir at the same time. If one moved, the other would also move. After watching this "sleep dance", I

became certain that something biologically healthy was going on besides just sharing space on the mattress.

- Then there was the *reach-out-and-touch-someone* phenomenon. The baby would extend an arm, touch Martha, take a deep breath, and resettle. Martha, without waking up, would reach out and touch the baby, who would move a bit in response to her touch. She would semi-awaken from time to time to check on the baby, rearrange the covers, and then drift easily back to sleep. I was amazed by how much interaction went on between Martha and our babies when they shared sleep. It seemed that baby and mother spent a lot of time during the night checking on each other.

With Ashton right next to me, I am always aware of her temperature. If I wake up a little chilly, then I know she must be cold and I cover her up more. If I feel myself getting a little too warm or wake up sweating from heat, then I know to check her to see if she needs less covers.

Next, I noticed that our babies fed at least a couple of times during the night, usually without mother or baby completely awakening. The next morning when I asked Martha how often our baby fed, she replied, "I don't know, as often as he needed to, I guess." (I later learned why frequent night feedings are so physiologically healthy for mother and baby.) These observations were teaching me to re-evaluate the nighttime parenting advice I was teaching medical students and parents in my pediatric practice.

sailing asleep

Dr Jim Sears, an avid sailor, offers a father's viewpoint on sleep-sharing sensitivity: "People often ask me how a sailor gets any sleep when ocean racing solo. While sleeping, the lone sailor puts the boat on autopilot. Because the sailor is so in tune with his boat, if the wind shifts the sailor will wake up. Co-sleeping mothers seem to have the same kind of awareness of changes in their baby."

our co-sleeping experiments

To study the physiologic effects of co-sleeping in a real-life environment rather than in an artificial sleep laboratory, in 1992 we set up equipment in our bedroom to monitor eight-week-old Lauren's breathing while she slept in two different arrangements. One night Lauren and Martha slept together in the same bed, as they were used to doing. The next night, Lauren slept alone in our bed and Martha slept in an adjacent room. Lauren was wired to a computer that recorded her electrocardiogram, her breathing movements, the airflow from her nose, and her blood oxygen level. The instrumentation was painless and didn't appear to disturb her sleep. Martha fed Lauren down to sleep in both arrangements and sensitively responded to her nighttime needs. (The equipment was designed to detect only Lauren's physiologic changes during sleep. The equipment did not monitor Martha's changes.) A technician and I observed and recorded the information. The data was analysed by computer and interpreted by a pediatric pulmonologist who was "blind" to the situation – that is, he didn't know whether the data he was analysing came from the shared-sleeping or the solo-sleeping arrangement.

Our study revealed that Lauren *breathed better* when sleeping next to Martha than when sleeping alone. Her breathing and her heart rate were more regular during shared sleep, and there were fewer "dips", low points in respiration and blood oxygen, from slower-breathing episodes. On the night Lauren slept with Martha, there were no dips in her blood oxygen. On the night Lauren slept alone, there were 132 dips. These results were similar in a second infant, whose parents allowed us to study in their bedroom.

Since this was the first study of sleep sharing in the natural home environment, in 1993 I was invited to present our sleep-sharing research at the 11th International Apnoea of Infancy Conference. Certainly our studies would not stand up to scientific scrutiny, mainly because we only studied two babies. We didn't intend them to. It would be presumptuous to draw sweeping conclusions from studies in only two babies. We meant this only to be a pilot study. But we learned that with the availability of new micro technology and in-home, non-intrusive monitoring, our belief about the protective effects of sharing sleep was a testable hypothesis. We hoped this preliminary study would stimulate other SIDS researchers to scientifically study the physiological effects of sharing sleep in a natural home environment.

science says: co-sleeping is healthy

Infant developmental specialists all agree: togetherness, not separateness, is the healthiest state for babies. Mother and baby are both biochemically better off when they co-sleep. Here's a summary of what science says about sleeping with your baby:

Stress hormones are lower. Studies in both infant animals and humans have shown that infants' attachment to their mothers affects their cortisol balance. A baby's body needs just the right amount of cortisol at the right times. Too much or too little, and the body is not in tune, sort of like an engine trying to run with the wrong mix of gasoline and air. Separation anxiety causes prolonged elevation of the stress hormone, cortisol, which may diminish growth and suppress the immune system. Prolonged elevation of the stress hormone, cortisol, may diminish growth and suppress the immune system. Cortisol balance contributes to thriving.

Besides studies in human infants, studies in animals show that separation from the mother affects the infant's physiology. For example, studies have shown that the longer the infant animals were separated from their mothers, the higher the cortisol levels, suggesting that frequently separated babies could be chronically stressed. The mothers also experienced elevated cortisol levels when separated from their babies.[1, 2, 3, 4]

With all this evidence for beneficial effects of babies and mothers being together, the "cry it out" sleep-training advice begins to look downright unscientific. Talk about high stress hormone levels. Wow! We can't imagine a more stressful situation for a baby than being left alone, in a dark room to cry herself to sleep. This baby has stress hormones surging through her body, and she gets a booster shot of stress hormones every time she wakes up. This can't be of any biochemical benefit to baby – or to mother. When mothers say, "It just doesn't feel right for my baby to sleep in another room", she may be responding to more than just mental images. Her body is telling her to keep her baby close.

Growth hormones are higher. Growth hormones are secreted during sleep. Babies grow while they are sleeping. Growth hormone not only makes your baby grow, it also stimulates hunger. Waking up to feed is a baby's way of getting the fuel needed to pack on the pounds. Endocrinologists have discovered that human infants deprived of sufficient closeness to the mothers have lower levels of growth hormones and fail to thrive. Studies in experimental animals showed that those infants who stayed close to their mothers had higher levels of growth hormones and enzymes essential for brain and heart growth. Separation from their mothers, or lack of interaction with their mothers when they were close by, caused the levels of these growth-promoting substances to fall.[5, 6]

Babies sleep more peacefully. Research shows that co-sleeping infants seldom startle during sleep and rarely cry during the night, compared to solo sleepers who startle frequently throughout the night and cry four times more than co-sleepers. When babies who routinely slept solo were changed to a co-sleeping arrangement, they cried less. When babies who routinely co-slept were studied sleeping alone, they cried more. Startling and crying releases stress hormones, which increase heart rate and blood pressure, interfere with restful sleep and can lead to long-term sleep anxiety.[7]

Babies enjoy a more stable physiology. Studies show that infants who sleep nearer to their parents have more stable temperatures, more regular heart rhythms, and fewer long pauses in breathing compared to babies who sleep alone. This means baby sleeps physiologically safer.[8, 9, 10, 11]

Decreases risk of Sudden Infant Death Syndrome. Worldwide research shows that the SIDS rate is lowest in countries where co-sleeping is the norm, rather than the exception. Babies who sleep either in or next to their parents' bed have a four-fold decrease in the chance of SIDS. Co-sleeping babies actually spend more time sleeping on their backs or sides, which also decreases the risk of SIDS. Further research shows that the carbon dioxide exhaled by a parent actually works to stimulate baby's breathing.[12, 13, 14, 15, 16, 17, 18, 19, 20, 21] In infants separated from their mothers, there is a decrease in REM sleep, the stage of sleep that seems to be most influential in brain growth and the state of sleep in which protective arousals (which you learned about on page 58) occur.[22, 23]

Current sleep research validates the hypothesis that we first proposed in 1985 in our book *Nighttime Parenting:* "Co-sleeping and breastfeeding can lower the risk of SIDS". We believe that mother's presence during the night helps regulate baby's breathing, which can reduce the risk of SIDS. Studies of co-sleeping mother-baby pairs have shown that they share many interactions during the night. On a broad scale, recent studies in Japan have shown a further decrease in SIDS as the rates of co-sleeping have increased in an already co-sleeping culture. A saying in Asian countries, where they enjoy some of the lowest SIDS rates in the world, is: "If you are sleeping with your baby, you always sleep lightly. You notice if baby's breathing changes. Babies should not be left alone. Babies are too important to be left alone with nobody watching them."

Seems safer than cot sleeping. A recent large study concluded that bed sharing did not increase the risk of SIDS, unless the mum was a smoker or abused alcohol.[24] Even though The Consumer Products Safety Commission in America published data that described infant fatalities in adult beds, this same data, however, showed more than three times as many cot-related infant fatalities compared to adult bed accidents.[25] (See related discussion on the pseudo-science of the CPSC study, page 116.)

Co-sleeping promotes long-term emotional health. Compared with solo sleepers, long-term follow-up of children who co-slept with their parents show they tend to be happier, less anxious, have a higher self-esteem, less likely to be afraid of sleep, show fewer behavioural problems, tend to be more comfortable with intimacy and their own sexual identity, and generally grew up to be more independent.[26, 27, 28, 29, 30] These long-term behavioural benefits may be attributed to more than just co-sleeping. Since co-sleeping is part of an overall increased parental nurturing package, it's often difficult to separate the effects of co-sleeping from other nurturing attachment tools. The above are findings which simply shed a favourable light on co-sleeping, but it should not be concluded that co-sleeping alone, in the absence of other attachment tools, is responsible for these effects.

My observations of Martha and our babies led me to conclude that co-sleeping mothers and babies seem to enjoy a mutual awareness without a mutual disturbance. As a pediatrician, I learned that co-sleeping and night feeding was a recipe for health. Over the past decade, studies in sleep laboratories have confirmed these observations: when mothers and babies share sleep, their movements and arousals are synchronized. It all seems like common sense to us now. Scientific research is validating what human beings have known instinctively for millennia: something good and healthy happens when we sleep with our babies.

nine benefits of co-sleeping

Remember, the goal of this book is to help you and your baby get more restful sleep. If practised safely and with the right attitudes and strategies, sleeping with your baby can be a wonderfully simple way to accomplish this. Here's why:

1. Babies sleep better. When we sleep we move from light sleep to deep sleep and back again several times during the night. As babies go from one sleep state to the next, they go through a transition period in which they are vulnerable to waking. Babies with easy temperaments, or "settlers", are sometimes able to soothe themselves through this restless period and move on into the next sleep cycle. Others, or "wakers", will feel more anxious during this sleep-state transition and will not be able to put themselves back to sleep – especially if sleeping alone. However, the presence of a parent can ease baby through this transition. Your warmth, closeness, heartbeat, and breathing all convey the message, "It's okay, you're not alone, you can go back to sleep …" Reassured by your presence, baby resettles and goes back to sleep. A co-sleeping mother often senses when her baby needs a little help in going back to sleep, and she intuitively offers a reassuring and familiar touch or a short feed. Often neither one totally awakens, and they both drift back to sleep easily. In a way, co-sleeping is a type of sleep training because it trains the baby to do what the parents do – sleep. Children get the message that when they lie down in the bed, they're expected to sleep.

Whether it is during the day or at night, Ashton sleeps much better when she is next to me. This could be lying in bed, or in the sling. I also see a difference if I am in the room while she sleeps. Noise or commotion does not bother her. But, if I put her in another room and leave, she often won't stay asleep as long.

Many parents have been led to believe that babies "sleep better" when sleeping alone. Science says otherwise. Studies at the University of California, Irvine, comparing co-sleepers with solo sleepers revealed that co-sleepers enjoy calmer and less restless sleep. In these studies, the infants who slept alone exhibited many signs of nighttime separation anxiety. Even though they appeared to be asleep, they startled frequently, went through periods of irregular breathing, and made more unpleasant sounds, such as squeaks and moans – which were interpreted by the observing researchers as signs that they were unhappy. The researchers noted that the physiologic responses they observed in the solo sleepers probably reflected an increase in production of stress hormones, especially in infants who cried themselves back to sleep. In our sleep counselling practice, we use the term *anxious sleepers* to describe these babies. (In contrast, just look at the face of a co-sleeping baby, and you'll see how happy he is.)

Another interesting observation that came out of this study was that when the co-sleeping babies woke up, their mothers seemed to engage more instinctively in nurturing behaviours to get baby back to sleep. The mothers of solo sleepers showed more annoyance at their babies' night waking. They perceived it as a "problem" and were not as naturally nurturing.

Not only do co-sleeping babies sleep less anxiously, they go to sleep more easily. They learn to associate familiar, enjoyable scenes and activities with sleep, so they relax and fall asleep easily when the simple, familiar pattern is repeated. Imagine that you are your baby. At the first hint that you are tired, Mum picks you up and lies down beside you. You feed and drift off to sleep. What baby could resist that!

Our two-year-old tells us when she's ready for bed ("Night-night, Mummy"). She and I have a wonderful routine: we go upstairs and get into bed together and read a few books. Then she climbs down from the bed and turns off the light. She then quickly falls asleep engaged in a wonderful nighttime hug. This gives her a positive association with sleep, and we avoid evening battles.

2. Mothers sleep better. Not only do co-sleeping babies go to sleep more easily and sleep more peacefully, so do mothers. In general, what's good for babies is good for mothers, and vice versa. Here's where sleep-sharing shines. When mother feeds her baby off to sleep, there are hormones at work in her body that help both of them sleep better – a kind of biochemical mutual giving. Mother gives baby her milk, which studies have shown contains natural sleep-inducing substances. Baby's sucking triggers the release of lactation hormones in the mother's body that, as a perk, help her relax. In effect, Mummy puts baby to sleep and baby puts Mummy to sleep. Both members of the feeding

pair sleep more easily when they do what comes naturally.

Martha notes: I regard sleeping with my baby as a "lazy mum" option. I like my sleep. Since she sleeps right next to me, I don't worry, and I don't have to get out of bed and wander down the hall when she wakes up to feed. Besides, she likes nestling next to me. That makes me happy. Feeding my youngest child in the late afternoon was like having someone inject a relaxing drug into my arm. After half a minute of feeding, this wonderful warm relaxed feeling would flow through my veins. I often fell asleep.

Many co-sleeping mothers and babies share what we call *nighttime harmony* – their sleep cycles are in sync with one another. Mother partially awakens as baby is going through the vulnerable period of night waking (as described on page 55), yet because baby is just inches away she can comfort or feed baby back to sleep without fully awakening. Because her sleep cycles follow a pattern similar to that of her baby's, mother is seldom awakened from a *deep sleep* to attend to baby. It can be harder to get back to sleep when you are jolted out of a deep sleep stage.

Martha notes: I would waken seconds before my baby. When the baby started to squirm, I would lay on a comforting hand, and she would drift back to sleep. Sometimes I did this automatically and didn't even wake up.

With a welcoming attitude about co-sleeping and a little practice, most, but not all, mothers

the hormonal helpers of co-sleeping

As you have learned in the science of co-sleeping (page 106), something biochemically healthy happens to mothers and babies when they co-sleep. It's those hormones again! Besides stress hormones being lower and growth hormones being higher in babies, here are some other hormonal perks for mothers.

Feel-good hormones are higher

When the body is biochemically right, the mind is more likely to be emotionally right. Studies on the neurochemical basis of mother-infant attachment suggests that being close to mother can stimulate the infant brain to produce feel-good hormones, called endorphins. Frequent feeding and lots of contact with mother, as happens while co-sleeping, stimulates the release of hormones that help mothers feel more relaxed. Prolactin and oxytocin, the hormones released when babies suck at the breast, not only help mother's body to make more milk, they also help her feel more relaxed and nurturing.

As I fed her off to sleep, I would feel those great sleepy hormones kick in, and we would both drift off to sleep.

There is an interesting biochemical quirk about these mothering hormones that tell us a lot about co-sleeping. Most of these hormones have a short half-life. In simple terms, this means they don't last very long in the bloodstream. They enter the bloodstream, do their job, and quickly exit. This suggests that babies and mothers need frequent doses of attachment to keep these hormones active. Co-sleeping gives mothers and babies frequent booster shots of these hormones, which helps them stay in tune with each other.

As an added hormonal perk, these increased hormonal levels that co-sleeping mothers enjoy suppress ovulation and promote child spacing.

---

achieve this nighttime harmony, and get a restful night's sleep while being there for their babies. Achieving this nighttime harmony may depend on a mother's ability to let go of her preconceived ideas about infant sleep. In fact, studies show that parents who have less flexible expectations about how their baby is supposed to sleep often have children with more sleep problems. The parents' expectation becomes a self-fulfilling prophecy: when their child's sleep pattern deviates from how the parents believe a child should sleep, the parents perceive it as a problem.

When Ashton needs to feed in the middle of the night, I look next to me and see her rooting around like a little birdie. She is only half awake. Because I can start feeding her before she starts crying, she usually doesn't ever have to fully wake up. Her sleep is not disturbed, nor is mine as much. I find that at seven months she sleeps longer stretches between feeding when she is curled up against me. Maybe my body presence allows her to stay asleep longer.

Another perk of co-sleeping is it helps make child spacing easier. Night feeding is essential if you are relying on breastfeeding alone for natural child spacing. Since co-sleeping and breastfeeding babies feed more often, co-sleeping mothers are less likely to have another baby in the bed soon. Frequent breastfeeding delays the return of ovulation and menstrual cycles. But there's much more to it than just co-sleeping and breastfeeding. You must breastfeed exclusively (and frequently) day and night, not use pacifiers or bottles, delay starting solids, and so on. Please read the whole story on natural child spacing in *The Baby Book* (Thorsons, 2005).

3. Babies grow better. Over my three decades as a pediatrician and baby watcher, I have noticed that co-sleeping babies grow better. They thrive. In our medical practice we have noticed that babies who are "trained" to sleep through the night at too early an age often show slower weight gain and lag behind in their development. They don't thrive, because their need for closeness and security is not being met. We call this condition the *shutdown syndrome* (see explanation of this condition, page 84).

There are several reasons why we think co-sleeping helps babies grow and develop better:

- Co-sleeping is an energy saver not only for mother, but also for baby. Instead of wasting energy crying at night, baby can use that energy to grow.
- It has been known for decades that extra touch stimulates brain growth. Co-sleeping babies get lots of touching at night.
- Co-sleeping makes breastfeeding easier. Babies who sleep with their mothers get more milk at night. They are also likely to enjoy a longer duration of breastfeeding. This is not only good for baby's body, it also benefits baby's brain. Recent research has shown that breastfeeding babies grow up not only to be healthier, but also smarter. This may be because of the extra brain-building fats in mother's milk.
- Co-sleeping is particularly therapeutic for babies and mothers who were separated for the first few weeks after birth because of a medical situation, such as prematurity. Co-sleeping gives you extra touch time and extra opportunities to feed. Premature babies and those who have struggled with other health problems naturally benefit from enjoying a "womb environment" a little longer – both day and night. When we notice a distance developing between a mother and baby who were separated in the first days after birth because of a medical situation or when we see a baby is not developing optimally, one of our prescriptions is: "Take your baby to bed and feed."

4. Mothers "grow" better. What's good for babies is good for mothers. As the extra milk helps your baby thrive, the extra feeding helps you thrive and grow as a mother. A co-sleeping mother is

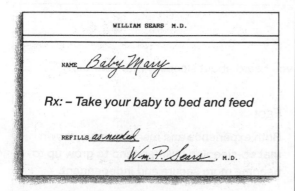

WILLIAM SEARS M.D.

NAME *Baby Mary*

Rx: – Take your baby to bed and feed

REFILLS *as needed*

Wm. P. Sears, M.D.

literally "in touch" with her baby for eight more hours than if she slept separately. Co-sleeping, night-feeding mothers enjoy higher levels of prolactin, one of the hormones that not only make milk, but also make mothering easier.

Co-sleeping, like breastfeeding, teaches baby reading. These mothers learn to know their babies very well. The many extra interactions with their baby that they enjoy while falling asleep, during the night, and when awakening boost their intuition. If baby fusses or has difficulty falling asleep at night, co-sleeping mothers are able to work out why and what to do about it. They instinctively know when a baby can comfort himself and when mother needs to step in. Because bed-sharing helps parents feel so close to their baby, their daytime parenting style is likely to be one that is very responsive to baby's needs. They will want to do the other Baby B's that are part of the whole attachment parenting package, such as babywearing and breastfeeding. Because they are intuitive parents, they are able to adjust to their baby's changing needs.

Ashton is the happiest when she first wakes up in the morning. After some big stretches and yawns, she starts smiling, chattering, and squealing. It's almost as if she is trying to tell us about the great dreams she had. This tells me that she had a good, restful sleep. Plus, we are there to enjoy her morning enthusiasm. If I was not there when she woke up, who would she tell? Coffee is nothing compared to the effects of Ashton in the morning. No matter how tired I am, I can't help but catch her enthusiasm, and we both end up cuddling and laughing. My husband, who loves to sleep like no one else, is often the first one to reach out and take her. I look over and she is in the air above him as they both squeal with joy.

5. Fathers "grow" better. Many fathers do not get to have a lot of time with their children during the day. Co-sleeping gives dads extra hours of closeness at night.

I think that being a dad in the family bed is akin to being a breastfeeding mother. There is an intimacy that comes with sleeping with your children that is about as close as a dad can get to what a mother experiences through the feeding relationship. I work long hours and having our children in our bed helps me spend quality time with them, even though we're all asleep.

6. Night feedings are easier. Breastfeeding and co-sleeping naturally go together. Because breastmilk is digested more rapidly than formula, breastfed babies need more frequent feedings. They are not able to sleep as long a

myths about co-sleeping

How many of these erroneous admonitions have you heard about sleeping with your baby?

Myth	Fact
"Your child will become too dependent!"	Both experience and research have shown that co-sleeping children tend to grow up to become more secure and independent.
"Co-sleeping is unsafe!"	As long as you follow the sensible precautions for safe sleep-sharing (listed on page 74), co-sleeping may actually be safer than solo sleeping. (See the science, page 106).
"Co-sleeping children have more sleep problems!"	We have found that children who co-sleep as infants and toddlers tend to have fewer sleep problems as they get older – though it depends on how you define a "problem".
"They'll never get out of your bed!"	Yes, they will. So what if it takes a while. How many parents have you ever talked to who wished they had spent less time with their children when they were younger?

stretch at night without feeling hungry. When co-sleeping, a breastfeeding mother's sleep cycles are more likely to be in sync with her baby's, so that she can partially awaken just in time for a feeding and easily drift back to sleep. If the baby is sleeping alone, mother may be awakened from a deep sleep for feedings, which is a lot more jarring. Getting back to sleep will be harder, too.

Just before my baby wakes up for a feeding, my sleep seems to lighten and I almost wake up. By being able to anticipate his hunger, I usually can start breastfeeding him just as he begins to squirm and reach for the nipple. Getting him to suck immediately keeps him from fully waking up, and then we both drift back into a deep sleep right after the feeding.

Co-sleeping often helps breastfeeding work better. When we counsel mothers who feel they don't have enough milk or who seem anxious about breastfeeding, we find one of the most effective "treatments" is again the time-honoured "take your baby to bed and feed". Mother and baby are more relaxed while lying down at naptime and nighttime. Baby settles in for a long, comfortable feeding, and the milk seems to flow better.

(See "Fifteen Ways to Make Night Feeding Easier", page 134 and "Twenty-three Nighttime Fathering Tips", page 166, for more night feeding tips.)

7. Co-sleeping is contemporary. Because many mothers work outside the home and are therefore separated from their baby during the day, co-sleeping seems even more necessary in today's lifestyles. Breastfeeding at night helps to perk up a mother's milk supply, which can dwindle away if she is pumping rather than feeding during the workday. Sleeping with your baby at night allows you to reconnect and make up for the missed touch-time during the day. Babies of working and feeding mums often fall into a pattern of breastfeeding a lot at night to make up for not being able to feed during the day. (See related section in chapter 12, "Night Waking after Mother Returns to Work", page 230.)

8. Co-sleeping babies tend to be better behaved. We have noticed, and long-term studies have confirmed, that co-sleepers tend to be easier to discipline. In fact, co-sleeping could be considered part of discipline. "What?" you say, "Letting your child sleep in your bed is good discipline?" Yes, it is, but first you have to understand what we mean by discipline.

Traditionally, discipline has been equated with being in control of your child. Parents had well-behaved children if they were strict about enforcing rules and careful about not "spoiling" infants and young children. The idea was that if you did not indulge a child, that child would soon learn to be more independent and to have more self-control. Better insights into children's emotional development have shown that this idea is wrong. When children are forced to become independent too soon, they end up being more needy instead of less. When parents do not respond to a child's needs for closeness and comfort from others, they increase the chances of the child becoming angry and difficult to discipline.

In the journey to nighttime independence, infants need to go through an early stage of dependence on their caregivers – which usually means some form of co-sleeping. When parents meet their needs during this dependent stage, children learn to feel secure, and in the long run, they become more independent, and even better behaved children.

co-sleeping for bottle-feeders

Co-sleeping also makes bottle-feeding easier. When baby wakes up or is about to wake up, you can quickly reach for a bedside bottle and help baby feed back to sleep before both of you are too revved up. Or, you can quickly send your partner for the bottle while you and baby stay snuggled in bed.

The challenge for co-sleeping parents is that this independence may not emerge as soon as they would like it to. Your baby is not going to suddenly decide that he's ready to sleep in a cot at 6 months – or even 2 years – of age. The friends who said "You'll never get him out of your bed" are now saying "We told you so." When you decide to co-sleep with your baby, you are making a commitment to allow your child to reach nighttime independence on his own inner timetable. When children feel secure and self-confident in their relationship with their parents, they gradually learn to sleep alone. As they mature, they learn to use the sense of security they experience in the parents' bed to help them sleep in their own beds. This same inner security helps them behave better in the daytime too. They obey their parents because they trust them, not because they are afraid of being punished.

9. Co-sleeping is safer. In recent years stories in the media claiming that co-sleeping is dangerous have confused and unnecessarily alarmed parents. Certainly, your infant's safety while sleeping is the top priority. For this reason, we have personally researched the issue of infant safety while co-sleeping, and we have also consulted with experts on infant sleep.

When mothers' intuition and "scientific" studies don't match

Why do so many of the people who advise new parents warn them that co-sleeping is dangerous for their babies? And how is it that these advisors claim to have science on their side, when so much of what behavioural scientists and parents know about infant needs and how mothers can best meet those needs suggests that co-sleeping is the norm for the human species?

When there is a conflict between scientific studies, or between science and common sense, suspect that somewhere there's a fault in the science. This is the case with the U.S. Consumer Products Safety Commission (CPSC) study that is cited by the "experts" who scare parents away from sharing sleep with their babies.

The CPSC study entitled "Hazards Associated with Children Placed in Adult Beds" was first published in the October 1999 issue of the *Archives of Paediatrics and Adolescent Medicine*, a professional journal for physicians, but it was widely and prominently reported in the American popular press. Front-page headlines in newspapers warned that babies should not sleep in the same bed as adults, and television news programmes across the country played up the story and alarmed viewers. In response, sleep researchers, such as Dr James McKenna, and breastfeeding advocates, spoke out against the study. As a well-known advocate of co-sleeping, I was interviewed by *The New York Times, The Washington Post*, CNN, and ABC's news programme *20/20*. We had a strong case against the results of the CPSC study and the Commission's recommendations, but somehow the rebuttals never have as much impact on readers and viewers as breaking news. I fear that many, many people – parents, soon-to-be parents, and health professionals – absorbed the alarming message about the risks of co-sleeping, without questioning the study or knowing anything about the benefits of sharing sleep.

Here's a summary of the study. Researchers looked at death certificates in the U.S. for the years 1990 through 1997 and found 515 cases in which a child under two had died in an adult bed; 394 of these deaths were caused by entrapment in the bed structure, for example, wedging of the child between the mattress and side rail or wall, suffocation in a water bed, or the infant's head becoming trapped in bed railings. The other 121 of these deaths were reported to be due to overlying of the child by the parent, another adult, or a sibling sleeping in the bed with the child. Most of these deaths occurred in infants under three months. Based on this review of death certificates, the CPSC issued a recommendation that parents should not sleep with babies under two years of age. They stated that the only safe place for an infant to sleep was in a cot that met the CPSC's regulations.

The study certainly highlighted the need for safety precautions when infants are put down to sleep in adult beds. (Read more about safety when co-sleeping on page 74.) *But the study does not prove that co-sleeping itself is dangerous.* The CPSC sleep study estimated that in the U.S., 64 deaths per year occurred in infants sleeping with another adult, but there is no way to determine the actual risk of co-sleeping since the study did not determine the total number of infants who sleep with their parents some or all of the time. Nor did the study examine how many infants each year die while sleeping alone in cots. While the researchers were quick to raise the alarm about co-sleeping, the study did not actually demonstrate that co-sleeping was more dangerous than solo sleeping. The gold standard of science is to do matched controls; that is to examine the cases of infants dying in cots over the same period of time. This study failed to use matched controls. The fact is that many more infants die when sleeping alone in a cot than when sleeping in their parents' bed. This includes approximately 5,000 babies who die of SIDS annually in the U.S., most of them while sleeping alone. A different study, one that would also have examined death certificates of infants dying alone in cots, might well have produced headlines such as "Hazards Associated with Infants Sleeping Alone in Cots". Instead of making parents afraid to sleep with their babies, a more valid approach would be to teach parents who choose to co-sleep to do it safely.

In Great Britain, experts are not taking such a hard line on co-sleeping, perhaps due to the influence of the UNICEF baby friendly initiative on maternity units, where rooming in and bedsharing are seen as practices which support the initiation and maintenance of breastfeeding. (See www.babyfriendly.org) The CPSC data has not influenced policy here; instead the large retrospective investigation into cot deaths in the U.K. did use matched controls, and this study concluded that sharing a room with a parent halves the risk of death. The study also found that bedsharing was fine when done safely. So in the UK it is recommended that babies share their parents' room for at least the first six months. The government has not yet stated publicly that bedsharing is fine, but they are under pressure to do so by UNICEF and other pro-breastfeeding organizations.

The truth is that babies have slept with their mothers for thousands of years and slept in cots for only a century or two – and then only in certain "civilized" parts of the world, in families well-off enough to buy cots and furnish nurseries. Wise mothers and fathers should not go against their instincts and their knowledge of what works for their families because of a single faulty study. As anthropologists, sleep researchers, and behavioural scientists continue to study mothers and infants who sleep together, we are certain to learn that this practical and responsive approach to nighttime parenting is, on the whole, good for everyone involved.

During the first six months of Leah's life, I noticed some dramatic differences in her sleeping when I wasn't sleeping next to her. In the morning I would often get up while she was still sleeping. Since I had the monitor on, I would hear loud and irregular breathing patterns rather than the quiet and regular breathing patterns she had when we slept together. There was a definite change in her breathing patterns after I would get out of bed. I think that I actually helped her breathe. Maybe I was her "pacemaker". I also noticed that when she was five months old and I would get out of bed that after a while she would roll over onto her belly. She never rolled onto her belly when I slept next to her. She was always on her side or back.

One of the experts I talked with was Dr James McKenna who said, "Their conclusion is backwards. The question that should be asked is, 'Is solo sleeping safe?'" Dr McKenna went on to explain that he had come to the same conclusions that we had: "If you thoroughly look at all the studies about sleep safety, it's impossible not to conclude that solo sleeping is the most dangerous of all sleeping arrangements." Dr McKenna and others have questioned the CPSC's interpretation of the data in their study. A critical look at the CPSC's report shows that the data in the study simply do not support the headline-grabbing claim that co-sleeping is dangerous. When parents pay proper attention to their infant's sleep safety, co-sleeping is as safe as, or safer than, cot sleeping.

True confessions. Ok, so co-sleeping is wonderful and healthy for parents and babies. But is it always so peaceful and magical, every single night? Of course not. Co-sleeping is not problem-free, and it's not always "easier" than solo sleeping. Having slept with many of our babies and counselled thousands of co-sleeping families in our pediatric practice, honestly, we have learned that there are challenges associated with any sleeping arrangement, and co-sleeping is no exception. Sometimes beds get a little crowded, sometimes baby disrupts the parents' sleep. Dr Bob relates what was happening with his two-year-old Joshua during the writing of this book:

Of course we wouldn't give up co-sleeping for the world. But for the last two weeks straight the little guy (now not so little) has started turning sideways in our bed with his head toward me. You'd think his head would gravitate toward his favourite food source, but no. Every morning around 6am I feel his little fingers gently stroking my chest, or his big head squished up against my tummy. I wouldn't mind at all if this occurred at 6:30 or 7 when I normally get up. But 6am is too early, and it's tough to go back to sleep on the narrow piece of real estate that's left to me. If I shove Joshua over towards Cheryl, he wakes up (and that's a big minus for me on the good husband rating scale). Of course this little annoyance is minor compared to the joy Cheryl and I share in having Joshua sleep with us. It will change all too soon.

nine ways to make co-sleeping easier

Many things happen while baby is in your bed. Some are funny (well, maybe they're not funny in the middle of the night when you'd rather be sleeping, but they're funny later.) Some things make wonderful memories. Others are annoying nuisances that come with the territory of nighttime parenting. Here are some tips that will help you use co-sleeping to help everyone in the family sleep better.

1. Be sure both parents agree. Whatever nighttime parenting style you choose, it should bring partners closer together, not divide them. Many modern fathers are actually proponents of co-sleeping, yet others may hesitate to jump into this nighttime parenting style. If you want to co-sleep but Dad doesn't, read together the benefits of co-sleeping in the beginning of this chapter. Suggest to him that you give co-sleeping a "30-day free trial". Many initially

sceptical dads get hooked on co-sleeping and find it brings them closer to baby. If your partner is concerned about sex, convince him that you'll do what you can to keep your sex life alive and healthy (see suggestions, page 125). Often, it's just a matter of getting your partner to trust your intuition, that here is where mother knows best. You could also point out to him that his sleep is less likely to be interrupted if baby is in your bed rather than in a cot down the hall – especially if it's *his* job to get out of bed and bring the baby to you for breastfeeding.

My partner initiated sleeping with our baby because he was tired of getting up to get our baby out of the cot to bring him to me for breastfeeding.

2. Start early, be happy. Attitude is everything, in life and in nightlife. We have noticed that parents who embrace co-sleeping as a natural part of the whole parenting package and begin co-sleeping with their baby from birth on usually come to regard it as not a big issue. And co-sleeping seems to work better for them than for parents who really don't want their baby in their bed but who give co-sleeping a try because they sure aren't getting enough sleep with baby in the cot. Parents who co-sleep for sheer survival often regard nighttime parenting as a chore rather than a bonding experience. Everything about co-sleeping becomes a big issue for them.

If you are a parent who is sleeping with your baby mainly so you can survive and get some rest, try to get past the feeling that co-sleeping is a big imposition that you are putting up with for the sake of your sleep. See if you can find reasons to enjoy co-sleeping with your baby. Look upon this as a joyful experience that will soon pass. Take a few minutes at night and in the morning to gaze at your sleeping baby, who is so content and secure when nestled next to you. You make everything right with his world, just by being close. Anyway, grumbling about your baby's presence in your bed won't make anyone sleep better.

3. Forget the "what ifs …" Parent in the present. Don't worry about next month or next year. Enjoy each night and solve problems as they occur. "But what if he gets dependent on

sleep science says: be happy where baby sleeps

Researchers at the University of California compared two groups of co-sleepers: "early co-sleepers", families where the parents began bringing their baby in their bed right after birth and regarded co-sleeping as a natural part of parenting; and "reactive co-sleepers", parents who reluctantly took their child into bed once night waking became a problem. In contrast to the early co-sleepers, reactive co-sleepers perceived co-sleeping as a solution to a problem rather than a natural extension of their daytime parenting. We wonder if the reason why co-sleeping sometimes doesn't work as well with reactive co-sleepers is that the babies perceive that the parents really don't want them there, but have them in their bed as the last resort.

sleeping with me and will never sleep in his own bed?" you may wonder. Of course your baby will come to enjoy sleeping close to the people he loves. What smart baby wouldn't? Once babies settle into a sleeping arrangement that feels so right to them, they're not going to suddenly one day wake up and say, "Let's go cot shopping." But babies change and grow. As newborns, their days and nights are mixed up and their brains are immature. As that first year goes by, they learn to sleep at night and play during the day. In the second year, they become more confident in their ability to handle the world. As they acquire new self-settling skills, they won't need to co-sleep anymore. Some day, with a little creative marketing, you will be able to ease your child out of your bed and into his own, and he will take a healthy attitude toward sleep into his new life as an independent sleeper. We can't tell you exactly when this will happen. Every child is different. Yet we can promise you that your baby will not be in your bed forever (just like we can promise you that your baby will stop breastfeeding – someday). You don't need to worry that you'll be buying your child his own bed as a wedding present.

The "authorities" dispensing sleep advice need to lay off the timelines.

Dr Bob relates:

I often wonder why my older kids sleep so well (they are now 8 and 11). Starting at about the age of six, we have been able to tuck them into bed, turn off the light, and be done with our parenting duty for the night (except, that is, for putting their younger brother to bed). They never try to procrastinate by asking for water. They never get

observations from our pediatric practice

Co-sleeping is not always romantic and problem-free. Over our combined forty years in pediatric practice, we have cared for thousands of co-sleeping families. We have seen co-sleeping work, and we have seen it not work. In the overwhelming majority of these families, we've noticed the following outcomes:

- These infants thrive, that is they grow optimally physically, emotionally, and intellectually.
- The parents are closer to their children. They are better able to read and appropriately discipline their children.
- The parents are more confident in giving intuitive and appropriate care to their children and need to rely less on outside advice (even *our* advice!)
- These children tend to be happier and healthier.
- These children grow up to be appropriately independent, that is *interdependent*. This may be a new term to you. Interdependence is the most mature stage of independence in which a child learns that he can do something by himself, but he can do it better in cooperation with another person. Mastering interdependence is one of the hallmarks of successful chief executives. People who are interdependent strive to cooperate with others. Relationships, not just personal power, are what matter most.

A common phrase we use in describing attachment-parented kids during a check-up is: "He/she seems nurtured." Over my years in pediatric practice, I have noticed a remarkable difference in children who are co-sleeping and night-feeding graduates. More often than not, these children radiate happiness. Often while examining a baby I will notice that there is something unique about that baby. He's happy, not anxious, and seems connected. I'll often say, "I bet you breastfeed and co-sleep!" Mothers will usually respond, "How did you guess?" The baby makes it obvious.

On the other hand, co-sleeping problems, if not addressed early and appropriately, can lead to mother burnout. The most common problem we see is the conditioned night feeder (see page 147), whom we dub the "all-night sucker". Some mothers simply cannot get enough rest when their babies feed every hour or two all night long. They end up feeling sleep-deprived and this affects not only mother, but the whole family. In the next chapter you will learn sensitive, appropriate ways to prevent a baby from becoming a conditioned night feeder, as well as ways to correct the problem if a mother is on her way to burnout because of lack of sleep.

up to come get us to tuck them in again. They seldom complain that it's bedtime. They never have nightmares or sleep terrors. They never wet their bed. They simply fall asleep quickly and peacefully, every single night. I don't know, maybe they're just genetically perfect kids, and it has nothing to do with how they have been parented to sleep at night. Yet, I would like to think growing up in a stress-free sleeping environment had everything to do with it.

Yet, if you do like to think in the future, consider this. One of the most precious memories you can give your child is to recall how they were parented to sleep and how they woke up each morning and the first people they saw were the people they loved. Is this a memory you would like your child to store? Or, imagine your child remembering waking up in his room in a wooden cage, peering out through bars. We still remember awakening to that beautiful face next to us and imagining that if babies could talk they would say, "Thanks, Mum and Dad, for sleeping so close to me."

4. Use a king-size bed. A big bed is not a luxury, it's a necessity. Take the money you would ordinarily spend on a fancy cot and all that cute bedding and buy a king-size bed. That tiny bundle snuggled next to you in a tiny space doesn't stay tiny very long. As baby grows, the nighttime gymnastics may begin. If you have a small bed, your baby will soon outgrow his allotted space. Bed sharing is more comfortable when there is a big bed to share. "But they're just too expensive!" you say? Well, don't buy a luxury one; just get one that will last a few years

(because of course you won't need it longer than that, will you?)

Sears' Sleep Tip: If you begin co-sleeping when your baby is a bit older, be prepared to go through a warm-up period before you start experiencing the biological benefits mentioned earlier. Eventually, you and your baby will get used to this new closeness at night.

5. Try different sleeping positions. Some parents and babies sleep best with baby in the middle, others prefer to have baby sleep between Mum and a side rail. The baby-on-the-outside position is usually less disruptive, especially to Dad, since baby can feed without waking Daddy up. Babies sleeping between Mum and Dad have been known to wake and try to "nurse" from Dad – which is a little disorienting for both of them. But Martha remembers feeling "penned in" being in the middle. It was awkward getting out of bed without disturbing the other two co-sleepers.

I don't know if other mothers have felt this way, but I hated sleeping between Dad and the baby, and especially between Dad and the toddler. Too confining. Too claustrophobic. Too many people needing a piece of me.

6. Make night feeding easier. Breastfeeding and co-sleeping go together, so be prepared for extra nighttime feeding. Read the night feeding made easier tips on page 147.

7. Try a co-sleeper. Some mothers believe they will feel too anxious to sleep well with their baby right next to them. These mothers do better with baby sleeping in a co-sleeper, a baby bed that connects to the parent's bed and gives baby his own sleeping space. Some babies sleep better in a bedside co-sleeper than they do in the parents' bed, where they may wake up every time Mum or Dad stirs. If you are uncomfortable with your baby in your bed, you might want to try a co-sleeper. Both you and your baby will have your own separate sleeping spaces, yet baby is within arm's reach for easier feeding and comforting. As an extra perk when using the co-sleeper, you don't have to worry about keeping your pillows and covers away from your baby's face.

Our co-sleeping toddler sometimes seems too stimulated by having Mum and his "yum-yums" so close.

Another alternative is to put baby's cot next to your bed. There may be bars between you and baby, but this may work for you. For some parents the term "co-sleeping" doesn't necessarily mean sharing the same bed, it could be just having baby next to the parent's bed or in the same bedroom. Here's what mothers noticed after moving baby's cot from a separate room to alongside their bed:

He used to stand up in his cot and wake up when he couldn't see me. Now he sees me and goes right back to sleep.

I wake up less frequently to check on her because I can hear her, since she's in our room and so close to us.

8. Try a mattress or futon on the floor. There reaches a time in the nightlife of every co-sleeper that you want to still sleep close to your baby, but not so close. It may be that she's squirming and keeping you awake, or you know that she'll crawl off when you're not there and

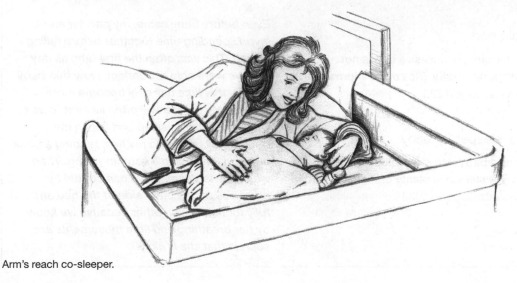

Arm's reach co-sleeper.

fall off the bed. In this case, try putting a futon or toddler-size mattress at the foot of your bed and co-sleep with her briefly to get her to sleep, and sometimes back to sleep. Here is an arrangement that our daughter, Hayden, and her partner, Jason, tried with their baby.

At nine months, I knew Ashton would crawl off our bed, so we took our mattress off the box springs and put it on the floor. We put it in the corner of the room so that walls surrounded two sides of the bed. We put her in that corner where she would be safe.

co-sleeping made easier for dad

Co-sleeping is often easier for mums than dads. Fathers don't enjoy the relaxing biological effects of breastfeeding, and their sleep cycles are not in sync with baby's like Mum's are. This biological fact of parenting nightlife naturally may make dads less enthusiastic about sharing a bed with baby. To keep Dad from having to move into the guest room to get enough sleep, try these alternatives:

Get a big bed

For co-sleeping, a king-size bed is not a luxury, it's a necessity. (See extra information on big beds, page 122.)

Try a co-sleeper for baby

Mother and baby can sleep close to one another, yet still leave plenty of room for Dad. (See co-sleeper, page 123.)

Get a "co-sleeper" for Daddy

Leave mother and baby in the big bed and Dad sleeps in an adjacent twin bed.

Make sure you get your "couple time"

Try putting baby to sleep earlier or take advantage of the time you do spend putting baby to sleep to be together.

Even before baby came, my partner and I loved spending time together before falling asleep. This was often the first time all day that we were able to connect. Now that baby is here, this time has only become more special. My partner will often lie next to us while I feed her to sleep and join in the bonding by caressing my hair, reading a book out loud, or singing a soothing song. Then when she is sleeping, we can cuddle by ourselves on the other side of the bed and fully focus on each other because we know by her breathing and little movements and sounds that she is okay.

9. Try part-time co-sleeping. Co-sleeping doesn't have to only be an all-or-nothing arrangement. As baby gets older and willingly accepts sleeping alone, try putting your baby down to sleep first in his cot (or on that futon) and then taking him into your bed the first time he wakes up. This arrangement gives you some privacy at the beginning of the night and also means you don't have to worry about your baby crawling off your big bed in the hours before you retire. (See related section, page 126.)

Sometimes part-time co-sleeping means that baby sleeps most of the night in the cot and comes into the parents' bed in the early morning, after Dad awakens. Mum and baby then enjoy co-sleeping for a few hours in the morning. This works well in situations where Dad does not sleep well with baby in the bed, nor does he want to sleep alone in another room. And it may keep an active toddler from wanting to get up and play at dawn.

common co-sleeping questions

Co-sleeping when sick

Our two-year-old went through a period when he had lots of ear infections. He would wake up a lot during the night, so we took him into our bed so we all could sleep better. Now we can't get him out. Help!

Nighttime is scary for little people, especially when they are hurting. A child wakes up in physical pain, and being in a dark room alone intensifies the fear and the pain. Naturally, this child is going to wake up. Enter Dr Mum and Dr Dad, nighttime comforters and soothers of both physical and emotional pain. The child naturally feels safe and secure and less bothered by discomfort when snuggling next to his parents. Even after the source of pain is removed the child still thinks, "Hey, this is pretty neat! I like this!" A smart child is not going to willingly accept a downgrade in accommodations and go back to sleeping alone in the wooden cage in the dark room.

Now that you can understand the situation from your child's standpoint, use the co-sleeping-made-easier techniques listed on page 124, or try the sensitive night weaning rom the family bed strategies, listed on pages 153–62.

Sex and the family bed

How can we enjoy a normal sex life and continue to sleep with our baby?

Romance doesn't need to end when a baby enters your family – and your bed. In the early months, babies are not aware of lovemaking going on in "their" bed, so if you're comfortable, don't worry about baby. However, many couples feel inhibited by a third (little) person in the bed, even though he is sleeping. We have found that nighttime parenting actually encouraged us to be more creative in our sex life. Try these tricks:

Baby goes in the cot first. Put baby in his cot during the first part of the night, enjoy private time together, and then welcome baby into the family bed after his first night waking.

Play musical beds. The master bedroom is not the only place where lovemaking can occur. Every room in the house can be a potential love chamber: another bedroom, the living room couch, in front of the fireplace – wherever the mood and the opportunity allows. (Our favourite love nest was our walk-in wardrobe, complete with futon and soft music.) If you prefer your bed, carry your sleeping child into another bedroom while you enjoy your privacy. If baby is co-sleeping when the mood hits, you either move baby or move yourselves.

Enjoy morning sex. Relaxing sex can help you sleep; tension sex can keep you awake. Most new mothers are so tired after a day of baby tending that all they want to do is sleep. As one mother so aptly put it, "My need for sleep is usually greater than his need for sex." If you can feed baby back to sleep in the early morning, go for it when *both* of you are in the mood and better rested.

father tip: enjoy daytime sex

Initiate sex during the day when baby is napping. Let her know that you are still interested in her and understand that she might be more "available" in the middle of the day rather than at bedtime. Also, there would be more time to get *her* interested, say by helping with some chores to free up some couple time.

In deciding when to enjoy sex, take a tip from your basic biology. The body is actually programmed for sex in the morning when more REM sleep occurs. REM sleep naturally stimulates erectile tissue in both men and women, setting the body up for more pleasurable sex in the morning.

Settle baby first. We figure that babies must have a built-in romance alarm. As soon as your intimacy starts to heat up, baby's radar goes off, she wakes up, and suddenly things aren't so hot anymore. Even if Dad is in the mood to continue, Mum's mind is with the baby.

Feed baby first. Trying to make love with full breasts is not only uncomfortable, it may be messy.

One night during sex my milk went off like sprinklers.

Trick inquisitive toddlers. When children get older, it's important they get two messages concerning their parents' bedroom: the door is open to them if they have a strong need to be with their parents, yet there are private times when Mum and Dad need to be alone. It's healthy for children to see affection between their parents, so don't hold back on hugs for your partner when your kids are around. And, if the bedroom door suddenly swings open and your child catches you in the act, don't worry. (It's also a good idea to keep the covers on – just in case.) It's better for a child to see his parents making love than arguing. If this happens, resort to the old standby: "go and watch TV", unless your child is really frightened by what he has seen and needs your attention. And teach your toddler that when your door is closed you need him to knock first.

Cover up if you co-sleep. Mothers will often ask, "My partner likes to sleep nude. Our baby sleeps in our bed. At what age could this be a problem?" To help your children develop healthy sexuality, you want them to learn that the body is good. That's why there is no need to panic and dive for cover when your toddler runs into your bathroom as you exit the shower in your birthday suit. Just casually reach for a towel. Yet, it can be overwhelming for a child to see a parent nude in other settings. To avoid this happening, it is prudent for dads to start wearing boxers, if they don't like pyjamas, well before the time that an older baby would be observant, and maybe by eighteen months, two years at the latest. Mums, too, may use this minimum of cover-up.

Overcrowded family bed

Our four-year-old and two-year-old love to sleep in our bed, with no signs of wanting to move out. How can we ease them into their own bed?

Too many people in one bed means that nobody gets enough room. The kids usually don't mind. This is what they're used to. But parents can only take so much. Here are your options:

Extend your bed. Put another bed, such as a twin or queen-size bed, next to your bed, and you have one big family bed. Tell the kids that

a note to dads: be sensitive during sex

Hearing your baby cry will instantly kick your partner out of lover mode and into mother mode. Don't try to compete with baby for her attention. You'll lose. Above all, don't get angry. Don't slam your fist down on the mattress and snarl, "Curses, foiled again!" (Of course, if you can do this and get a laugh, that's another story …) Instead, be a loving sensitive dad and go get baby and bring him to mum to feed. Offer some reassurance, "Feed the baby and we can make love later." The sensitive approach is a far more effective way to keep your partner in the mood.

the nighttime rule is, "If you want to sleep in Mummy and Daddy's bedroom, you need to sleep in this bed …"

Make special beds. You can get a lot of mileage out of the word "special". Put a futon or mattress on the floor at the foot of your bed. Encourage your four-year-old to sleep in his "special bed", and then gradually move the two-year-old into his own "special bed" next to his sibling. When they both become comfortable with this arrangement, move their "special beds" into their own room. Then, make a fun trip to a children's furniture store and let them pick their own "big boy" or "big girl" beds. Children are more likely to use the bed they choose.

Consider weaning your kids to a double bed in their own room. Since they are accustomed to sleeping with other people, they may sleep better together than in separate twin beds. Plus, you can lie down with both of them at the same time to read stories at bedtime. (See illustration of various sleeping arrangements, page 154.)

Making room in bed for new baby

We're expecting a new baby soon. How can we ease our two-year-old out of our bed?

It usually does not work – nor is it safe – to have a young baby and an older child in the family bed at one time. If you do, be sure that the new baby sleeps between Mummy and the wall or rail, and the toddler next to Daddy. Children should not sleep next to babies under nine months.

To ease your toddler out, try the "special bed" suggestion mentioned above. Or, have Dad sleep next to your toddler in the "special bed" or in another room, while you sleep with your new baby. As the older child gets used to sleeping without being next to you, Dad can re-join Mum and baby. It's best to try these easing-child-out strategies well before the new baby enters your bed, so your toddler doesn't feel displaced by the little "intruder". If you do wait, be sure he sees the positive spin and do what you can at other times of the day to reassure him that he hasn't lost his importance to you.

Fear of rolling over on baby

I want to sleep with our new baby, but I'm worried I'll roll over and smother her. Is this possible?

Each night all over the world millions of parents sleep with their babies and their babies wake up just fine. The same subconscious awareness of boundaries that keeps you from rolling off the bed prevents you from rolling onto your baby. Mothers we have interviewed on the subject of co-sleeping report that they are so physically and mentally aware of their baby's presence, even while sleeping, that they know they would be extremely unlikely to roll over onto their babies. Even if they did, their babies would put up such a fuss that mother would awaken in an instant (unless, of course, they should happen to be under the influence of alcohol, drugs, or medication). Experiments have shown that even newborns vigorously fight to remove a cover placed over their heads during sleep.

Fathers, on the other hand, may not always have the same keen awareness of baby's presence while asleep. So, it's possible that Dad might throw an arm out onto baby or roll over onto baby. Because of this possibility, it's safest not to position a tiny baby between mother and father, but rather baby should be next to Mummy and Mummy next to Daddy.

The controversy about the safety of co-sleeping goes back to studies done in New Zealand in the late 1980s. The data seemed to show that co-sleeping babies were in greater danger of dying during sleep than babies who slept solo, because of the risk of a parent "overlying" the infant. But when researchers went back and re-examined the data about overlying, it was found that in almost all of the cases where this happened, there were other factors involved, such as the co-sleeping parents being under the influence of drugs or alcohol.

humour in the family bed

My partner always slept with his top off, until our son started scooting around the bed in his sleep. He woke up frantically to discover, much to my amusement, that our infant son was trying to latch onto his nipple and was getting very frustrated when it wasn't working! My partner has slept with his top on since then.

I woke up and frantically started shouting to my partner to find the baby. He pointed to our son and said "He's right here," but I continued to shout at him to find the "other baby". I was dreaming about having twins and I couldn't find the second twin! It took a few minutes for my partner to calm me down and convince me that we only had one baby and he was happily sleeping right there between us.

"Fathers, please evolve and lactate", pleaded an exhausted mother of a frequent night feeder.

A few nights after our baby was born, our dog was the one keeping us awake! Every time the baby whimpered or rustled the sheets, our dog would jump to attention and start barking at us while running from one side of the bed to the other. It seemed as if the dog was letting us know that the baby needed attending to. She was so excited about the baby and wanted to "help" us. At one point we did lock her out of the bedroom, but that was worse because she sat on the other side of the door whining and crying. She was very stubborn and knew she absolutely had to look out for the baby's best interests just in case her masters were a bunch of idiots. Luckily, by the third night the dog settled down and realized that we did know how to take care of babies. The dog now sleeps in her own room.

When the data was re-examined and families with these dangerous sleep-sharing practices were excluded, it was found that co-sleeping was actually safer for babies than solo sleeping.

Sleep researchers use the infant car seat analogy when evaluating safe co-sleeping studies. If you looked at all the traffic deaths and injuries of infants in car seats, it would be alarmingly high. Yet, if you separate out from the statistics infants who were not properly and safely secured in their car seats, or who were in unsafe car seats, the stats would be much, much lower. Rather than discouraging car travel with infants as unsafe, better to teach parents how to travel more safely with their babies.

Ditto this approach to co-sleeping. Rather than discourage co-sleeping, *teach parents how to do it safely.* (See related sections: Safe

Co-Sleeping, page 74; "Science Says Co-Sleeping is Healthy", page 106; and "When Mothers' Intuition and Scientific Studies Don't Match", page 116.)

Pets in the family bed

We have a cat who likes to curl up with all of us at night. Is it dangerous for the cat to be in bed with our baby?

Yes. Pets and babies should not co-sleep. The pet needs to sleep in another bed, preferably in another room. If your pet nestles next to baby, its fur could interfere with baby's breathing enough to be concerning. Also, animal dander from all kinds of furry pets is a potential allergen that could irritate a baby's sensitive breathing passages, causing congestion and difficulty breathing. You don't want to set your child up for a lifetime of pet allergies.

Toddlers, on the other hand, often love to sleep curled up next to their pets. Providing the older child is not allergic to her pet, this is a safe arrangement; and sleeping next to a favourite pet as a "soothie" helps some children enjoy a more restful night's sleep.

chapter 6

night feedings and nightweaning
– when and how?

"Why does my baby wake up so frequently to feed?" This is the number one nighttime parenting concern we hear about in our pediatric practice. Young babies need to feed at night, and smart babies – especially high-need babies, or those with persistent personalities – are reluctant to give up night feeding as they get older.

As babies become busy toddlers (especially if paired with a busy daytime mummy) they enjoy the *private time* of night feedings. In this chapter we'll discuss why babies feed at night and how to make those night feedings easier. We'll also help you work out what to do if baby's all-night feeding is keeping you from getting the sleep you need to be a happy mother during the day and you are really ready to have the night feedings come to an end.

ages and stages of feeding at night

Breastfed babies need to be fed often, which keeps mother close by. Babies love to breastfeed, and the relaxing hormones released during feedings make it a pleasurable experience for mothers, too. Breastfeeding is an important part of how mothers get attached to their babies. Is it any wonder that you can't shut off this wonderful relationship just because it's time to go to bed? Since you're going to be spending time feeding your baby at night, you need to understand why your baby wakes up to be fed. The reasons change as your baby matures.

Birth to four months. Young babies breastfeed a lot. They are seeking both food and comfort at the breast. The sweet milk fills their tummies, and the sucking, combined with close contact with mother, calms their bodies and minds.

Tiny babies have tiny tummies, about the size of their fist, so they need to feed frequently around the clock. Breastmilk is dubbed an "easy in, easy out" food because it leaves the stomach quickly and is digested easily and efficiently. Less wear and tear on the intestines is why breastmilk leaves babies with a "good gut feeling". Formula and solid foods take longer to digest. A formula-fed baby may feel fuller longer, but may have more "pain in the gut" from wind and allergies. In the first four months expect babies to need at least two feedings during the night (midnight to 6am).

Breastfeeding also helps young babies organize their behaviour. Newborns are not very good at paying attention or staying calm, but breastfeeding helps them pull themselves together. It also eases the transition from being awake to being asleep. Some babies will even feed themselves awake again. The best thing is that this tool babies use to keep themselves happy has a human being attached to it. When baby breastfeeds, he learns to associate mother with all kinds of good feelings.

Four to six months. By this time, baby has become conditioned to this pattern of association: wake up, need comfort, breastfeed, feel better, go back to sleep. It works! Babies depend on breastfeeding at night to cope with more than just hunger. When teething pains, stuffy noses, and other physical causes disturb baby's sleep, he looks for the breast to help him feel better and go back to sleep.

Naturally, babies come to regard feeding as the best source of comfort, so they think, why not use it? Here is where sleep trainers and others who believe that parents must be in control of their babies' behaviour start to issue warnings: "If you feed your baby for comfort, he is going to want to feed all the time. He's got to learn to take care of himself." If babies could voice an opinion, they would say, "Nonsense! I'm not ready to handle life on my own, not yet." And they are right. Eventually babies do learn other ways of calming themselves and dealing with discomfort. But for now, they are learning about trust and security while feeding at the breast. These are important lessons that, later on, will help your child be happier, confident, and yes, more independent.

Six to twelve months. Separation anxiety comes into play at night as well as during the day. As babies become able to hold an image of mother in their mind, they begin to worry and fret when this important person is not there. We believe that separation anxiety is a built-in survival mechanism. As babies develop the motor skills to move away from mother, their bodies say, "let's go", yet their minds worry and say "not too far". Breastfeeding is an important way to reunite with mother, especially when babies feel anxious and alone in the dark of night. By this time, baby regards breastfeeding as a wonderful connecting tool, so that naturally, when he feels separation anxiety, how does he spell relief? B-R-E-A-S-T!

Some babies are more separation sensitive than others. High-need babies – those whose brains are wired in such a way that they need a lot of assistance from parents in staying calm and making transitions – may stick like glue to Mum at night, and feed often, some almost continuously. (Don't panic – there are things you can do to help your baby not need to feed *that* much). When one of our high-need babies was going through one of those clingy stages, we dubbed her "the Velcro baby". Other babies may be more laid back and will want to feed at bedtime and once or twice before morning.

How breastfed babies sleep. How babies are fed affects how they sleep. If your formula-feeding neighbour is boasting that her four-month-old is sleeping through the night, while your breastfeeding six-month-old is still waking two or three times a night to feed, you may be wondering what's going on here. If breastfeeding is so good for my baby, how come she's not a better sleeper? The fact is, breastfed babies tend to wake up more often than artificially fed babies, especially breastfed babies who sleep with their mothers. This isn't just an impression we have formed over the years. Researchers have documented this by comparing sleep patterns of breastfed and formula-fed babies and of babies who co-sleep and babies who don't.

Is this a hidden disadvantage of breastfeeding – something people kept from you when you signed on to feed and nurture your baby at the breast? Actually, not sleeping so soundly is a good thing for your baby. Remember what you learned about protective arousals on page 58? Babies need to be able to wake up easily. What if they were hungry in the middle of the night, but didn't wake up? They would miss out on feedings they need in order to grow. What if a baby who is left alone at night couldn't easily wake up and cry for someone to take care of him? A baby who cries or wakes up when he is out of mother's arms keeps mother close, which ups the odds that he's going to thrive.

The all-night feeder. If you suspect that breastfeeding and co-sleeping have something to do with how many times your baby wakes up at night, you are probably right. It takes longer for breastfed babies to get to the point where they sleep a good four to six hour stretch at night. Hopefully, the inconvenience of waking up more often to feed your baby at the breast is offset by how easy it is to feed at night. If you can get baby latched on and go right back to sleep as baby breastfeeds, you may find that you are getting the sleep you need and breastfeeding is actually helping you do this.

It was Snoozeville for me during night feeding.

But what if you have a baby who is nine months old, twelve months old, even eighteen months and still likes to feed all night long? And what if this means that you feel sleep-deprived, depressed, and cranky during the day? Most babies' nighttime feeding starts to taper off in the second half of this first year, and they learn to sleep more soundly. As toddlers gradually wean from the breast, they also wean from night feedings and from co-sleeping. But some babies continue to feed frequently all night long.

This can take its toll on Mum. At some point, mothers have to decide whether they're going to continue to feed whenever baby wants to at night, or if they are going to find ways to encourage their child to feed less or stop feeding at night. We often see mothers in consultation who have never been given tools to make night feeding easier on themselves. Baby is thriving, but mother is barely surviving. It is to these sleep-deprived mums that we devote this chapter.

The rest of this chapter is full of suggestions about how to make night feeding easier with both younger and older babies, and how to get older babies who are very persistent about feeding at night to feed less or not at all. It's up to you to work out what combination of night feeding and co-sleeping allows everyone in your family to get the rest they need. And as with so many other features of nighttime parenting, your approach to night feeding will probably change as your baby grows.

fifteen ways to make night feeding easier

In the early months babies need to breastfeed at night in order to grow well. Throughout the first year and beyond, there may be medical conditions, family situations, growth spurts, or other reasons why a baby continues to feed once or twice at night. High need babies, who need more of everything may breastfeed several times during the night, even in their second year of life.

Mothers who both survive and thrive with night feeding find efficient ways either to feed

without completely awakening or to go back to sleep easily after feedings. Here are ways to manage night feeding without setting yourself up for sleep deprivation:

1. Co-sleep. Most women who breastfeed for more than a few months sleep with their babies. Some of them make this decision before baby is born. Some experiment with different sleeping arrangements and gradually realize that co-sleeping is much easier on everyone in a breastfeeding family. Some night feeders learn "self service". They find the nipple without waking up mother. Co-sleeping mothers often lose track of how many times their baby feeds at night, since they are sleeping too well to be certain or even care. (See page 113 for more on the breastfeeding benefits of co-sleeping.)

I would be comatose during the day if I had to get up every couple hours at night, lift my baby out of the cot, rock and feed her back to sleep, somehow get back to sleep myself, and then have the whole process start all over again in a few hours.

2. Master the art of feeding while lying down. First, here's some pillow talk. Pillows are the key to comfortably feeding a new baby while lying in bed. Place two pillows under your head, a pillow behind your back, and one under your top leg, much like you did when you were trying to find a comfortable position to sleep in while pregnant. Does this seem like a lot of pillows? You're worth it! Night feeding should also be relaxing for Mum. Put your baby on her side facing you and nestled in your arm. Then latch her on, just as you do when you are sitting and holding her in your lap.

Have a breastfeeding counsellor or an experienced friend show you how to feed lying down early on. Some mothers and babies get the hang of this side-lying position right away. Others take a little longer. Keep working at it until it's comfortable for you, and your baby can latch on and nurse well enough to get a satisfying amount of milk and fall asleep.

Mastering side-lying feeding is the key to surviving night feeding. Side-lying feeding is much more restful than sitting up in bed and waiting 45 minutes for your infant to finish feeding before you can go back to sleep. Feeding lying down lets you fall asleep while baby feeds. Getting out of bed and sitting up to feed has many drawbacks for Mummy and baby. You have to fully wake up to retrieve the baby and find the chair, and if baby falls asleep at the breast, you have to work out how to get baby off

the breast and into bed again without waking her up. When you feed while lying down, all you have to do is drift off.

Martha notes: My sleep really improved when I finally figured out that I could feed from either breast while lying on one side rather than flipping us both around every time she switched sides.

3. Encourage a longer latch-on. When baby wakes up to feed at night, encourage her to feed long enough to fill her tummy. If she keeps popping off the breast, you're likely to get sore nipples and she's likely to wake up hungry in a very short time. Try these suggestions for longer latch-on:

Be sure your baby is latched-on well. She should get a good-size mouthful of breast. Once your milk lets down, you should see baby's jaw moving and notice her swallowing as she gulps down milk.

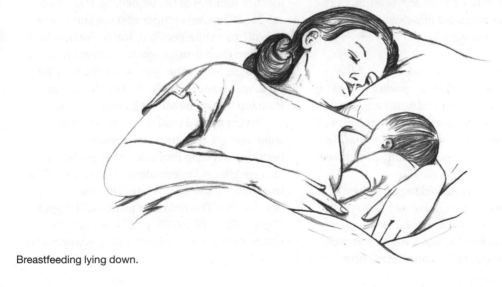

Breastfeeding lying down.

Cuddle your baby in close to you as you feed her in the side-lying position. If she has to reach and crane her neck to stay on the breast, she'll get less milk.

Curve her body towards you by bringing her knees toward your abdomen. Bending baby discourages back arching, which leads to un-latching.

When baby finishes the first side, place her on your chest and rub her back to gently bring up any air bubbles in her tummy. Then roll to the other side (reposition all those pillows!), and offer the second breast before she falls asleep. Once you get the hang of it, you can try staying on your first side to let baby feed from either breast just by angling your torso toward baby to present the top breast.

4. Make the breasts more easily available. Some mothers sleep better when they make their breasts easily available (baby sleeping near topless Mummy) to baby for self-serving. Even newborns can navigate themselves toward the nipple if they are close enough.

I slept with my breasts available to her. If she latched on, she could often do so without waking me when I was exhausted. I slept on my side, facing her, and her head was at nipple level, with my arm positioned above her head. I found she was happier with her head touching something.

5. Pre-hydrate yourself. Waking up to feed is one thing. Having to get out of bed to go to the bathroom while baby fusses for a feeding is another. Yet you need lots of water to stay well hydrated while you're lactating. Here's one strategy: drink a lot of water a few hours before bedtime. Then before you go to bed, be sure to empty your bladder well using the triple-voiding technique: after the urine flow stops, bear down with your pelvic muscles to squeeze out any urine that remains in your bladder. Do this three times.

6. Give a big bedtime feeding. Called "cluster feeding", try to feed baby every couple hours during the evening, beginning after the late-afternoon nap. Then do the "tank up feeding". Encourage your baby to feed actively for a long time before he falls asleep. We call this the *dream feed*. By active feeding, we mean the kind of sucking where you can see a wiggle at baby's temple and baby is swallowing milk after every two or three sucks. Gentle comfort sucking puts babies to sleep, but it doesn't fill tummies. You might want to start this bedtime feeding before he gets too tired, so that he doesn't nod off after just five minutes of breastfeeding. If he does start to fall asleep at the breast too soon, take him off, burp him gently to wake him up a bit, and then latch him on again. Let him finish the first breast, so that he gets lots of the high-fat milk, which will help him feel full longer, and then top him off by offering the other side.

Trying to load babies up with formula or solid food (or even too much breastmilk) before bedtime may help them sleep longer, but it can also backfire. An overstuffed tummy may allow irritating stomach acids back into the oesophagus. The pain that results will trigger night waking. (See GER, page 214.) Yet, increasing the before-bed feeding is worth a try.

I tried to load and reload. I would feed him just before his usual bedtime and then wake him for another feeding before I went to bed. This combination helped both of us sleep for longer stretches.

7. Keep the bed dry. If you produce an overabundance of milk, put a few absorbent towels under yourself, since you're likely to soak through breast pads and nightshirts. A waterproof pad under baby will protect your mattress if his nappies leak.

8. Dress for the occasion. Wear whatever attire keeps you the most comfortable at night, with the least fumbling when it's time to feed. Pyjama pants and a loose top work well. Some mothers like feeding nighties, with special openings for breastfeeding.

I used a bedrail cover that had pockets in it so I was able to put everything I would need during the night in the pockets – a change of clothes, burp clothes, nappies, wipes. That way I wouldn't have to physically get out of bed.

martha's de-latch

Some babies need to stay latched on at night to stay asleep. They startle awake when they lose the sensation of holding onto the nipple. If your baby falls asleep with the nipple clamped in his mouth, or he continues to "flutter suck" as he would on a dummy, this can be irritating. If you can't drift off to sleep that way, how do you get your breast back? Here's what Martha discovered and wrote about twenty years ago. Wait until baby is barely sucking. Then use your finger to gently pry his jaws apart, ease your nipple out, and let him finish sucking for a while on your finger. It is easier to sneak your finger away than it is your nipple. But babies older than around two months may not accept sucking on a finger any longer. With an older baby, use a finger to release the jaws and slowly draw the nipple out of his mouth,

keeping your finger there to protect your nipple in case he suddenly clamps down. If he gropes for the nipple, he is reacting to the change in pressure sensation in his mouth. So push firmly inward and upward under his lower lip or on his chin with the length of your index finger, keeping his mouth closed and applying enough pressure to keep him from awakening. Hold the pressure with your finger until he settles back to deep sleep. (You can also lay your other hand on his tummy to help him settle.) If he does wake back up, quickly give the nipple back to him, and try again after he is back to a deep sleep. You may have to do this three or four times before he stays still, but it usually works on the first try if the baby really is in deep sleep and you have been patient enough not to rush it.

9. Get comfortable. To get yourself back to sleep after feeding, lie in the position you find most sleep inducing. Also, pull your baby toward you to feed, rather than arching your back or contorting your body to get to baby. Falling asleep in a twisted position can cause you to wake up with a sore back.

10. Burp baby the easy way. Soon you'll find that traditional burping is no longer needed and you can do it "in your sleep" (so to speak). Simply prop baby up over your tummy or hip as you relax on your side and pat his back. After a few months, burping usually isn't necessary. Babies feed in a more relaxed manner at night and so swallow less air.

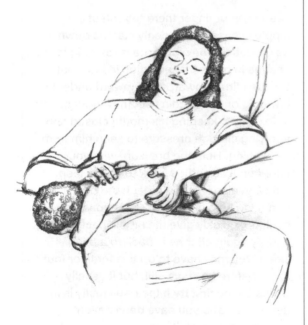

Night burping.

After she's finished feeding and needs to be burped, I lay her on my chest, while I lie with my back propped up with a couple of pillows. This enables me to stay in bed so that I don't fully awaken. If she awakens, I give her a finger or dummy, and that helps her go back to sleep without more feeding. Sometimes Dad does the burping duty.

11. Change feeding positions. Muscle and backaches are sometimes a side effect of night feeding and co-sleeping. It's possible to *feed from both breasts without turning over* to lie on the other side. But if you find this leaves you feeling stiff and achy in the morning, try to change positions during the night, so that your baby sleeps on your right side part of the night and on your left side the rest of the night. Or switch off from one night to the next. Be aware of your body position as you lie there feeding your baby. Are your shoulders tight? Are your fingers tingling because of the position of your arm? Are you tensing muscles in your neck, your back, or your legs? Relax into that pillow supporting your lower back. (What? You're not using one? Trust us, it makes a difference.) Allow your body to sink into the bed and the pillows as you fall asleep. Ask your partner for a back rub while baby feeds to help release any tension. Do some gentle stretches or some yoga during the day to counteract any tightness in your muscles from the way you sleep at night.

I fed the baby on the first side, changed his nappy, and then lay down on the other side and we fed to sleep. This way baby was already in position for the next feeding. This was a huge help.

12. Read baby's cues. Remember, our goal is to get you and your baby back to sleep as quickly as possible – no messing, no fuss. Reading baby's cues will tell you what to do to accomplish this. Most of the time, when babies wake up at night they need to feed – at least in the early months. If you can respond to baby's pre-cry signals (squirming, sputtering sounds, etc), you will get her back to sleep more quickly than if you wait for her fussing to escalate into a full-throated angry cry. You can offer to feed her right away, or hold off for a minute or two and see if she goes back to sleep. She might settle with just your loving touch or a few soothing words. If this doesn't do the trick quickly, offer the breast – or you may be awake for much longer than you'd like. When in doubt, err on the side of being more responsive rather than waiting to see if baby can soothe himself back to sleep without breastfeeding.

13. Offer a substitute. As baby gets older, you'll find that he is able to settle himself more and more of the time. You could also try offering a substitute for breastfeeding when baby is less likely to be hungry at night. Dad can comfort baby, or you can pat baby's tummy or sing to her. This will help her learn that she can go back to sleep without always breastfeeding.

14. Seek out night-feeding friends. Don't complain about your baby's night feeding to friends and family members who find it hard to understand why you continue to breastfeed. They'll offer an easy solution – just stop feeding. Your 'misery' needs the company of like-minded mums. Join your local La Leche League group and/or hang out with parents with a similar nighttime parenting mindset. Veteran mothers who have "been there and done that" can usually offer you some helpful tips and you can gain some perspective on the challenges of nighttime feeding.

Each time my child woke at night to feed, I would vow to wean him at night. Then in the light of day I would realize that I didn't feel that bad and that night weaning would be very difficult on both of us. Somehow when daylight hit, some kind of adrenaline kicked in and it didn't seem so bad. I also had some friends who were in the same boat and it helped to know that I was not alone.

15. Adjust your attitude. Night feeding is a season of parenting. All babies need to feed at night, especially in the first six months. Since it's inevitable that your sleep will be disturbed, you might as well adjust your attitude and approach night feeding in a positive way. You can allow feeding to relax you and help you get more sleep – rather than dreading each night feeding and filling your system with stress hormones that just keep you awake. (See the attitude-adjusting tips that mothers offer on page 64.)

Once I let myself enjoy the hours of rocking and feeding, the private time, and I regarded it as a passing privilege and not a chore, it became easier. I began to look at it as an opportunity for relaxing and getting close to my baby. It's a time in your life when your baby is in-arms, at-breast, and will drift off to sleep easily in your arms. That time will soon pass. Celebrate it while you can.

nighttime bottlefeeding made easier and safer

Formula-fed babies tend to wake up less often than breastfed babies. Formula is digested more slowly than breastmilk, so tiny tummies stay full longer. Also, we suspect bottles and formula are not as strong a motivation for waking up as the breast and mother's milk.

I have fallen into the habit of giving our 15-month-old a bottle as a way of putting her to sleep at night. She also wakes up in the middle of the night asking for her "ba-ba". Should I break this routine? And, if so, how?

Many infants need to suck to relax themselves into sleep. Going to bed with the bottle is not what's potentially harmful; it's what's in the bottle that counts.

Before putting baby to sleep, try to give him an extra ounce of formula in his last nighttime bottle. For example, if he takes five ounces at most feedings, see if you can get him to take six ounces. Don't force it though – if he gets too full it could backfire by causing discomfort. Try giving your child nutrient-dense solid foods as before-bed snacks. Nutrient dense foods are those that pack a lot of nutrition in a small volume and keep the tummy full longer. Try the filling before-bed snacks listed on page 40.

Prepare the nighttime bottle early in the evening. Put it in the refrigerator, so that it gets nice and cold. Place the cold bottle next to baby's bed just before you go to bed, along with an electric bottle warmer. When baby awakens for a feeding, you can warm and feed without making that long trip to the kitchen.

Share night feedings with your partner, when possible.

I pumped once in the morning when I had extra milk, and my partner used this milk to feed her at 9 to 10pm on those days that I went to bed earlier. Our son slept longer because he got some of my 'morning milk,' which seemed to satisfy him more than the before-bed feed when my milk supply was lowest.

Remember, there should always be a person at both ends of the bottle. Don't prop the bottle and let her suck herself to sleep unattended. Also, though it is tempting to leave a bottle in the cot for a 3am self-serve, don't! Not only does this practice contribute to tooth decay, baby can choke on the contents with no one there to help. Also, lying down during formula feeding allows formula to enter the middle ear through the Eustachian tube and triggers ear infections.

Try to gradually wean your baby from nighttime bottles between one and two years. Bottles of formula or juice are not friendly to a sleeping baby's teeth. When baby falls asleep, saliva flow decreases, diminishing its natural rinsing action on the teeth. The sugary stuff bathes the teeth, resulting in severe tooth decay called "bottle mouth". To ease baby off the nighttime bottle, try *watering down:* gradually dilute the bottle contents with increasing amounts of water until baby figures out it's not worth waking up for a bottle of water.

After giving her the bottle of milk or formula, brush her teeth gently, trying not to awaken her if she has drifted off to sleep. Toothpaste is not necessary. Use either a baby toothbrush or a piece of gauze wrapped around your finger, whichever method is easier. You may then need to walk her around to resettle her without the bottle. If your baby still needs a middle-of-the-night bottle, be sure to brush her teeth as soon as she wakes up in the morning.

Don't give a juice bottle before naptime or bedtime. Reserve juice bottles for times when the child is wide awake (juice should always be served diluted with half water). In fact, it's best to serve juice out of a cup, so baby doesn't get used to walking around with a juice bottle during the day and wanting it at night. Besides, juice is not as filling as milk or formula, so it serves little purpose for satisfying nighttime hunger.

If baby is hooked on a nighttime bottle as a comforter rather than a source of nutrition, try feeding her with a cup instead of a bottle before bedtime. Then offer a friendly comforter, such as her thumb (see teaching thumb sucking for self-soothing, page 26) or a cuddly. If she is old enough to understand, show her how her teddy bear goes to sleep without a bottle: "See Bear-Bear doesn't need a bottle to go off to sleep."

As we have previously said, night feeding is good for you and good for your baby. It may seem like a burden at times, but it also has benefits. During sleep, your levels of prolactin and of growth hormone go up, and both of these increase your milk production. Babies get substantial amounts of the milk they need to grow from feeding at night. (We call the milk you produce at night "grow milk".) As an added hormonal perk, the higher level of prolactin has a relaxing, de-stressing effect. Also, researchers have discovered a sleep-inducing protein in mother's milk. So, night feeding helps both the baby and the mummy sleep.

Cherish this time. I remember that age like it was yesterday, yet my son is now two years old. It will be gone before you know it. Listen to the breathing of your little one, replay pleasant memories, and so on. Take a nap the next day when baby naps if you feel short on sleep. Forget the household chores or other tasks calling you. Your baby will only be a baby for a short time.

Here are some other tips from seasoned night feeders on how to stay sane during the time your baby is waking to feed at night:

- Don't look at the clock every time baby wakes up. Don't count the minutes (or hours) of sleep you're missing. An exact record won't make you feel any less tired. In fact, you'll feel worse.
- If you've been awake at night, be kind to yourself and make some adjustments in your plans for the next day. Grab a nap. Don't cook. Don't worry about the housework when you're overtired.
- If you find yourself lying awake during or after a night feeding, don't fuss and fume and don't worry about tomorrow. Do something to take your mind off the fact that you're not sleeping. Read a paperback that will amuse or relax you. Keep a pad and pen handy so you can do some writing or meal planning. Listen to music (keep the stereo remote control next to your side of the bed). Enjoy watching your baby sleep. Turn this problem into an opportunity to enjoy some "me time".
- Pick a relaxing favourite movie and turn it on at night when you night feed. This makes the feeding time seem shorter and gives you something to look forward to.

Just as medications come with both benefits and side effects, night feeding has its good points and its drawbacks. Certainly the benefits outweigh the side effects. The benefits are: baby is secure, thrives and grows well, and gets to enjoy all the health, nutritional, and developmental benefits of breastfeeding. Besides this, quite honestly, babies *love* to feed at night. For mothers, night feeding helps them maintain an adequate milk supply, which is especially important for mums who work outside the home during the day. Night feeding also prolongs the period of time in which a lactating mother doesn't have menstrual periods and has less chance of getting pregnant again. The "side effects" of night feeding are that baby learns to associate sleeping with feeding and may not want to go back to sleep any other way. This is okay with some families – they're happy to have a guaranteed way of getting baby to sleep – but may not be okay with others.

thinking about cutting back on night feeding?

"Weaning" does not mean a *loss* of a relationship, but rather a passage from one relationship to another. A child can be weaned from mother's breast at night, yet still be "nursed" in other ways.

Remember Sears Basic Parenting Advice: "To understand why infants and children do what they do, put yourself behind the eyes of your child and ask: "If I were my child how would I want my mother/father to act?"

Imagine you're your baby. Night feeding feels so good to you. And some little voice inside says, "This is good for me!" Imagine you're a toddler. You're so busy during the day that you forget to feed. Then at night you make up for these missed daytime feedings, especially if your favourite all-night café is open and easily available. It's no wonder a smart baby doesn't give up night feeding without a protest.

Yet, mothers who breastfeed all night (or what seems like all night), every night, can get very tired and burned out. Even the most on-fire mother needs sleep to keep going. If you are the burning-out mother of an all-night feeder, you need to make a change. It may be time to work out how to get baby to feed less at night or how to wean baby from night feedings completely. If you wean your baby partially or totally from night feeding (you can still feed during the day), your baby will probably wake up a lot less, since there's no longer anything pleasurable to wake up for at night.

Baby's need for night feedings usually lessens with time and maturity. Yet, some babies become toddlers who are very reluctant to give up night feeding. Because they have always been breastfed whenever they awoke at night, they've been conditioned to expect this, and they won't settle for anything less. They may be feeding more out of desire or habit than need.

What's the difference between a habit and a need? Habits can be changed. Needs don't go away so easily. If you give some night weaning techniques a try and baby adapts fairly easily, you'll know that night feeding was a habit he was ready to lose. He may protest a bit. He may be unhappy for a couple of nights. But then he will settle into the new way of sleeping. If night feeding is filling a genuine need, baby will protest strongly. He may also become more clingy or anxious during the day. You'll know you are dealing with a need, because baby will become much more needy.

If multiple nighttime feedings are leaving you burned out on breastfeeding and mothering, it's time to change something. Here is a sensitive approach to easing off nighttime feeding. We want to help you meet both your child's need for closeness and your own need for sleep:

How much of a problem is it? Be honest!
Remember, babies need happy, rested mothers. If night feeding is disrupting your sleep to the extent that you can't function well the next day, mentally or physically, your body and mind are telling you that you need to make a change (and not feel guilty about it). Listen to these signals! If you've tried many strategies to help you sleep better and to catch-up on your sleep during the day and you're still sleep deprived, that's even more evidence that you need to make a change and try something else. If you dread going to sleep because it's work rather than rest, you know that something's got to give. If your health, your marriage, and your ability to care for your family during the daytime are being negatively affected by your efforts to meet your baby's needs at night, you need to get some balance back in your life. Many kids ago we learned a valuable survival principle:

If you resent it, change it!

I love her dearly, but I'm tripping over the bags under my eyes. My mother once told me, "If Mum isn't happy, nobody's happy."

At fifteen months I decided enough was enough! She was getting me up to feed every two hours. So, my partner took over the job of comforting her when she woke at night. It was very hard to listen to her cry on that first night, but I knew that she was just angry, not lonely, scared, or alone. She caught on very quickly and now sleeps consistently from about 8:30pm to 6:30am. Then I feed her and have a morning cuddle until she falls back to sleep. She sleeps for another two hours.

(Comment: babies may give up the middle-of-the-night feedings more easily if they know they're going to get some feeding and snuggle time in the morning – sort of like skipping a midnight snack when you know you're going to go out for breakfast the next morning.)

If, on the other hand, you are coping reasonably well with your baby's night feeding, then there is no reason to change. You may be tired occasionally because your baby has kept you awake more the night before, but most of the time you manage to get enough sleep. While you are wondering if your toddler will *ever* sleep through the night, at the same time, you find that meeting his nighttime needs with feeding works pretty well in your family.

Once I got her used to other ways of going to sleep, I felt less pressure and actually enjoyed breastfeeding more. I knew I didn't HAVE to feed her to sleep.

Also, don't feel pressured by peer group norms. When mothers talk among themselves, some tend to exaggerate how long and how well their babies sleep, instead of being honest about their babies' sleep patterns. They want to make themselves look good, in their own eyes as well as yours, but as a result, mothers often end up believing that everyone else's baby is sleeping through the night at age three or four months. (If they really are, there is probably a lot of night crying that went on.) This is not the norm, even for formula-fed babies and those who do not co-sleep.

On the other hand, anthropologists tell us that prolonged night feeding is actually the norm in most human societies outside of Western cultures. Babies seem to be "wired" for it, and these other cultures are more accepting of how dependent babies are on their mothers. In Western cultures we value independence and push children to act independent at an early age. But we fail to recognize that babies have to go through a prolonged period of being dependent on others to achieve the kind of emotional security that is the foundation of later independence. We think of weaning as a goal we must strive toward, whether it's weaning from the breast, from the parents' bed, or from childish behaviours. Yet in ancient writings, the term "weaning" means "filled" or "completed". For example:

My soul is stilled and quieted, like a weaned child with his mother.
Psalm 131:2

Children are not truly ready to move on to the next stage until the needs of this stage are filled.

Many mother-infant pairs continue to night feed throughout the first year or two without Mum getting overtired and baby becoming over-demanding. Baby's needs for closeness, security, and nourishment are met and mother gets enough sleep because she doesn't wake up completely while baby feeds, or she goes back to sleep easily afterwards. In fact, some mothers feel night feeding helps them sleep better. Some of the physically and emotionally healthiest children we have met through the years are those who have been allowed to wean from their mother's breast and their parents' bed in their own good time.

I became a sleep feeder. Some people walk in their sleep and don't remember it. I was able to feed in my sleep. I remember the first time I realized he had fed during the night and I didn't remember it the next morning. I woke up and my PJ top was up and my bra flap was down.

We would advise you to keep checking on yourself to be sure that you are mostly happy with your nighttime feeding situation. Also, think about how you can help your child accept other forms of comfort. If you meet all of your child's nighttime needs at the breast, you may not be giving him opportunities to learn other ways of falling asleep. This may be fine if your baby is only a few months old, but if your "baby" is a fifteen or eighteen-month-old toddler, he may be able to wean a bit at night. Just as you encourage him to learn to eat solid foods, to walk around on his own two feet, or to solve problems as he plays, it's also your job to show him more grown-up ways of falling asleep and back to sleep. Some of the tips listed below will help you do this, and you will be able to make a gradual transition to bedtimes and nighttimes without feeding. Knowing that you aren't going to be breastfeeding at night forever can make it easier to enjoy night feeding now.

Consider what you may "lose" by night weaning. A word of caution: we're talking about older babies and toddlers here. Trying tricks to lessen night feeding in the early months can lessen your adequate milk supply, so that baby fails to thrive. Besides "losing" the milk baby needs to grow, you lose the relaxing and sleep-inducing perks of night feeding, which you may have got used to. Some mothers find that during the first three days of night weaning, they miss the sleep-inducing effects of night feeding and have more trouble falling asleep and staying asleep. Finally, you lose the ovulation-suppressing effects of those night feeding hormones.

I actually feel more tired now that my baby is weaned. Feeding helped me drift quickly back to sleep. I can't imagine settling a baby in the middle of the night (or indeed any time) without recourse to feeding.

Balance your needs with baby's. Sometimes we see babies who are thriving, with mothers who are just barely getting through the day. This is why in the last few years we have added another B to the Baby B's of attachment parenting – BALANCE! If baby is doing great, but Mum is marginal, things are out of balance. Does this sound like you? Does the message playing inside your head say, "My baby needs me so much, I don't have time to take care of myself"? Many mothers have this "baby-first, Mum-whenever" mindset, especially in the early weeks of parenting a newborn. A healthier mindset for mothers is "I need to take care of both of us." As we say throughout this book, a thriving baby and a barely-surviving mummy is not a healthy combination. If achieving balance means that Mum has to get more sleep, some nighttime changes may be necessary.

It helped to cut out the night feedings once we knew he wanted them out of habit and not hunger.

"But if I try to cut out night feeding, my baby will cry! And I can't just let my baby cry, can I?" One of the tenets of Attachment Parenting is to *respond* to baby's cries. Some take this to mean that parents must do whatever it takes to *stop* their babies from crying. Yet, what we really mean is this: don't let your baby cry *alone*. To expect an avid night feeder with a persistent personality to give up without a protest is unrealistic. Crying in itself isn't a bad thing. Babies often need to cry to release frustration and other negative emotions that are a part of everyday life, just as adults do sometimes, though of course a lot less! It's the message that baby gets from parents while he cries that matters. This is why we feel that the cry it out-alone sleep-training method is bad for babies. Baby feels abandoned, left alone to solve big problems by himself. But what about using techniques at night that might involve some crying, just not alone, or at an inappropriate age? As an obvious example, even breastfeeding parents have nights when baby is fussy, won't feed, and all they can do is carry baby around the house and hope that the motion will lull baby to sleep while she cries. Baby is getting the message that you *are there* with him to help him through this fussy time. This is a sharp contrast to the message that a baby gets when left to cry himself to sleep *alone* in a cot.

"Oh my gosh, I can't believe the Sears are saying that I should let my baby cry at night!" We are saying nothing of the sort. We aren't saying you *should* or *shouldn't* do anything. We are saying that *if* you are at the point where you need to wean baby from night feeding, and *if* your intuition tells you that it would be okay for your baby to go through some periods of fussing to sleep in Mum or Dad's arms, and *if* you feel this is the right thing for you and your baby right now, we believe that you *can* gently and humanely wean your baby from night feeding without endangering your baby's trust in you, because *you are still going to be there.* However, if you feel that it will harm this trust, then you shouldn't do it.

We love co-sleeping, yet my nine-month-old uses me as a dummy. She sucks while she sleeps. In the early months I didn't mind, but now I'm not sleeping well. I find her constant sucking irritating. How can I break this annoying habit?

When it comes to night feeding, it's important that both of you enjoy it. The key to enjoying it is to night feed your baby because you *want* to, not because you *have* to. Your lack of sleep and your annoyance at your daughter's all-night feeding are signs that you need to make a change. Your baby may be very comfortable with feeding while she sleeps, but it is no longer working for you. We'll now offer some suggestions on slowing the all-night sucker.

twelve tips for getting baby to feed less at night

Night weanings are often difficult for mother and baby because you both have become *conditioned night feeders*. Baby wakes, you are programmed to feed, and it works. Because it works so well, it won't be an easy behaviour to change. (One *really* conditioned mother shared with us, "I heard the cat meowing and I tried to latch my infant on while she was sound asleep. Another time I tried to latch the cat on when she climbed into the crook of my arm during the night.") If you are a conditioned night feeder and it's working for you, no need to change, as your baby will wean in due time. Yet, if you are an *exhausted night feeder* and baby is conditioned to night feed, expect the re-programming process to take some time. Realize your baby is adjusting and resisting a change to a new pattern, not starving from giving up night feeding. Understand that night weaning will not occur overnight. It will be a gradual process over several weeks. How strongly your baby protests depends on his personality and the length and frequency of his previous night feeding.

1. Tank your baby up during the day. Many toddlers get so busy during the day that they forget to feed. They make up for the food and closeness they miss during the day by feeding more at night. Or, Mum may be too busy during the day to pay much attention to baby, and night feeding becomes a baby's way of reconnecting. Many babies feed more at night after their mothers return to work. Infants will "cluster feed" (feed more often) at night because the breasts are actually more available at night. When possible, try to reverse this pattern and help baby cluster feed during the day.

When we say "tank baby up" we don't mean stuff your baby with solid foods right before bedtime. This rarely helps babies sleep better and could even backfire, since a windy baby with an uncomfortable tummy is more likely to wake up at night. Yet we suspect that some babies who feed a lot at night aren't eating that well during the day. Many parents have told us that they notice their babies had little appetite for solid foods until they were weaned from night feeding. Snacking all night can depress baby's appetite during the day. If this sounds like your all-night feeder, try offering more food during the day. If baby is less than a year old, always offer solid foods in addition to, but not instead of, the more valuable breastfeeds. Offer more feedings during the day as well. Try to work in one or two extra feedings during late afternoon and early evening. If baby breastfeeds while falling asleep, be sure he feeds for ten or fifteen minutes before he drifts off.

Cluster feedings before bed made a big improvement on sleeping longer once we both got the hang of it.

2. Increase daytime touch. As babies get older and spend more time out of your arms, they get less touch-time each day. All-night feeding can sometimes be a baby's way of getting more of the physical contact he is missing out on during the day, either because he's busy crawling around on the floor, or because you are busy and not spending as much time with him. Night feeding reminds mothers not to rush their baby into independence. A child develops independence at her own pace. Baby leaves and comes back; lets go and clings, takes two steps forward and one step back, until he is away from you more than he is with you. Many mothers have noted that babies and toddlers show an increased need for feeding and holding as they enter a new stage of development or cope with a change in lifestyle. Changes such as learning to crawl, walk, or stay with a new sitter are stressful, and baby copes by feeding more.

To give your baby more touch time during the day, wear her in a sling when she's tired or needs a break from her active play. Use the sling rather than the stroller when you go out. Sit down and play with her. Cuddle together while you read stories. Give her a back rub at naptime and bedtime.

3. Change nap "feeding". As we have frequently reminded you, "nursing" implies comforting, not just breastfeeding. To help baby learn to accept alternative ways of comforting at night, introduce these other ways of falling asleep at naptime, when it's not dark and you are not exhausted from a long day of mothering. When Dad is home, encourage him to father "nurse" baby down for naps. On the other hand, some mothers find that if they feed less at night, their babies need to feed at naptime intensifies. Nap feeding also helps to tank baby up so that he doesn't get hungry at night. Do whatever works best for you.

4. Awaken baby for a full feeding just before you go to bed. This may help your baby sleep a longer stretch at night. If baby goes to bed at 8pm, you go to bed at 11pm, and baby wakes up hungry at midnight, you get only one hour of sleep before he wakes. If you wake baby and feed him at 11pm, the two of you can go back to sleep together and will likely get three or four hours of uninterrupted sleep. Feed him in a chair or someplace other than your bed so he'll feed longer. Then hand the almost-asleep baby to Daddy to add the finishing touch.

Yet, this strategy will work only if baby is in the state of *light sleep* and would be about to wake up anyway. Awakening baby out of a deep sleep can throw off his natural rhythm and actually cause more night waking. It's probably better to "let sleeping babies sleep". Yet, it's worth a try – it may work for you. An extra before-bed feeding is especially helpful during growth spurts when baby really needs that extra feeding.

5. Get baby used to other "nursings". Get your partner to "father nurse". (Tell your partner that when you are more rested, there's more of you to go around.) Try *wearing down*. After baby is fed, but not yet asleep, one of you wear him in a baby sling while you walk around the house or around the block. When he's in a deep sleep, gently lay him onto your bed and ease yourself out of the sling. Wearing down is a good way for dad to take over part of the bedtime routine. As your baby learns to associate father's arms with falling asleep, he may be more willing to accept comfort from Dad in the middle of the night as an alternative to Mum. Other ways to ease your baby into sleep without breastfeeding him include patting or rubbing his back while you walk with him, singing and rocking, or even dancing in the dark to some tunes you like or lullabies you croon. (See list of suggestions, page 14.)

My partner had me "dad nurse" him at night when he was a "little leech" and wouldn't let up.

6. Feed to sleep – but not completely. Help your baby learn that there are other ways to fall asleep besides breastfeeding. This works best when it's started when baby is young. Toward the end of the feeding, ease her off the breast *before she is completely asleep.* Then you or Dad can add the finishing touch with other sleep cues, such as "night-night" or finger sucking. She will associate these cues with the sleepy feeling she has and will learn to accept them during the night hours. (See suggestions for Dad adding the final touch, page 179.)

7. Offer a substitute. While a baby with discerning tastes is unlikely to settle for anything less than the softness of your nipple and the sweetness of your milk, other things can fill in for mother when she's not there or when she is trying to sleep. Here are some time-honoured substitute for a baby who has just been fed:

- Dad's pinkie finger to suck on. (Works for young babies, but not for older babies and toddlers.)
- Baby's own thumb or fingers.
- Water in a trainer cup. (A possible compromise for a toddler who wants to feed at night.)
- Dummy.

Let your child hold a favourite toy, such as a teddy bear, while feeding during the day and at night. Eventually he may go to sleep, or back to sleep, with a teddy bear only. It won't happen overnight, but at least he's getting the picture.

I let him gently play with my hair while feeding during the day, and at night he can touch my hair to get back to sleep without feeding.

8. Make the breast less accessible. Co-sleeping is a set-up for night feeding. It's a nighttime parenting package babies love. If baby is sleeping in his favourite restaurant, inches away from his favourite food, he's going to want to eat. (Wouldn't you?) It's hard to tell a baby he can't eat when he smells the milk. That's why babies who co-sleep often feed a lot at night. If you want to cut down on the frequency of night feeding but still enjoy co-sleeping, try to keep the food in the cupboard (as it were).

Put a barrier between breast and baby. A baby who doesn't sense the nipple readily may not be stimulated to think of it ("out of sight, out of mind"), though some babies with persistent personalities *will* keep searching and fussing until they find what they're looking for.

After I had fed him to sleep, I would "close up shop" (put the bra flaps up securely), pull my nightgown all the way down, and sleep covered up. This helped a bit.

Let baby sleep on the other side of Dad instead of next to you.

When our little boy wants me all night but I really need to sleep, we put him down next to my partner and I sleep on the other side of the king-size bed. This way our son still has a warm body to snuggle up to, but he is less likely to wake up wanting to feed. My partner loves this, and I get a good four hours or so of uninterrupted sleep. Then if he is really fussy, we switch back.

Turn your back on baby. Sleep facing away from baby to make your breasts less available.

Try a co-sleeper. To increase the sleeping distance between baby and breast, try putting your baby in a bedside co-sleeper. Or, put your toddler on a mattress or futon at the foot of your bed so that Dad can lie down beside baby to comfort him if he awakens.

Try creative positioning. With an older baby or toddler, especially in the summer when fewer or no covers are involved, you can arrange yourself so that baby's head is not at breast level. Maybe turn baby "upside down" so her head is next to your thighs. Of course, her feet will then be at your breast level. If she's a night kicker, this trick won't work.

Find a behaviour barrier. One mother told her two-year-old: "I have to brush your teeth every time you feed at night." That slowed down the night feeding.

So my breasts aren't so close to his mouth, I sleep with my head close to his abdomen, or even sometimes with my feet at the head of the bed.

9. Move out! No, not out of the house. If your toddler persists in wanting to feed too much, relocate "Mum's All-Night Diner" to another room and let baby sleep next to Dad for a few nights. Baby may wake less often when the breast is not so available and when he does wake, he will eventually learn to accept comfort from Dad. Naturally, baby is going to fuss when "his breasts" are not within reach. And his protests may start to escalate. That's why you are sleeping down the hall.

10. Just say no! One night when Martha was desperate for sleep I woke up to hear this dialogue between her and our two-year-old, Matthew: "Nee" (his word for feed) … "No!" … "Nee!" … "No!" … "Nee!" … "No, not now. In the morning. Mummy's sleeping. You sleep, too." A firm but calm, peaceful voice almost always did the trick.

I tried to reason with our 19-month-old by telling her that "Mama was tired and 'ma' (that's her word for breastfeeding) is night-night", but she started kissing my breast and telling me that she loves "ma," she loves "ma," she loves "ma"! She would literally crawl onto my head and roll around on my body begging for "ma". After three weeks of this craziness, I found I got a better night's sleep by just rolling over and feeding her on cue. We all woke up happier and more refreshed. Oh well, back to square one.

11. "Nummies go night-night." Around eighteen months your child has the capacity to understand simple sentences and the idea that *the breasts are sleeping.* Use simple concepts to explain to your toddler when she can feed and when she has to wait. Tell her, "We'll feed again when Mr Sun comes up." You can even show your child how it is dark outside. In the morning when she wakes up, show her that it is daylight outside and announce, "Mr Sun is up. Time for feeding."

When he was able to understand, I'd explain that he could have milk to get to sleep, but not any more until the sun came up. Yet, then he started to rise earlier (with the sun of course), which is the price I paid for getting him to sleep through the night without feeding. Guess you can't have it both ways!

Or try this routine: as your child feeds off to sleep tell her, "Mummy go night-night, Daddy go night-night, baby go night-night, and 'nummies' (or 'milkies', or whatever cute word you use) go night-night." When she wakes during the night the first thing she should hear is the same gentle reminder, "Nummies are night-night. Baby go night-night, too." You may have to do this for a week or two, but soon she will get the message that nighttime is for sleeping and she will stop waking up to feed at night. If "nummies" stay night-night when it's dark, hopefully baby will too. If sunrise comes too early for you, blackout blinds may buy you an extra hour of sleep.

Martha notes: "When weaning Erin, I showed her some picture books during the day of babies sleeping without the breast nearby, and I talked to her about how the babies sleep without 'nummies'."

12. Go off night call. Honour your partner with his share of "night feeding" so your toddler does not always expect to be comforted by your breasts. This gives Dad a chance to develop nighttime fathering skills and the child a chance to expand her acceptance of other nighttime comforters. High-need babies are not easily fooled; they don't readily accept substitutes. Still, it's worth a try. (See "Twenty-three Nighttime Fathering Tips", page 166.)

Martha notes: One of the ways we have survived toddlers who wanted to feed frequently during the night was for me to temporarily go off "night call". Bill would wear Stephen down in a baby sling, so he got used to Bill's way of putting him to sleep. When Stephen woke up, Bill would again provide the comfort he needed by rocking and holding him in a neck nestle position, using the warm fuzzy and singing a lullaby. Babies may initially protest when offered father instead of mother, but remember, crying and fussing in the arms of a loving parent is not the same as "crying it out". Mums, realize it will be really hard for you to hear your baby crying. But, if you "rescue" him, it will be harder the next night because he'll expect that again. Dads, realize that you have to remain calm and patient during these nighttime fathering challenges. You owe it to both mother and baby not to become rattled or angry when your baby resists the comfort you offer.

Try this weaning-to-father arrangement on a weekend, or another time when your partner can look forward to two or three nights when he doesn't have to go to work the next day. You will probably have to sell him on this technique, yet we have personally tried it and it does work. Be sure to use these night-weaning tactics only when baby is old enough and your gut feeling tells you that your baby is feeding at night out of habit and not out of need. It's best to wait until your baby is around eighteen months. By then he'll be old enough to manage that kind of frustration.

No, you are not going against what you said you'd never do: "let him cry it out …" As we've repeatedly discussed, we believe it's wrong to let baby cry *unsupported and alone*. Crying in the arms of Dad or another familiar and nurturing caregiver is different, especially when you consider the stakes are high here – a sleep-deprived and burning out Mum is not much good to anyone – Dad or toddler. Although *you* may be "crying it out alone in another room", try to give Dad and baby some time and space to work this out. You'll be surprised what creative strategies Dad can come up with.

Martha notes: Let baby be the barometer. When trying any behaviour-changing technique on a child, don't persist with a bad experiment. Use your baby's daytime behaviour as a barometer of whether your change in nighttime parenting style is working. If after several nights of working on night weaning your baby is her same self during the day then persist with your gradual night weaning. If, however, she becomes more clingy, whiny, or distant, take this as a clue to slow down your rate of night weaning.

chapter 7

moving out! tips for transitioning to a big kid's bed

Your older toddler is beginning to wear out his welcome in your room. Your bed is no longer big enough for three, especially when that third person seems to take up more than his fair share. It's time for him to move out (if not out of your room just yet, at least out of your bed). Or maybe your child has been sleeping well in his cot for a while, but last night you found him standing on top of the railing getting ready to dive off.

Wherever you are right now with your kids, you will reach a point when it's time for a big kid's bed. This age will be different for every family. Some parents enjoy sharing their room or bed with their kids for years, while others can't wait to reclaim their own private bedroom once again. There is no right age for this transition. You will know when it's time by your own instincts.

In this chapter we will discuss how to tell if your child is ready to move out, how to tell if you or your partner is ready for your child to move out, how you can actually make this happen in a stress-free happy way for everyone involved (usually the happiest person is Dad), and how to transition from cot to bed if applicable. We will also give you tools to use if your child begins resisting this change.

five steps to easing your kids out of your bed, out of your room, and into their own room

Okay, so you've been co-sleeping for a year or more, maybe two years or more. It probably looks to you like *all* your kids will be in your bed forever, and you'll be sleeping as a family until they go off to college. You're not too crazy about this, but you don't want to just shove them out of bed and say, "See you in the morning." Well, we've got some ideas that will help you teach your child to sleep independently at night. But

seasons of infant-child sleep

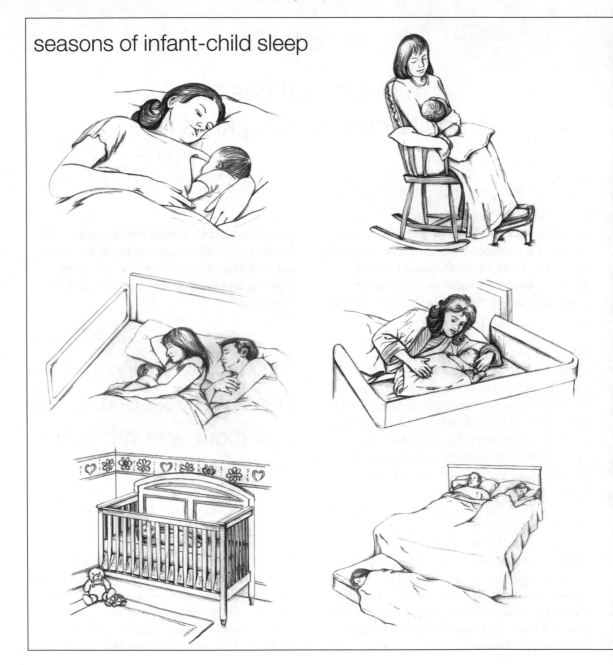

These seasons show a progression of sleeping arrangements from oneness to separateness. The age at which children develop various stages of sleep maturity varies greatly. The important point is that children go through this progression and develop a healthy attitude that sleep is a pleasant state to enter and a fearless state to remain in.

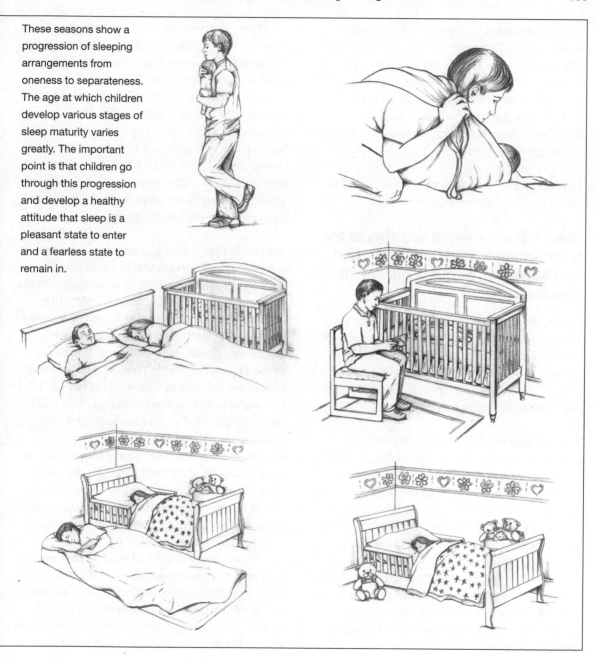

don't worry about turning them loose in the hard, cruel nighttime world at too early an age – this is going to be a verrrrrrrry looonnng process. By working through this chapter, your kids will get out of your bed and room and go to sleep without you, and they will do so happily. Eventually. Does that help? Do you feel a little better now? Okay, good.

Here is our Five Step plan to moving your kids out of your bed and out into the world.

Step 1: Decide when you should try to move your child out of your bed and bedroom, or out of his cot into a toddler bed.

Is your child ready to sleep by himself? Are you ready to have him sleep elsewhere? You may not have firm answers to one or both of these questions. That's okay. Learning to sleep alone is a process. It's not something your child will achieve overnight. Here are some points to consider:

Is your child ready? It can be very hard to persuade a co-sleeping, night-feeding toddler to sleep alone all night, every night. If you have chosen to co-sleep, and your child is still feeding frequently at night, you may find that trying to move your child out of your bed now will be near to impossible. What's more, it will create a great deal of nighttime stress for both you and your child. Since avoiding nighttime stress was one of your main reasons for co-sleeping, you may not find this acceptable, and you may want to concentrate more on decreasing baby's night feeding (chapter 6) first.

If your co-sleeping child is starting to *sleep longer stretches* without waking up to feed, this may be a sign that she is ready to sleep by herself for part or all of the night.

Realistically, you are likely to be ready before your child is. It's not like she is going to tell you one day, "Mummy, I'm ready for my big girl bed." You're going to have to sell the idea. Getting your child in his own bed all night will take some time. Just like weaning from the breast, weaning a child from his favourite place to sleep should be done gradually, and with love.

Are you ready? Before you decide to ease baby out of your bed, be sure you're doing it for the right reasons. Do you want to move baby into his own bed because you are wondering, "Will he ever sleep on his own?" Are you tired of criticism from friends, family, even your partner, who complain, "you're making him too dependent" or "you're spoiling her!"? The real question you should ask yourself is: "Is it working for us?" If it is, there's no rush to make a change. Your child will leave your bed when he's ready, or when you're ready to help him be more ready. Meanwhile, why mess with an arrangement that helps everyone sleep better at night? But if co-sleeping is no longer working for you, meaning one or more of you are not getting enough sleep, or you simply want the bed to yourselves, it's time to make a change.

Is baby becoming a bed hog? There comes a time when many co-sleeping toddlers become thrashers, and parents just can't take it anymore. You get poked and kicked throughout the night or you wake up with your toddler sleeping *on top* of you. Maybe you want to put some distance between you and a child who will feed all night long if mother's breasts are readily available. Remember our motto: *if you resent it, change it!*

Time to put away the cot? Most kids will transition out of a cot between 18 months and 2½ years. It's more a matter of the cot no longer being a safe place to leave a child unattended than it is a matter of a child wanting to move into a toddler bed. Watch for these ready to move out signs:

- Rattling the cage: baby stands up, holds onto side rails and starts shaking the cot.
- Trying to climb over the guard rail: if you have the mattress at the lowest height, yet baby is trying to climb out, take this as a sign that he's no longer safe in his cot and he's ready for a less confining space. Removing the padded bumpers will delay the escape artist, but your child will eventually monkey his way out of the cot.
- Baby wakes himself up when he scoots around his cot and bumps into the rails or end. He needs more room, so that he can stretch out like a giant starfish.

Step 2: Decide what type of bed you are going to use and where this new bed is going to be.

Decide if this new bed is going to be in your room at first or in a separate room for your child. The advantage of putting the bed in your room is that you are nearby when your child wakes during the night. The advantage of putting the bed in a different room is that you will not only have your child out of your bed, you'll have him out of the room as well. You'll have attained both objectives as part of the same project. Kids are comfortable changing to a new room, as long as you come along.

When it's time to get baby out of your bed or room or cot, where do you move him? And what type of bed do you transition into? This really depends on where he is sleeping now, and what his age is. Here are some ideas:

If baby is in your bed. The most logical next step is a small bed next to your bed. If your baby is still a baby (under age 18 months) then you should probably move baby into something cot-like for safety reasons. Here are the options:

- *A bedside cot or co-sleeper.* We call this the sidecar arrangement. (See illustration on page 123.) A co-sleeper clamped to your bed frame or a cot alongside your bed allows you and baby to each have your own separate bed space, yet you're within arm's reach of one another for easier feeding and comforting during the night. This alternative works well for parents who want their babies to sleep close to them, but not in their bed.
- *A cot in your room.* This gets baby out of your bed, so that you can enjoy some separate sleep – at least until baby wakes up. You can experiment with getting baby to fall asleep in the cot, or you can put baby to sleep in your arms and when he is sound asleep, transfer him to the cot. It will take some time for baby to adjust to sleeping solo. Be prepared and willing to take baby back into your bed for part of the night, if he wakes and needs your presence. Cots work

well for babies and younger toddlers, who need the bars to keep them from falling out of bed at night and from getting into trouble when they awake.

Sears' Sleep Tip: Gradually increase the distance. Once baby settles well in the bedside cot, gradually move it farther and farther away from your bed, not outside your bedroom. If you find you are all waking up more often as baby sleeps farther away, shorten the distance again.

If your toddler is in your bed. If your "baby" is no longer really a baby (over 18 months to two years), then moving to a secure cot isn't necessary. Here are your options for this age:

- *A futon or cot mattress on the floor next to your bed.* This is the easiest transition to make. It's conveniently next to your bed for when your child wakens, and it's close to the floor so there's no worry over injury when rolling out of bed.
- *An adult mattress on the floor next to your bed.* You may find this easier if you need to snuggle in this bed with your child during the night. Its size is one major drawback.

When she was 17 months I decided I would sleep in a twin bed beside her bed. The first few nights she woke up every hour and sat up and cried. I didn't get out of bed, but I would talk to her gently and say, "It's okay. I'm right here. Lie down and go to sleep" and she did! After a week, she would only wake up once or twice and then by a month she was sleeping through the night two to three nights a week.

Moving to child's own room. When you feel your child is ready for her own actual room, here are some ideas for choosing a bed:

- Cot mattress in a toddler bed frame very close to the floor. This is the standard choice that works for most kids.
- *Adult size mattress on the floor.* We strongly suggest not putting a young child up high on an adult bed with box spring and bed frame. Your child is likely to fall out.
- *Futon on the floor.* An inexpensive and portable option.
- *Keep a home base.* Keep a toddler bed set up in your room for a few months (or years) that your child can use when he wakens during the night and wants to come into your room. Your child *will* wake up during the night and want to return to the old nest. Let your child do this at first. Keep things positive and stress-free. You can expect children to take two steps forward and one step backwards as they make progress toward a goal. If you want to discourage your child from joining you in your bed, you could try taking him back to his own bed and sleeping with him there (a good reason for skipping the toddler bed and getting a big one). Or you can keep a futon on the floor by your bed and lie down with your child there as he (and you) fall back to sleep.

Step 3: Sell the idea

Make a special family trip to the "big girl bed" store. Like picking out a potty for toilet training, kids are more likely to use the bed they choose. Pick out special bedding too. Set the bed up at

discouraging the midnight visitor

Even when kids begin sleeping in their own room, they *will* on occasion want to return to the old nest. Nighttime can be scary time for little people, and a child's desire to be with you at night may be something she needs, not an annoying habit to be broken. This desire for nighttime contact may be particularly strong if your child has had little contact with you during the day and needs to reconnect with you at night. The need for nighttime contact also increases when a child is dealing with family stress during the day, for example, the birth of a sibling, a move, or problems in the parents' marriage, or if she is starting nursery or childcare. You need to handle this problem in a way that respects both your need for privacy and sleep and your child's need for nighttime security.

Above all, don't feel that you are spoiling your child or that she is psychologically disturbed because she can't yet sleep all night on her own. Many emotionally healthy children simply enjoy the nighttime security of sleeping close to their parents, especially when they are coping with challenges and upsets during the day. (What do you think makes them so emotionally healthy?) Remember, the goal of nighttime parenting is to nurture a healthy life-long attitude about going to sleep and staying asleep. One thing that helped us cope with our many midnight visitors was realizing that this time of nighttime closeness is a passing stage and that losing sleep is an inevitable part of parenting. If you invest some nighttime energy now in helping your child feel secure and happy, you'll probably end up sleeping a whole lot better when your children are teenagers.

(See chapter 2, page 45, for ways to deal with midnight visitors.)

home, but don't push your child to start using it just yet. Let her play at putting her dolls or toys to sleep in this bed. Read stories there. Try napping in the new bed. Get to know the new bed as a comfy, safe place to be. If you sense that your child is resisting the idea of this new bed, back off and try again in a week or two. Don't force the issue. Sit your child down by the bed some afternoon and explain to your child what the bedtime plan is going to be. Be upbeat and positive. Focus on what your child is gaining – her own place to sleep! – not on where she isn't going to sleep anymore.

Step 4: Continue your usual bedtime routine for a while

Just because your child has a new place to sleep doesn't mean he is happily going to lie down and fall asleep on his own. You are going to have to continue your previous bedtime routine, only now with a new ending location. Only when your child is sleeping well in his new bed can you begin weaning *yourself* from the bedtime routine.

Step 5: Fading away – beginning the long process of teaching your child to fall asleep without you there

Now the fun begins. Once your child is used to going to sleep in her new bed with you there, you can work on helping her go to sleep without you there. We have termed this process "Fading Away". It can be done as fast or as slow as you feel is right for your child. As you will later read, Dr Bob faded away over a five-year process. That was one looooooooooooonnnnnnnnngggggggggg fade out. Try these fade-away strategies:

- *Snuggle to sleep.* Lie in bed with your child while he falls asleep. If using a cot mattress, sit on the floor and lean over to snuggle with your child. Wait until your child is completely asleep. If you try to sneak away early, and your child wakes up, she'll realize you aren't actually falling asleep with her and she may become stressed about this new arrangement.

Dr Bob notes: One way I could tell that Andrew was completely asleep is that he would have muscle twitches. As soon as I felt those, I knew I could leave in another minute or two.

- *Camp out next to bed.* As your child becomes comfortable in the new bed, begin sitting on the floor next to your child while she goes to sleep. You may need to lay hands on your child during this time. This is an opportunity to read using a flashlight or small book lamp. When your child is okay with this set up, begin moving yourself away night after night until you are no longer in actual physical contact with your child or the bed.

Watching my daughter learn to fall asleep on her own has been so funny. At first, after her story, I would lie beside her and read my own book until she was sound asleep. She always knew what I was reading, and was always asking if I had finished it yet. Then we went through a stage where she pretended to "read" her own chapter books, which she brought home from the library by the armful, while I read my book close by. After a few minutes, she'd turn out the reading light, turn her face to the wall, and go to sleep. Now, because my reading light is broken and I borrowed hers, she goes to sleep with just a hug and kiss. There was no master plan behind any of this. It's just how it happened.

Sears' Sleep Tip: When baby isn't falling asleep "by the book", try not to become impatient – baby will sense that you are wanting to hurry things along and that will make it even more drawn out.

- *Move in and out.* Once your child is comfortable without being in physical contact with you while she falls asleep, begin leaving the room for brief intervals every five minutes or so. Tell her you have to check the washing, go and get your book, or anything else. Step out of the room for 5 seconds (longer if you know she can handle it), and then come right back and sit down again for a while. Over a few weeks gradually lengthen the time you step out of the room. Use a catch phrase each time you leave, such as "one minute" or "I'll be right back." If your child gets anxious during the seconds or minutes you are out of the room, sing a song while you are gone. Leave her door open so she can hear you singing.

Check on your child. You will eventually find that you are out of the room more than you are in. After you tuck your child in, tell her you'll check on her. Return every few minutes and peek your head in the door. You can even keep yourself busy in the hallway or the next room making quiet noises so your child knows you are near. Gradually lengthen the intervals at which you check on your child. Soon (maybe not soon enough) you will find yourself checking on your child every 10 or 15 minutes, and you'll find a peacefully sleeping child after only one or two checks.

This "Fading Away" strategy is perhaps the gentlest way to move your child into falling asleep independently. It may be too "gentle" and drawn out for some parents. You can go through each step fairly quickly if your child is willing. Just remember the important goal of creating a stress-free bedtime routine.

Parents have shared with us their own versions of Fading Away. Some parents find it helps to sit quietly in the chair and not move or make a sound, but try to sleep, or at least pretend to sleep until baby is asleep. When baby wakes up and seems not to be resettling, come into the room, issue a reminding sleep cue, "sleepy-sleep", and then quickly pretend you're going back to sleep yourself. Depending on your baby's sleep temperament and the persistence of her personality, you may have to occasionally compromise a bit and help her resettle by taking her into the chair and rocking her and then putting her back into bed. Ideally, you gradually lessen the number of responses needed until your visual presence alone is enough and you and the chair gradually fade toward the door and are eventually gone from sight.

My partner was responsible for getting our 2½-year-old daughter into her own bed. I was pregnant with our son and needed the extra sleep. The process took several months. First, he would read to her and sleep with her all night in her bed. Then he'd sleep on a futon next to her bed, but she'd sometimes wake up and need his reassurance. Gradually, he "crept" out of her room into ours – literally. At first he was sleeping on the floor next to her bed. Each night he'd sleep a little further from her bed, until just his toes were in her room. She'd sit up in bed and see him (even if just his toes) and be comforted by his presence. Then, he was on the floor outside her room, inching closer to our room each night. Eventually … she was used to sleeping by herself.

Here's another happy sleep ending story parents in our practice shared with us:

We brought our nine-month-old infant, Vikki, in for a sleep consultation because although she was a happy, wonderful baby, we were wiped out. After hearing our history that she used to be a colicky, restless sleeper, Dr Sears suggested that in the early months she probably had reflux and that she was conditioned to associate sleeping with pain rather than with pleasure. And, now that the reflux was over, she needed to be retrained to associate sleep with pleasure. That made sense to us since she never liked to sleep horizontally and she had so much pain in the first three months. Here's how we used the fade away strategy:

Days 1–3 we placed a chair next to her cot. We would console her through the bars and say, "Sleep-a, sleep-a, Vikki". We never picked her up. She would play and run around her cot, but didn't fuss hard. We would stand up to help her lay back down many times. By night three I put all six dummies in her cot because I noticed she would drop the one I would put in her mouth. It would take her about an hour to fall asleep.

Days 4–6 we moved the rocker to the middle of the room and verbally consoled her. By now it only took her about 20–40 minutes to fall asleep. She again would fuss a little, but play more than anything. Her biggest struggle was finding the dummy when it would drop or she would spit it out of her mouth.

Days 7–8 we stood or sat in the open doorway. She knew the routine enough that it took her only twenty minutes. At this time, we also moved her bedtime up to 8:30pm from 9pm. It got to the point that when we would move toward her bed, she would quickly fall into her sleep position.

Day 9 was our night to do the short routine and then put her in the cot and slowly walk away. We did just that and she slept from a little after 9pm to 6:45am. This was my first time to sleep through the night without interruption since she was born. She whimpered twice through the night, but never really cried, and fell right back to sleep.

getting your child to sleep independently: a case study

Dr Bob's experience with weaning his own three kids out of his bed and into their own rooms shows how differently even siblings can react, and how to make the most of your time with a higher-needs child.

At two years old Andrew had weaned from the breast, and bedtime was now my job. Despite the fact that he had slept in our bed for two years, in reality Andrew didn't care where he slept, as long as Cheryl or I fell asleep with him. So getting him out of our bed was easy. I just had to go with him. We set up a twin bed in our bedroom next to our bed. (As I was a junior doctor, it was a one-bedroom flat. Nobody got their own room.) Every night we read stories, brushed teeth, all the regular stuff, and then Andrew and I would snuggle into bed together. I would tell him a made-up short story that would continue night after night, and then he would fall asleep. I don't mean he would just fall asleep. He would actually take about a half hour to fall asleep. And I almost always fell asleep with him. Cheryl would come in and wake me up, and we'd enjoy the rest of the evening together.

Sounds easy, right? Well, there were a couple of problems. Often I was so groggy from dozing off that I was useless to Cheryl the rest of the night. (She'd just send me back to bed on those nights.) Other nights I would get very irritated when Andrew took longer to fall asleep. I wanted him to hurry up and fall asleep so I could get up and enjoy my evening with Cheryl. Even more annoying was when I'd think Andrew was asleep and I would start to sneak out of the room, only to hear, "Dad!" Rats. I was frustrated with the situation because I was losing anywhere from 30 to 60 minutes of my "finally the baby is asleep" part of the night. I had to change something. So I changed my attitude. I decided that by spending this time with Andrew I was making a commitment to his long-term happiness and self-confidence.

However, by the time Andrew was three (yes, this is a whole year later), nothing had actually changed. "Was he more independent?" you ask. Independence was still a long way off. For that whole first year of "me and him" Andrew wanted my arm around him as he fell asleep. But now I decided that since I was stuck here in bed for a while, I might as well make better use of my time. I love to read, and being married with a child, I didn't have much free reading time. So I brought a flashlight to bed, aimed it away from Andrew, and read every night. I persuaded Andrew that he didn't need to have my arm around him as he fell asleep (hard to do that and read). Instead, he snuggled up to my leg or my back. I actually loved this. Free time to myself! Sometime between age four and five, I moved myself and my book to the floor next to Andrew's bed. For a few months, I

had to keep one arm touching him, but I was able to wean him from that too.

When Andrew was six (many books and flashlight batteries later) child number two, Alex, was three years old and newly weaned, and he joined Andrew and me in a queen-sized bed for our nightly three-guy snuggle fest. I found myself once again back in bed because Alex needed snuggling. But this time the weaning went faster. Alex would fall asleep right away, and I would sit on the floor until Andrew fell asleep. By the way, that short bedtime story that I always told Andrew had turned into a never-ending adventure saga with a new chapter every night for both the boys.

Soon I started to leave the room for brief periods after Alex was asleep, telling Andrew I would come right back. Andrew took this just fine, and so did Alex (well, he was asleep – he really didn't have anything to say about it). I'd tell Andrew I'd check on him every five minutes. And then I'd come back to the room, lean over and kiss his forehead, and say "I'll be back in five minutes" over and over again until I'd find him asleep. He wanted to be able to hear us during this time, so Cheryl and I would be sure to make some noise. This five-minute check time turned into 10 minutes, then 15, and by age 7 years I was able to simply tuck Andrew in and leave. He'd fall asleep without any problem. I'd come and check on him 20 or 30 minutes later. Occasionally he'd still be awake. He'd just smile at me peacefully. I'm sure having Alex sleeping there in the room also helped.

Oh, and what about waking during the night? Of course, they still woke up from time to time. Between age 2 and 4 when Andrew woke up he'd climb into our bed (often without us even knowing – we'd wake up the next morning and there was an extra body). Between age 4 and 6 Andrew would come to our bed, tap us on the shoulder, and I'd walk him back to his bed and tuck him in or let him fall asleep on the futon on the floor next to our bed. From age 6 to 8 Andrew would just climb into the futon during the night without even waking us up. Alex almost never woke up during the night. But there was something about Andrew – he just needed to touch base with us, then he'd go back to sleep. After age 8, Andrew stopped waking up at night. Or if he did, we didn't know it.

Looking back, I realize now that I could have got through this weaning process with Andrew a bit faster. I could easily have started leaving the room when Andrew was four and had him falling asleep completely independently by age

avoid long-term sleep stress

One of the best gifts you can give your child is to grow up feeling that bedtime is a happy, peaceful, stress-free time to look forward to every night. You can achieve this goal by sensitively meeting your child's needs at bedtime and during the night. If a child is pushed too quickly into sleep independence before he is ready, he will grow up feeling anxious about sleep and may experience a variety of sleep problems.

5, but you know, it just never occurred to me. I really truly loved the closeness that Andrew and I developed, and I was in no hurry to change it. (Plus I got to lie around and read lots of books, all in the name of sensitive nighttime parenting.)

Now, at age 8 and 11 both Alex and Andrew get tucked in at bedtime, kissed goodnight (the made-up never-ending bedtime story, sadly, ended a couple years ago) and they fall asleep without a hitch. Unlike many kids, they aren't anxious sleepers. They never feel night stress, they never get up and ask for water, they almost never complain that it's bedtime, they never get up during the night, and they have never had problems with sleep terrors or bedwetting. I wouldn't have changed a thing. I actually look forward to this bonding experience with our third son.

As for child number three, when Joshua was two we put a cot mattress (the same one we bought eleven years ago for Andrew's cot that he never used – glad we kept it all these years) on the floor next to our bed and dubbed this his "big boy bed". Since he is at the age where everything is all about being a big boy, he loved this idea. Cheryl feeds him to sleep and lays him down in his little bed. He sleeps most of the night there, and we finally (Hallelujah!) have our king-sized bed to ourselves. Joshua wakes up and comes into our bed sometime during the night about twice a week. I actually look forward to being the one to snuggle him to bed once he is weaned (I've got a whole pile of science fiction books stacked up to read).

Okay, so you mums are probably thinking to yourself, "Wow, that would be so amazing if my partner would take over the nighttime routine." And you dads are probably thinking, "I can't spend an hour every night for five years putting my child to bed. I just can't." We're not about to tell you that it will take five years to teach your child to sleep independently. And you certainly don't have to do exactly as we did. Here are some points to consider:

If you want to hurry this weaning process along, you can. Just be sensitive to what your child needs from you and find a way to give it to him that works for both of you. Mum and Dad can share in the bedtime routine. You can take turns, or Mum can do one part and Dad the other.

Every parent and child combination is different. In our family, our second child always went right to sleep. Our first took longer. That was our experience. Your mileage may vary.

Besides, I didn't set out to spend five years putting my child to bed. It just happened. In the parenting business, it's smart not to think too far ahead. If you think about how many hours in total you'll have to spend watching matches, you may never sign your kids up for football. Just see what happens. You can make adjustments as you go.

chapter 8

twenty-three nighttime fathering tips

Dads, nighttime is where you can really shine! How often we have heard tired mums lament, "I wish my partner would help more during the night." Yet dads often develop an acute case of nighttime hearing loss after a newborn joins the household, especially when Mum seems to be so much better at getting baby to sleep.

Big mistake! Skip the earplugs and get ready to take an active part in nighttime parenting. When we look through our "survivor" files – the stories of parents who have made it through those early months without succumbing to utter exhaustion – one feature stands out: the presence of a sensitive and involved Dad. This chapter is all about how you can help your baby and your baby's mother get more sleep.

Mums, we want to say a quick word to you at the beginning of this chapter. We know that you are probably reading this chapter before your partner does. The second part of this chapter is all about how to get your partner more involved with nighttime parenting, if he hasn't volunteered already. We will give some helpful insights (from the male standpoint) about how you can tell your partner about your needs and your baby's needs in a way that he'll understand.

We will also help you understand what your partner is feeling during this time, in case he isn't effectively communicating this to you. Even if he is reluctant to read this whole book, we hope that he will read this chapter to understand why a sleep-refreshed partner is more pleasant to live with.

Now, back to Dad. Dads, if your partner is handing you this chapter to read, it's likely she is getting burned out. Take a hint!

part one – for dads

Here are 23 tips that will help you support your partner, be involved with your baby, and enable your whole family unit to function better at night.

Be a supportive father by day

Nighttime fathering starts with things you do in the daytime. The relationship you have with your partner and baby during their waking hours will carry over into what happens in the wee hours of the night.

1. Understand the switch to mother mode. As soon as that umbilical cord is cut, your partner moves into mother mode: all baby, all the time. All her energy is focused on nurturing baby, and she may forget her own needs. Mother mode is nature's way of giving little human beings the right start in life. After all, for your baby to thrive, he needs almost constant care. Your partner's intuition is to put baby's needs above her own need for sleep – and certainly above your need for sex.

In those early months of marathon giving, many mothers are on the verge of burn out, but won't admit it. What's the biggest contributor to mother burn out? Father walkout! By that we mean fathers who are not involved in their babies' care and who fail to be sensitive to their partner's needs. If you want your partner to go through the mother mode stage with romantic feelings about you, respect her need to nurture her baby and help her take better care of herself.

My partner does what he can to free me up to be a mother.

2. Keep the nest tidy. A neat, orderly home is more conducive to mothering than a home in which chores pile up, waiting for the woman of the house to do them. Because she already has so much to learn and worry about, you may find that the slightest mess easily upsets your partner. During the postpartum period, Martha was upset by even one dirty dish, though usually a sink-full of dirty dishes wouldn't have fazed her. An upset mother often translates into an upset baby. An acronym to remember is: TIDY – Take Inventory Daily Yourself. Don't wait for your partner to make a "to-do" list. You need to make out the list yourself – and then do the things on it! Hire some help if you can; otherwise take over the housekeeping yourself. Each day walk around the house and look for things you can do so that your partner has more energy for mothering. Sort out the junk mail. Wash the dishes. Clean the bathroom mirror. Put away the clean clothes.

If you are a night owl, use that time to make the house look tidier for your partner the next day. If you have older children, enlist their help. Show them how to pick up after themselves and remind them to do so. (Preschoolers will need hands-on supervision.) Tell them that it's an important time for them to care for Mum. Remember, you are bringing up someone's future mate, and some day that mate's partner will hug you and thank you for training your child to do housework. One day a grandfather in my office beamed, "My daughter-in-law gave me the supreme compliment: 'Thank you for bringing up such a sensitive man!'"

3. Be sensitive. Stan, a new father and professional tennis player, asked me how he could help with his newborn baby. I advised him: "Improve your serve!" Think about what you can do to help *before* your partner has to ask. Many new mothers are trying to do everything for the baby and everything in the household all by themselves. They are trying to be perfect mothers in their own eyes and in their partner's. This is completely unrealistic, yet their partners seem clueless about their need for help. As one mother told me, "I'd have to hit my partner over the head before he'd realize I'm giving out." Try to imagine how you can help and intervene before your partner is so drained that she begins to feel overwhelmed and depressed. For example, you notice mother and baby are sleeping. Take the phone off the hook and put a "Do not disturb" sign on the door. If baby wakes up before Mum, quickly pick him up and take him outside for a walk, so that your partner can sleep a bit longer. That extra bit of sleep will get you a big hug.

When your baby is born, take as much time off from your job as is economically feasible. Also, when you do return to work, cut back on evening meetings and out-of-town travel.

As one father summed it up: "I can't breastfeed, yet I can create an environment that helps my partner breastfeed better."

Realize that some mums will not ask for help, because they don't want to seem less than the Supermum they hope to be.

4. Change your attitude. Instead of dreading nighttime and viewing it as an occupational hazard of having a baby, change your attitude. Try a principle that we try to teach our kids as one of the keys to happy living: *view a problem as an opportunity*. Becoming more involved with your baby's nighttime care will earn you double rewards: you will deepen your relationship with

your baby and enjoy gratitude and admiration from your partner. It's going to be a while until your infant reaches the Promised Land of Nod, where she sleeps through the night. You might as well make nighttime fathering a positive experience.

It's normal to feel that you have the right to sleep at night. You work hard during the day to provide for your family. Maybe you are the sole breadwinner, and you need to be alert in the morning so that you can go to work and ensure your family's economic well-being. In some families mum shares this attitude that it's more important for Dad to get a good night's sleep. But some burned-out and sleep-deprived mums don't agree:

Don't make any comments about going to work the next day. Mums work, too. Imagine working 24 hours a day at your main job and living at the office. That's what full-time mothering is like.

I felt my partner worked all day to provide for me to stay home, so I was not about to wake him to feed the baby. I viewed this as my job. I did mine and he did his. Yet I would, of course, encourage him to care for her in the evening and change nappies, etc., so I could rest; and he delighted in it.

I think a lot of stay-at-home mums try to do it all at night. They don't realize that their sleep is just as important as their partner's.

Don't shush mum and baby when you're half-asleep. Get up and help. Otherwise, your attitude conveys that something is wrong with baby or

my partner will ...

"Nothing turns a woman on like seeing a man nurture her baby", a rested mother once told us. From our happy-family gallery, here are some inspirational quotes from mothers about sensitive fathers.

- ... My partner rubs my back or gives me a foot massage, while I feed, when I'm having a middle-of-the-night meltdown.

- ... My partner tells me (over and over) that I am doing a great job and that it will get better.

- ... My partner encourages me to go to bed when baby does, even if it's only 7pm.

- ... My partner brings me a midnight snack.

- ... My partner becomes a night-light. He holds a soft light for me to get our newborn latched on correctly for the night feeding in the first few weeks.

- ... My partner did the Daddy dance. He would take our twins downstairs and dance to his favourite CD in the living room. Years later these songs continue to calm them immediately. We call them "Daddy's songs".

- ... On the weekends my partner lets me SLEEP IN, which is like paradise.

- ... My partner and I put our baby to bed every night as a FAMILY. My partner lies next to us when baby feeds to sleep.

- ... My partner treats nighttime parenting as an EQUAL responsibility. None of that "I'm a hero for taking turns with a wakeful baby" stuff!

- ... My partner helps when our son is hyper and playful and doesn't look like he's going to sleep soon. My partner walks around the house and sings to him to wind him down.

- ... My partner got baby used to being comforted by him, which gave me a break now and then. At night we were a "feeding team". It was great!

- ... When my partner comes home from work he takes over baby duty so I can make dinner and do things that need to be done.

- ... My partner gets up and uses the "magic shoulder" to burp the baby for me.

- ... One night I woke up to find my partner sitting at his computer at 2am listening to rock and roll with the baby bouncing to the beat.

- ... My partner leaves the room with the baby when he's helping out. There is no point for both of us to listen to the screaming.

something is wrong with her method of getting baby to sleep. Your partner may feel that it's her fault that baby wakes up and that you think she's not a very good mother when she can't get baby back to sleep more easily.

5. Be a "share-holder". Don't wait until the middle of the night to learn how to comfort your baby. If you are comfortable holding and comforting baby during the day, it will be easier for you to work out what to do at night to ease baby into sleep. Baby will get to know your ways of holding and comforting and will learn to trust that Dad can make everything all better. Experiment with various holding patterns to get baby used to your unique way of comforting. Wear your baby in a carrier as much as possible throughout the day, so that baby gets used to your unique motion, scent, and voice; and you get used to ways of daytime comforting. The more baby is accustomed to your special ways during the day, the more likely he will be to settle for you at night.

If you have a toddler and a new baby, now is the time to strengthen your bond with the older child. Some nights you and your partner will do team nighttime parenting: Daddy snuggles the older child while Mummy feeds the baby. Or, baby is handed over to Daddy while the older child is snuggled to sleep by Mummy. If both of your children are comfortable with you, you will have more flexibility in solving nighttime problems.

My partner would walk with baby in a football hold. She loved this and would fall asleep easily.

Occasionally, Dad needs to sleep in another room and "freshen up" for work. Yet, we have settled into a sense of shared responsibility at night where we each respond to the fusses we hear. Often we are up together helping each other out – we are a family at night.

6. Get involved early. During pregnancy and in the first weeks after birth, most mothers worry, "I wonder how my partner is going to handle all of these changes?" The sooner you can alleviate this worry, the better. Don't be a distant dad – day or night. Be part of the parenting team right from the start. Newborns become creatures of habit very early. The sooner you give your baby the message that both Mum and Dad are going to care for him, the easier it will be for your baby to adapt to your style of nighttime fathering. And the sooner you start, the sooner you will gain confidence in your abilities to care for your baby. Learning how to comfort your baby at night builds Daddy-baby trust. Early on your child learns that mum is not the only one who makes "it all better".

Because our son was a marathon feeder and was attached to my breast much of the time, my partner was a little afraid in the beginning. He didn't know how to get involved. By the time we decided to get him involved in nighttime shifts, our son did not want a change in routine. It wasn't until he weaned at seventeen months that he began to want his Dad at night. With our next baby, we'll know better and start nighttime fathering earlier.

HOW DO YOU SPELL RELIEF? F-A-T-H-E-R

7. Support your partner's mothering style. Whatever nighttime parenting style your partner chooses, be supportive. Most new mothers are a bit shaky about trusting their own wisdom. Mum really does know best! Let her know that you support whatever she chooses to do. If your mother, her mother, or a friend criticizes the way she cares for your baby or starts pressuring her to do something differently (maybe they're telling her not to "spoil the baby by picking him up all the time"), do what you can to shield her from these bearers of bad baby advice. Don't bring home stories about friends' babies sleeping through the night after "only one night of crying it out". Your friends' baby is not your baby. Your baby has a unique temperament, and you and your partner have a unique parenting style. Besides, making comparisons like this gives your partner the message that you think your baby is waking up because of something she's doing or not doing. Don't pressure her to work out how to get baby to sleep better at night. Read this book together and discuss sleep strategies as a team.

The best fathering my partner does – besides some one-on-one time with our son – is when he supports me and our choice to co-sleep and night feed in the face of a lot of criticism of this choice.

Sears' Sleep Tip: "Nursing" implies comforting, not only breastfeeding. Fathers can "nurse"!

Support the tired mum at night

If your baby falls asleep at the breast every night and goes back to sleep by breastfeeding in the middle of the night, you may be thinking, "Hey, this is great! I don't have to do anything." You may be right. This style of nighttime parenting works for some families. But it may not work for yours. Mothers who breastfeed a couple times every night can get very tired. They may also resent a Dad who sleeps through it all. Here's some things you can do to make nighttime feeding easier on your partner.

8. Serve baby to Mummy. If your baby awakens in the middle of the night in her cot wanting a feeding, don't roll over, play dead, and incur your partner's jealous wrath. Instead, get up, get baby, and deliver her to Mummy. Murmur some sweet and encouraging words to your partner and enjoy this beautiful middle-of-the-night family moment. Baby, Mum, and Dad can all drift back to sleep while baby feeds. Often mothers prefer to let their babies sleep with them after the first night feeding. If baby needs to be returned to the cot when the feed is over, let sleeping Mummy lie there (she's zonked out on relaxing breastfeeding hormones) and you be the one who shuttles the sleeping baby back to the cot. This is just one example of the importance of learning how to handle baby on your own.

Don't "pretend" to be sleeping when baby cries. We know you are awake! Don't fake snore and roll over like you are so wrapped up in sleep that you can't possibly wake up and help.

We do team nighttime parenting. Daddy gets baby and Mummy nurses baby. So, in a way, Daddy nurses Mummy.

9. Support the feeding pair. You may feel that since Mum is feeding, there is nothing you can do at night, so you might as well sleep. There may be nights when, because of your work schedule, you need to sleep. Yet, as often as possible, be available during nighttime feedings. Even though you can't breastfeed, do what you can do to help your partner breastfeed more comfortably: fluff her pillows or massage her back. If she's lying on her side curled around the baby, wedge a pillow between the bed and her lower back for extra support. Keep her company. Just knowing you are there and that you care helps the feeding pair. If you tend to fall back to sleep quickly, as least give your partner an encouraging word of support as you drift off.

My partner would wake up when he heard the baby and I wake up. He didn't do anything, he just sat there in the dark with us. It was at those times that I loved him the most. He was providing nighttime fathering in the most unselfish way … by supporting his baby's Mum!

points – or rewards

A quick word about points. We use this word a lot in this chapter because we know that men think this way. The problem is, mothers don't. Or, if they do, they see your puny "point total" as laughable. What would happen if mothers kept score on how much they give to baby versus what baby gives back? In the first weeks of parenting, the score would be about a million to three. So if you think that eighty or ninety accumulated points are going to win you some rewards (i.e., sex), you'd better forget about it. Chances are, your partner will resent the fact that you are keeping score. Just keep on giving, and think of points as a way of accumulating long-term rewards, not gaining short-term victories. Your contribution to parenting your baby will give you a happy, well-rested partner and a close marriage. And yes, sex (eventually) will be part of that.

10. Offer a nighttime relief bottle. If your baby is bottle-feeding or going through a stage of marathon night feeding and you sense your partner is giving out, offer to give baby a bottle (of pumped breastmilk if breastfeeding) once in a while in the middle of the night, so that Mum can get a few uninterrupted hours of sleep. Notice we only advise an occasional relief bottle when Mum is on the edge of nighttime burnout. Don't try this until baby is at least six weeks old and Mum's milk supply is well established. Substituting a bottle for the breast on a regular basis can interfere with the balance between baby's demand for milk and the breasts' ability to make milk. Also, mother may wake up uncomfortably engorged.

Not all breastfed babies will accept a nighttime bottle. It might be easiest to get baby accustomed to the occasional bottle during the day first, before you try to offer one at night. It's common for an avid breastfeeder to protest both the milk's container and the milkman who is delivering it. Try these tricks.

- Warm the bottle teat under warm water to make it more supple.
- Hold your baby in a position similar to how he is used to being held during breastfeeding. If that doesn't work, hold him in a position that is completely different from breastfeeding.
- Walk around or rock with your baby as you offer the bottle.
- Don't force the bottle teat into your baby's mouth. Instead, encourage baby to open wide and latch on as he does at the breast.

A policeman dad in our practice offered this tip: "I hold the bottle under my arm like I hold my flashlight and let baby feed on the bottle that way. That's as close as I could come to doing it like she's used to at the breast."

Getting Dad to give the 2am bottle of pumped breastmilk sounds attractive, but since I had to get up and pump anyway to keep from getting engorged, what's the use?

11. Be the water boy! While your partner is feeding, bring her water, juice, a snack, or whatever she needs for comfort. Ask, "What do you need?" or "How can I help?" Be the "go-fer", fetching nappies or a change of baby clothing. Do whatever you can so mother does not have to leave her nest. If she needs to get up and go to the bathroom, hold and comfort baby while she does and keep her side of the bed warm. Even though you're tired and would rather be sleeping, try to do night chores with a willing attitude. Resenting the loss of sleep won't help you feel any more rested, and it won't "make points" with your partner.

Breastfeeding and night feeding was my job. My partner would change baby's nappy before and after feeding and I would assume the job of burping the baby. Many times I would wake up starving in the middle of the night from all the feeding and he would go down to the kitchen and fix me some toast and juice.

12. Be a weekend warrior. On weekends, holidays, and other days you don't have to work, care for your infant when he wakes up in the morning and allow Mum to sleep in. After baby feeds in the morning and is wide awake and eager to play, whisk him away to another room, or even outside, so your partner can stay in bed and sleep. Take the phone off the hook as you go out the door. Put baby in a carrier and stroll around the block for a nice baby-daddy walk. If your walk puts baby back to sleep, keep him with you instead of laying him down next to Mummy. Let her enjoy a morning of waking up baby-free. If your work schedule permits, try this arrangement on the occasional weekday, too – especially days when baby wakes up early. Keep baby with you in another part of the house and let your partner catch another hour of shut-eye.

When Matthew was eleven months old we both enjoyed going for a walk around the neighbourhood right after his morning feed. Eventually, Matthew got so used to this habit that after feeding he would give me the cue "go!" Then he crawled toward the baby sling hanging near the door.

My favourite thing that my partner did was that every Sunday he would take the baby in the morning and go and get croissants and coffee, go

should you complain to your partner that you need more sex?

Okay, let's talk about sex. While the doctor may have okayed having sex six weeks after childbirth, the doctor is not the one recovering from childbirth. It may be many *months* before your partner has sexual feelings again. The reason for this is her body chemistry is telling her, so to speak, "Recover from childbirth, make milk, and don't even think about having another baby." So even if your partner actually begins having sex with you again six or eight weeks after the birth, the reality is she may not really feel like it. When wives are not sexually attracted to their men, it is a blow to the male ego. But should you complain to your partner about this? You go right ahead, if you think it will do any good. At least she could reassure you that, of *course*, she still loves you and thinks you're hot. She's not too worried that you'll cool down before she starts warming up to the idea.

Men don't understand hormones, but at least it's something to blame the lack of sex on. Here's what happens to hormones after becoming a mother. Before pregnancy and birth a woman's hormones to mate are higher than her hormones to mother. After birth, a reverse occurs, and here's why. Not only do babies do what they do because they are designed that way, but mothers also act the way they do because they are designed that

way. A shift from mating hormones to mothering hormones seems to ensure survival of the young of the species. Face it, guys, according to the rules of nature, babies can't thrive without their mothers, but Dads can survive without sex for a while.

Another reason for your partner's apparent disinterest in sex is just plain old fatigue. After being drained by a needy baby all day (and other demands in the household), all they need to do is sleep. Mothers describe this end-of-the-day feeling as being "all touched out" or "all used up". So you can see, the best way for her to have any energy left over for you is to pitch in and share the baby care and household chores.

Want to make points the affectionate way? In the first few months after birth, "sex" does not have to equal intercourse. Many times your partner simply wants holding, loving words, or even a soothing massage. After a bit of postpartum courtship all over again, you may be surprised that your partner is more ready and willing to go all the way. Also, acting like a sexually thwarted male who is ready to pounce is a guaranteed turn-off.

Be open about your partner's sexual feelings and your frustrations. Have sex, but don't expect it to be the "bouncing off the walls" kind of sex you may have enjoyed during your couple phase. Tell your partner that you love her and understand the state of her body and mind right now. Tell her you simply want to have sex every so often and you understand that in time (in a very long time) your sex life will return to its B.K. (before kids) status. No pressure, no expectations, no problem, right? Well, not always. Some men get more frustrated about the temporary loss of great sex than others, just as some women get their desire for great sex back sooner than others. If you feel she is neglecting you too much, tell her so in a very, very understanding and patient way, preferably when she is well rested and not feeding the baby. Do not blame her because her postpartum hormones are keeping her from feeling sexy (that's partly *your* fault anyway – *you* helped make the baby). If you are open and understanding about this whole subject, who knows, maybe your partner will surprise you one night. (See related section, "Sex and the Family Bed", page 125.)

to the supermarket, the DIY store, or anywhere he could go. He tried to stay away until noon most times, and that 6am till noon was the longest stretch of sleep I would have all week. I LOVED that!

You can also take over naptime duties on the weekend. This is a good time to practise your getting-baby-off-to-sleep skills. Meanwhile, your partner gets a chance to enjoy some "just for me" time.

13. Encourage earlier bedtimes and morning sleep-ins. Couples often want to stay up late to have some private time after baby is in bed. But this can backfire. Baby's longest stretch of sleep is likely to come during the *first part of the night,* say from 8pm to midnight. If Mum goes to bed at 11:30pm, she may have to wake up thirty minutes later, and every two hours thereafter to feed the baby. She has missed out on her chance to get four solid hours of sleep. In the early months, encourage your partner to go to bed when baby does, at least a couple nights a week so she can catch up on her sleep. Or, if Mum is tired but baby isn't, encourage her to go to bed while you tend to baby for another hour or two. If some night you discover that Mum has drifted off to sleep while feeding, but baby is still awake, ease baby away from sleeping Mummy and enjoy some baby-and-Daddy time until baby is ready for sleep.

Encourage morning sleep-in. In addition to becoming a weekend warrior, try to do Daddy duty during an occasional weekday morning. Once a week try to schedule your work so that you can care for baby for a few hours when he first wakes up, which allows your partner to sleep in.

The best thing my partner has done is an early morning thing. When our son was six months old and I was suffering from severe sleep deprivation, he started getting up with my son for "guy time" in the early morning. This allowed me to catch an extra hour or so of "private" sleep. This truly made me love him in an all new way. He and my son have an incredibly close bond, and when our son wakes in the morning he automatically says: "Dad!" and wants to go play.

14. Actions speak louder than words. Don't just tell your partner to get more rest. Make it happen. Your reminder to "nap when baby does …" sounds pretty lame if you are also complaining about the house being a mess or if you are expecting your partner to entertain your toddler while caring for the baby 24/7. Hire some help with the housecleaning. Pay a teen to come in and look after your toddler so that your partner can nap. When she starts to worry about "getting something done", remind her that she is doing the most important job in the world right now – raising a human being. It's okay to let other things go for a while. Lower your standards. Easy meals and quick clean-ups are the norm when there are small children to care for. If your partner is going through one of those "I don't have time for myself" phases, make time *for* her. "I've scheduled an hour for you at the spa and have already paid for it, and I can't get our money back. I'll drive you there and look after baby while you enjoy yourself …" One time when Matthew was going through a high-need stage, Martha said: "I don't have time to take a shower. My baby needs me so much." I lovingly reminded her, "Martha, our baby needs a happy, rested mother."

My partner is what we call "Daddy magic" with our son. If I hand our son to him so I can do something, I will often return to find that he has simply fallen asleep. I think part of it has to do with my partner's voice and calm demeanour (and his lack of lactating breasts!). My partner always had greater success putting our son to sleep when he was a newborn. I think that it is simply a Dad thing, but I can't explain why.

15. Exude confidence. You and your partner both know that baby settles down easily when Mum breastfeeds her, but Mum is wearing out. It's time for you to take over at naptime or nighttime. Your partner may be wondering, "Can he really handle this?" Put on your coping face (even if you have to fake it) and give your partner (and baby) the message "Relax, I can do this!" (We call this the Caribbean attitude, "No problem, mon!") Try to be calm and confident. When you exude confidence as a nighttime father, Mum and baby will both relax and you'll do a better job. Eventually, your partner will be more willing to leave you to it, because she knows she can count on you to get the job done.

    This man deserves a medal. He sees nighttime parenting as part of his "job" too.

Our baby is adopted and once a week he would sleep with the baby in our room while I slept in another room. He would take over night feedings just to give me one full night's sleep a week.

Try our favourite nighttime fathering strategies

We feel that fathers have a unique and different way of holding and comforting babies. It's not better or worse than Mum's – just different. And babies enjoy that difference. While there is no way Dads will ever beat the breast as baby's favourite nighttime pacifier, they can use the assets they do have – stronger arms and a deeper voice – to "nurse" the baby.

Okay, so your partner's breasts are like a magic button for putting baby to sleep or stopping baby's crying. This doesn't mean that you can't find your own way to comfort your child and get your child to sleep. Babies need to be able to count on both parents for comforting, even if, in the early months, they settle down most easily when put to the breast. There's no dishonour in coming in second to breastfeeding. You, your partner, and your baby will all know that baby can often trust Dad to help him calm down and feel better.

So how do you comfort a breastfeeding baby when you don't have lactating breasts? Early on, help baby learn to associate other kinds of comforting with falling asleep. As you learned in chapter 1 (You did read this chapter, didn't you, Dad?), babies should have more than just one sleep association. Here are some of our favourite ways to help babies fall asleep:

16. Use the "neck nestle" and "warm fuzzy" holds. *The neck nestle.* Hold baby in your arms or in a baby sling against your chest with her head snuggled into the curve of your neck and your chin gently touching the top of her head. Baby's head will then rest against your voice box and she will feel the comforting vibrations as you talk or sing in a low voice. Here's where Dads shine, since the male voice is lower and the vibrations of the larynx are stronger. Just before naptime, bedtime, or even during the night, I would put Lauren in the neck nestle position and in a low droning voice sing (to the lullaby tune):

Go to sleep, go to sleep,
Go to sleep my little baby.
Go to sleep, go to sleep,
Go to sleep my little girl.

Often, my little girl and "big girl" would go to sleep to this tune. Double points!

My partner and I had a deal. If I could comfort baby without getting out of bed, I did it. Most of the time this was the case. If he needed to be walked, then my partner would do it.

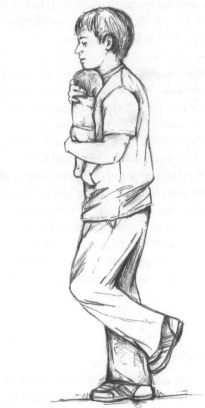

Neck nestle.

The warm fuzzy. While lying down on the bed or relaxing in your favourite recliner, drape your nappy-clad baby over your bare chest with his ear over your heart. The combination of your heartbeat, the rise and fall of your chest as you breathe, and the warm air from your nose flowing over baby's scalp will soothe and lull him into a sound sleep.

From the start, our baby loved to snuggle up against Daddy's chest and feel him breathe. I think she immediately knew the difference between her small, soft Mummy and her big, strong Daddy. She seems to also need Daddy. It's amazing what both parents, being so different, individually offer the baby they love.

17. Be a hands-on dad. Dads, the comfort of your loving hands on an awakening baby can often lull her back to sleep. We call this baby calmer the "laying on of hands". Use it to help baby stay asleep as you transfer her from your arms to the mattress. Use it again during the night when baby fusses in her sleep and seems like she might wake up. Put your hand gently on baby's chest for a minute or so. You can gently pat baby, if this seems to be what she needs. Gradually ease your hand away, even letting it hover for another minute an inch or two over baby's chest. Baby will get used to that special touch to go to sleep, and it will also help her go back to sleep.

read the rules!

Dads, now that you are team co-captain of the Nighttime Parenting team, you must read the sleep safety rules listed on pages 72–9.

If she wakes up when we put her back down to sleep at night and I know she's not hungry, my partner ever so gently puts one hand over her chest and the other on her stomach and softly holds them there. She feels like she's being held, even though she's in her cot, and she nods off. She has moved from the bedside Moses basket to the cot only recently and seems to need this extra reassurance. It is also great for my partner, because he's a loving, hands-on father and this gives him the feeling of being able to really nurture and comfort her.

Dad in motion. Adults lie still to fall asleep. Babies like to be in motion. Some babies need you to get up out of your chair to help them sleep. Snuggle your baby into a comfortable position in your arms or put her in the baby sling, then get moving. You can take a walk outside, stroll through the house, or do the "Daddy dance" around the living room. Babies fall asleep most easily when you move in all directions – back and forth, up and down, and side to side.

18. Try motorway fathering. If your baby is so wound-up that he won't wind down with any of your usual techniques, secure him safely in the car seat and take a ride, preferably on a long, monotonous road that has no stop signs or curves. Babies are usually lulled to sleep by the motion and sound of the car. When you return home, carry sleeping baby, car seat and all, into the house for naptime or nighttime. Years ago when our son, Dr Jim, was seventeen years of age, he was babysitting for two-year-old Erin, who was asleep when we left and asleep when we got back. In between, Jim told us that he had to do some "motorway fathering" while we were gone to get her back to sleep. Years later when he became a dad himself, he remembered learning and using this technique.

Stay cool. Some babies adapt more easily than others to alternatives to Mum's breast. Those with persistent personalities may fight your clever tries at nighttime fathering. Other more easygoing infants may actually enjoy Dad's novel approach. Try not to take baby's protests personally. If baby is looking at you with an expression on his face that says "There's something really wrong with this picture", stay calm and keep reassuring your baby that all is well.

Take baby out of earshot of the mother, so she can get some GOOD sleep and not just lie there awake listening to Daddy try to calm the baby.

My partner, left to his own devices, has been great at finding innovative and successful ways to get our son to sleep.

19. Add the finishing touch. You and your partner may decide that you want your baby or toddler to learn to fall asleep without always breastfeeding. You can make the transition from breastfeeding at bedtime to going to sleep with Dad easier on your child by doing it gradually, using the *finishing touch* technique. Baby continues to be breastfed at bedtime, but *without feeding completely to sleep.* When baby's tummy is full and she is getting drowsy, your partner can ease baby off her breast and into your arms.

Now what does Dad do? We hope you are prepared with some comforting tricks that have worked for you during the day. Try all of the strategies we listed above, or whatever else you think might work. Your goal is to soothe and comfort your baby until she is in the state of deep sleep, when you can put her down without her up waking.

If baby sleeps in a cot. After mother has rocked or fed baby, add these finishing touches before putting baby into her own bed. Use:

- Your *voice:* say a sleep cue (such as "sleepy-sleepy" or "Nighty-night") or sing a gentle, repetitive sleep song.
- Your *body:* snuggle baby into the neck nestle or hold her against your chest in the warm fuzzy position.
- *Motion:* rock baby in a rocking chair, or if baby begins to wake up, start walking around with baby in the neck nestle position while you continue your sleep cue or sleep song.
- If baby wakes up from the almost-asleep state, put her in a baby carrier and wear her around the house. (See wearing down, page 19.)

If baby sleeps with you. If baby is sleeping between you and your partner in the same bed, then Mum simply eases baby off her nipple (see how to suggestions, page 137), rolls over, and Dad adds the finishing touch by patting baby's tummy and softly repeating a sleep cue or sleep song. Baby should sleep on her back, or you can cuddle her in your arms and pat her back and bottom as she lies on her side. Continue humming and singing until baby is in the state of deep sleep (see signs to recognize this sleep state, page 19). If baby is beginning to wake up instead of drifting off, give her more body contact. Lay her on your chest, tummy to tummy, and continuing the patting and humming. If this doesn't do the trick, you may have to get up and add motion to the mix. When baby finally drifts off into a deep sleep, ease her onto the mattress to sleep on her back.

If baby is still young enough to need night feedings (most do under six months), add the finishing touch after each feeding instead of having Mum feed baby all the way to sleep.

On weekends my partner would put our baby on his side of the bed (between him and a guard

switch places!

When baby becomes a toddler and your partner is working on cutting back on night feedings, after baby is sound asleep do a *quick switch in sleeping positions.* If baby wakes up next to Mum, he will gravitate to Mum's breast like a heat-seeking missile. Instead, if baby wakes up next to *you*, it's easier to get him back to sleep without waking Mum to feed. Move baby over to your side of the bed, between you and the guardrail (or move baby into the co-sleeper, if that's what you're using), and then get yourself into position to sleep between baby and Mum. Sometimes if baby doesn't settle for Dad, Mum may have to wake up and move to your side of the bed, which you have pre-warmed for her. Make points! (And did you notice that your partner is now sleeping next to you, without baby in between? Clever, eh?)

rail). On those nights, I felt a bit of relief and could focus on sleeping. When she woke to feed I would feed her on my side and after he burped and changed her, she went back to his side of the bed. Oh, how I looked forward to weekends!

When baby wakes and wants to feed at night, use the same combination of sleep cues, body contact, and gentle patting that you used at the beginning of the night to get her back to sleep.

My partner always uses the same song to put our son to sleep, "Barbara Ann" by the Beach Boys. I'm even singing it now, and our son asks for it by name. It's very sweet!

20. If bottle-feeding, take turns doing bedtime. With bottle-feeding, you and your partner can take turns covering the nighttime shift. Work out a routine that fits your family's nighttime schedule and your individual sleep needs. Try this shared feeding arrangement so that baby gets used to being bottle-fed at nighttime by both Mum and Dad. If baby learns to go to sleep when the father gives a bottle, he is more likely to go back to sleep for Dad in the middle of the night. Teach your baby other sleep associations besides bottle-feeding. Use the finishing touch technique after feedings but before baby falls asleep.

My partner helps me by taking the baby just before bedtime. This allows me to be ready for my shift.

21. Enjoy fathering-to-bed rituals. There's more to getting baby off to sleep than adding the finishing touch. Older babies and toddlers depend on bedtime rituals to get them in the mood for sleeping. These bedtime rituals can be a wonderful way to enjoy special time with your child, especially if you are apart all day long. Bedtime is primetime for dads. Even if your baby usually breastfeeds to sleep, you can get him ready for that last feeding while Mum rests or has some time to herself. A bedtime ritual might include a bath, saying "night-night" to everyone and everything, story time, prayers, or other quiet activities.

My partner is so good at it we call him "Daddy Night-Night".

Be prepared for your infants and children to string these rituals out as long as they can. Take this as a compliment. It means that your child wants to spend more time with you, especially if he hasn't had you around during the day. Expect your toddler to prolong the bedtime ritual after a new baby comes into the home, as if he's thinking: "This is my special time with Dad before bedtime and I'm going to get the most out of it."

22. Help transition your child into a big bed. Dads have the starring nighttime role when it's time for a toddler to move from Mummy and Daddy's bed or a cot into a big bed of his own. Refer to the transitioning tips listed on pages 153–62. Dad is especially important if this transition is part of preparing for a new baby. Realistically, dads need to take over the nighttime parenting of the toddler so that Mum can feed the newborn at night.

23. Just be there! There may be nights when you've tried all these strategies and nothing is working and baby needs Mum. That's just the way it is, and mothers understand this.

Having my partner up with me in the middle of the night was unbelievably comforting. Even if he didn't physically do anything, just having him next to me was wonderful. Eventually, we settled into a nighttime routine of Daddy = nappies and Mummy = milk. He's in charge of changing nighttime nappies and I'm in charge of feeding. It works for us.

part two – for mums

Mums, you have, of course, read the first part of this chapter just so you'd know what we are telling your partner. We are not going to give another 23 long points to read. We just want to tell you a few things that we, as dads and partners (along with Martha as partner/mother), think you should know as you work together in your shared (or not) nighttime parenting career.

1. Get Dad involved early. For bottle fed babies, this is easy. Simply ask your partner to share in the bedtime and middle-of-the-night waking duties. Sure, you (Mums) will probably end up doing most of it (unless you married Super Dad), but it's helpful to get your baby used to being fed and bedded down by Dad early on before baby gets completely hooked on you at night.

For breastfeeding mums, however, it is all too easy to take on all the nighttime duties yourself. You may feel that the only way baby will go to sleep is by breastfeeding. If this *is* the only way baby is put to sleep in the early months, then you are right – you *will be* the only person who will be able to put baby to bed at night. If, on the other hand, you do want your partner to help at night, let him get started early. Baby may not like it quite as much, but over time you may find the occasional night off a blessing.

I didn't "sleep through the night" while our baby was learning his father's comforting style. I was so used to waking up at every little sound, plus I thought I'd better stay "on call" just in case I was needed. I usually wasn't.

2. Allow your partner to help. What? Let your partner help? You are probably saying, "Of course I'd let my partner help. It's *he* who doesn't want to do his share of night duty." Ask yourself this question: are you allowing your partner to develop his own techniques, instincts, and ways of being with baby? Are you giving your partner some time and space in which to master nighttime fathering? Or are you hovering nearby to rescue baby at the first fuss? Are you getting exasperated when your partner can't calm baby after 30 seconds? If you constantly give your partner the message that he can't comfort baby as well as you can, then he will probably gladly let you have all the nighttime duty for the years to come. Even if he can't comfort baby as well as you can in the beginning (and believe us, he knows this), if you are patient, supportive, and encouraging he will get better at it. You will come to appreciate his baby-comforting skills, and *you* will both sleep more.

3. Don't be too quick to rescue baby. When you hear your baby crying in Dad's arms, of course you want to come to the rescue, for your partner's sake as well as baby's. But before you rush in to help, use your knowledge of your baby to decide if you are really needed. A baby who is screaming hysterically *does* need you. Rather than persist with a bad experiment, this would be the night to intervene and feed baby and encourage Dad to try again the next night. (You don't want either one of the pair to start associating this hysterical screaming with bedtime.) You and your partner can even agree beforehand about how he will decide when enough is enough. That way he can develop the instincts he needs to decide when it's time to bring baby to you. But if baby is simply fussing and taking a while to settle down, without growing more and more upset, let your partner be a Dad and do the job.

5. Don't be a martyr. Tell your partner what you need. It's very easy to start feeling like a martyr when your baby is waking you every two hours and your partner just rolls over in bed, or worse, doesn't wake up at all. But if you don't tell your partner about your feelings and your needs, he may just assume that you're doing okay and you don't need his help at night.

6. Talk openly about sex. Sex (or lack of) is a common frustration dads reveal to us during sleep counselling. We have been through this with our wives (and one of us has *been* the wife) many times, and we've found that the best way to approach the topic of post-natal sex is to be very open and talk about it now and then. We

when to rescue dad

There will be times when baby just won't settle for anyone but Mum. Here are some clues that you need to intervene:

- Baby's protests are escalating instead of winding down.
- You sense Dad is becoming frustrated and angry.
- Your gut instinct says you need to help (unless you're a control freak!).
- It's a night when you're more rested than Dad.

During times when we were sure he was not hungry, Daddy would take him and rock him to sleep. If he didn't go to sleep, he was probably hungry and I would feed him.

My 21-month-old son woke up one night and my partner went in to try to soothe him and give me a little break. Our son continued to wail, so I finally went in. He stopped crying immediately, smiled, and said: "Mummy!" throwing his arms around my neck. Then he said, "Daddy, out! Mummy, in! Bye Daddy!" It's pretty clear that even when the *vocabulary isn't all there, your kids still know how to communicate their needs. Also, it's a good illustration of how bossy your sweet child becomes at this age!*

There may be times when it's actually easier and more restful for Mum to get up with baby than to have Dad do it. Some parents take one week on and one week off night duty.

My partner is an extremely heavy sleeper, and early on it became very frustrating to try and rouse him to help me out. And, truthfully, since my sleep is in sync with baby, it's a lot easier for me to wake up.

My son never did anything as quaint as "fussing". He screamed. It's all well and good to say "Daddy needs to learn to comfort baby," but when the baby turns purple from crying, it's time for the Mum to intervene.

---

told your partner (on page 174), which you've probably already read, that you may not feel like having intimate sex for a while, and that he should be sensitive to this. We want to say a few words now to you mums so you can understand how guys might be feeling about sex during the months after a new baby comes along.

Remember, your partner's hormones don't change after childbirth like yours do.

We know that you know that your partner is probably feeling neglected. He is trying to be patient and deal with it. What can really help him is for *you* to acknowledge that he feels neglected. Men get frustrated when they think that their wives don't even know (much less care) about their sexual needs. A new dad is likely to feel "all she thinks about is the baby. Doesn't she know that I have needs, too?" Try telling your partner every few days, "Sweetheart, I know you really miss sex, and I know you wish that I would feel sexual toward you. I will again someday, I promise" and it will mean the world to him. That way your partner can grumble about not getting enough sex, instead of grumbling to himself that you are oblivious to his needs. At least he'll know that you understand.

Can you actually give your partner *enough* sex during the first year after you have a baby? Probably not. So what *can* you do – besides talk about it? Let him know that you are aware of and sensitive to his needs, by actually giving him sex – maybe not as often as he'd like, but at a frequency that you are comfortable with. Sometimes you may find that once you get started, sex is actually pretty nice. Other times,

you may feel like you just aren't into it and that you're having sex just for your partner's sake. If he's being too demanding, let him know.

One sure way to get him to back off a bit is for *you* to occasionally initiate sex yourself. Nothing will make him feel more appreciated. Such an experience will probably last him (and his sexual ego) a good week or two.

When our new baby was going through a frequent night waking stage, my partner suggested that we bring her into our bed. I slept better, but he didn't. So, he began sleeping in another room. Sometimes, after quickly feeding baby back to sleep, I would sneak into the other bedroom and "surprise" my partner.

Hopefully we have given you new dads a lot to think about and do, and you mums some ideas about how to help your partner become a member of the nighttime team.

chapter 9

naptime strategies
that work

It's hard to say who needs naps more: children, or the grown-ups who take care of them. Tired parents need babies and small children to take naps during the day so they can tend to needs of their own, or sometimes, so they can nap too!

Napping habits vary tremendously from one child to the next. How well babies and children nap depends a lot on their temperament. An easy-going baby will tend to nap longer. High-need babies will take short naps (unless you hold them and carry them around while they're sleeping – then they'll sleep for hours!)

In this chapter, we will share practical tips for getting the most out of naptime. We will help you work with your child's individual nap needs. We want naptime to be a pleasant oasis in the middle of a busy day – not a time when you have to struggle to get your child to fall asleep.

creating healthy nap habits

Don't you wish that babies came equipped with a sleep switch, that you could use to put them in sleep mode at naptime and bedtime? You could put your baby to sleep the same way you turn off your computer, with just a click of the mouse. Too good to be true? Yes. You can't force a baby to nap, just as you can't force a baby to sleep at night. Yet, you can create conditions that allow sleep to overtake your baby when it's time for a nap. Babies are creatures of habit. Develop regular sleep conditions around baby's naptime and you will have the next best thing to a nap switch. Here's how:

Observe baby's need-to-nap signs. Babies who are not tired will not nap, no matter how hard you try to help them fall asleep. If you want your baby to nap at more predictable times, you need to know when he will be sleepy. Watch for clues that your baby needs to nap. Just as you learned to read your infant's need-to-sleep signals at bedtime, learn to recognize the signs that your baby or toddler is ready for a nap. As you notice that certain behaviours lead to napping, record them in the nap chart, on page 189, to help you remember and identify these signs in the future. Also note the time of the day and anything else that might shed light on baby's need for sleep (a busy morning, outdoor play, not enough sleep the previous night).

Pre-nap signals might include:

- A change in behaviour, for example, a wiggly baby slows down, a toddler stops his active play and wants to cuddle.
- A change in mood from happy to cranky.
- Nodding head, drooping eyelids, yawns.
- Baby wants to feed, but more for comfort than for food.

Seize the opportunity. As soon as baby gives you clues that she is tired, put her down for a nap without delay. If you wait a few minutes (because you want to finish what you are doing), you may miss your window of opportunity. Baby will rev herself up again and will be much harder to wind down into sleep. If you help your baby fall asleep as soon as you notice that she is tired, you will set up *patterns of association* in her brain between feeling cranky or drowsy and drifting off to sleep. The more you strengthen these associations, the easier it will be to get your baby to nap. Even better, begin putting her down *before* she shows

tired signs, as we recommended on page 85 for nighttime.

Set the scene. Retreat into the bedroom. Dim the lights, pull the shades (or put blackout shades on the windows), turn on soothing music and set the tape or CD player for *continuous* play. Use background white noise from a fan or air conditioner. Cut out distractions. Turn off the phone ringer, put tape over the doorbell, and set your other kids up with a quiet activity. Read, rock, or feed your baby to sleep. This nap-enticing scenario is called a *setting event:* baby recognizes these changes in his environment as the prelude to naptime. Circuits in his brain learn to connect the dim lights and the quiet music with rest and sleep. The more often you follow this pattern the easier baby will go down for a nap.

Try to create a nap routine that *you* enjoy. You are more likely to use the routine if it is something you look forward to each day. Play music that you enjoy, or use this time to relax and read a book.

Don't sneak away until baby is fully asleep. If baby falls asleep in your arms or cuddled up next to you on the bed, be sure he is in the state of deep sleep (see limp-limb sign, page 19) before you put him down or try to leave. If baby is still in light sleep when you try to exit (recognize this by baby's tight fists, flexed limbs, facial and limb movements, and squirming) he may wake up a few minutes later. You can forget about doing whatever it was you were sneaking away to do. Also, place an item of your clothing with your body scent next to your sleeping baby.

Co-nap. If your infant or toddler fights naps or won't stay asleep for very long, pick one or two times during the day when *you* are the most tired, and snuggle up in bed with your child. Use this special time to enjoy napping together.

Most mothers discover that their infants sleep longer when they co-nap. Get behind the eyes of your tired baby. Wouldn't you sleep more peacefully if you were nestled next to your favourite person? Wouldn't you be content to stay there and sleep longer? Even toddlers sleep better knowing that mother will be there at the nap's end just as she was there at the nap's beginning.

Okay, so you won't be able to "finally get something done". You will get the rest you need, and you get to enjoy a special time of touching and quietly being close to the baby or toddler who keeps you hopping the rest of the day. Trust us, this stage passes all too soon. You won't get to enjoy high-quality naps like these in the years to come, when you are busy driving your child to football matches, gymnastics, and piano lessons. Enjoy co-napping while you can.

Another solution if baby sleeps better with you nearby is to stay in the room and still do something for yourself, like read, write letters (remember them?), catch up on email (wireless internet access is amazing!), make shopping and to-do lists, sew or knit … She may sense your presence and sleep better than if you are not in the room.

When he sleeps by himself, he naps only twenty to thirty minutes. When we co-nap, he will sleep one to two hours.

Use a motion simulator. What is the number one thing that keeps a baby asleep? Motion. That's why your baby will nap for hours in a baby sling or swing, in a moving vehicle or buggy, or in your arms. Most of these motions involve *you*. Of course on some days you don't mind being the motor that drives your baby's nap, even for the whole nap. But when you need a break, call on some non-human motion sources for help. Try settling baby into a baby swing. Wind it up and let it rock baby back to sleep each time baby stirs. Some babies, however, don't sleep well in swings. They need more than back-and-forth motion to keep them asleep. When you walk, you naturally move in all three directions: back and forth, up and down, and side to side. That's the style of motion baby was used to in the womb.

A "hands free" alternative that best simulates being carried is a swinging hammock bed. This little Moses basket hangs from a spring, so each time baby stirs, the bed gently moves in all directions – side to side, up and down, and back and forth. Baby may nap longer.

Enjoy nap feeding. If you are breastfeeding, you will discover that your baby likes to nap and feed. He will feed a little, sleep a while, wake up and feed some more, and then drift off to sleep again. This is a great a way to get more milk into your baby, especially if baby is easily distracted during daytime feedings. Nap feeding is good for mums, too. When baby feeds, your body responds by producing hormones that relax you and help you drift off to sleep.

"Wear down" to nap. When you know your child is ready for a nap (or you need him to nap), snuggle your toddler into a baby sling and wear him around the house while you do simple jobs. Or just stroll around your home, your backyard, or your neighbourhood until baby is lulled to sleep. Keep baby in the sling until he drifts off into a deep sleep, then walk slowly to his bed, bend over, and ease the sling over your head while you put baby down on the mattress. This *wearing down* technique has been very useful in our families. We find it's especially helpful when the toddler is hyper stimulated and is so wound up that he can't relax and nap. Nestling baby in the sling contains his energy. The rhythmic motion of your walk, while he is snuggled against your chest and you are gently patting his back will all help him relax. Wearing down will help you relax, too, since you know wearing down almost always works! A great tool for dads as well.

nap needs

Here are some general age-and-stage guidelines for naps. Keep in mind that children vary greatly in their nap patterns. Some are born nappers and take long, regular naps. Others are cat-nappers.

Newborn:
Three naps daily; 1–2 hours each; or frequent, irregular, short catnaps

1–3 months:
Two to three naps daily, 1–1½ hours each, with some predictability

3–6 months
Two naps a day, 1–1½ hours each

6–12 months
A one-hour morning nap and a one-to-two-hour afternoon nap

12–24 months
Drops the morning nap; one-to-two-hour nap in the afternoon

2–4 years
One-hour afternoon nap daily

Enlist Dad as nap coach. If your baby gets used to Daddy putting her down to nap, when he's available she may more willingly accept Dad putting her to sleep at night.

It helped transition our son into falling asleep without feeding by having Daddy work on putting the baby to sleep at naptime. He was usually more calm falling asleep during the day and was more willing to fall asleep with my partner. Once he got more used to the idea that Dad could comfort him to nap, Dad was able to help more with nighttime duty.

getting baby to nap at predictable times

While we don't often advocate strict scheduling, the truth is that if you want easy consistent naptimes, you are going to have to work at some form of routine. Many parents will just have baby nap whenever she seems tired. If this isn't working, then we suggest you try nap scheduling. There's something to be said for consistency. If baby's lunchtime is always followed by twenty minutes of quiet play and then an opportunity to lie down and go to sleep, you may soon be able to count on a predictable naptime every afternoon. If more consistent naptimes sound like a good thing to you, here's how to plan them:

Get to know your napper. Don't just jump right into nap scheduling. You first have to get to know your baby's natural nap schedule, since this will be the starting point for the nap schedule you create for your baby. Keep a nap log for a week or so. Don't try to make baby take naps at certain times during this week. Just chart how your baby naps on her own. Fill in the log below.

Make this nap chart:

Day	Time of first nap	Duration (hours or minutes)	Time of second nap	Duration
1				
2				
3				
4				
5				
6				
7				

So, do you see any pattern? Is your baby naturally getting sleepy at a certain time each day? Are your baby's nap needs similar to those in the chart in the "Nap Needs" box? Or are they different? Don't worry if your baby isn't napping long enough or often enough compared to the numbers in the chart. These are just averages. What counts is *your* baby's nap pattern.

Looking at your nap log will show you one of two things. Either your baby is already napping at a fairly predictable time each day, and you just never noticed it before, or your baby's naps are truly unpredictable. In the first case, voila!

There's your nap schedule. Just keep putting baby down for a nap at those times. (If you want to modify this schedule, see changing baby's nap times, page 195.) If your nap log doesn't show much consistency, then let's work out why.

Are you interfering with your baby's naps? Perhaps baby would take predictable naps, but you are out gallivanting around town and baby can't get some shut-eye. If this is true, then try to take a week off from your busy life and concentrate on naps for a bit. (You realize, don't you, that if you want your baby to take naps on schedule, you are going to have to shape your day *around* baby's naps, instead of letting baby catch a nap around *your* busy day?)

Are you trying to put baby down for naps independently before she is ready? Often parents will try to teach baby to fall asleep on her own for naps, but baby just isn't taking well to that idea. Baby falls asleep stressed, then has a short, restless nap. If you *first* teach baby to fall asleep (and stay asleep) in a way that is more comforting to baby, she will learn to crave these long, comfortable naps. This may involve feeding baby to sleep, then holding baby while she sleeps, for a few weeks. Don't worry. Once baby learns to nap well, you can then teach baby more independent ways of napping.

Are you missing baby's tired signs? Perhaps your baby is showing some signs of needing a nap at predictable times each day, but you are missing them or can't stop what you are doing at that time to get baby down for a nap. By the time you get around to naptime, baby has a second wind.

Is baby sick or teething? Don't try to meddle with your baby's nap pattern in the middle of a stressful time like this. Wait until this complicating factor is out of the picture, then try again. What? Your baby is always teething? Well then, do the best you can. It may take every nap tip in this chapter to get a stressed-out baby to nap when you want him to.

Is your household simply too busy? If you have older kids, this can be a problem. One way around this is to create a daily pattern for your older kids where they are engaged in quiet play at baby's naptime every day. They don't necessarily have to be quiet for baby's whole nap, just while you get baby to sleep. See what you can do to eliminate the factors that are getting in the way of your baby's naps. Then try another week of keeping a nap log.

Establish a set nap schedule. Once you have discovered predictable sleepy times, you can create a nap schedule by first doing whatever it takes to get baby to nap at those times every day. Breast or bottle-feed baby down for naps if this is a sure-sleep method for your baby. Once you have the sleepy times established and set into baby's natural sleep rhythm, baby will more easily fall asleep at naptimes using whichever method of falling asleep you choose.

In order for a nap schedule to sink in, you will not only need to programme in the nap times, you will need to get baby to take long naps. During the learning stage this means doing whatever it takes to get baby to nap longer. For some babies this will involve holding baby, wearing baby in a sling, or lying down with baby for the entire naptime.

If your baby starts to wake up prematurely, try to soothe him back to sleep before he has a chance to become fully awake. Pat him, talk soothingly to him, offer the breast – whatever you did to get him down for a nap in the first place. We know this may not be how you want to spend baby's naptime. This is just temporary. The idea is to programme a nap routine into baby's mind first. Once this routine is set you can start working on other, less hands-on ways to keep baby asleep longer (see page 198).

My baby would nap longer if I held her. I made sure I had books, drinks, the TV remote control, a phone, and sometimes the computer keyboard handy. Sometimes she'd stay asleep if I moved her from my arms into her car seat, even though we weren't going anywhere. The car seat didn't upset her like the cot did.

Sears' Sleep Tip: Sleep research has shown that babies usually enjoy longer naps and deeper sleep in the afternoon than in the morning. So, consider napping *with* baby in the morning, and plan some time for yourself during baby's *afternoon* nap.

Schedule the afternoon nap – the key to a consistent bedtime. Some babies go to sleep every night at a predictable time, no matter when their afternoon nap takes place. For most babies, however, bedtime depends on what time that afternoon nap happens, and how long it lasts. Find your baby's tired time. In order to create a consistent and predictable tired time each evening you need to have baby nap at a predictable time each afternoon.

So how do you achieve this? For a few weeks do whatever it takes to get baby to nap at a

sleep science says: naps are healthy

Like nighttime sleep, naps are restorative. When babies and children awaken from naps they are happier, calmer, and ready for another go at life. What makes just an hour or two of sleep (twenty minutes for power nappers) so healthy? Babies enjoy a lot of REM sleep during naps. While non-REM sleep mainly benefits physical well-being, REM sleep improves emotional well-being. And, as you learned on page 54, REM sleep improves brain maturation.

Napping also reduces levels of stress hormones, such as cortisol. This is why naps cure crankiness, and why children who skip their usual naps are irritable and unhappy until bedtime. When it is finally time for bed, the child who has not napped may have trouble falling asleep. That unrelieved build-up of stress hormones makes it harder to relax. This explains why keeping your child from napping during the day is not a helpful strategy for getting your child to sleep longer at night. Children who have not had a chance to relax and unwind during the day bring all that fitful energy to bed with them. They have trouble falling asleep and don't sleep as peacefully.

certain time. What afternoon naptime is right for your baby? Here are some ideas:

- *If you want baby to have an early bedtime.* If your desire is for baby to go to bed around 8pm, then the afternoon nap should be from around 2pm to 4pm (for a baby who is taking two naps). This gives baby enough energy to get through dinner in a good mood while leaving him tired by 7:30 or 8pm. Of course, with baby going to bed so early, she'll probably be up at sunrise. Baby will probably take a late morning nap around 10am. As baby gets older and changes to one nap, you will find this one nap will best fit in right in the middle of the day, around noon or one o'clock. These times are guidelines only. Working the naps in as close to baby's natural tired time as possible is best.
- *If you want baby to stay up late.* If you enjoy late evenings with baby, then time the afternoon nap to occur right before dinner, around 4 to 6pm. Baby will likely sleep late each morning, then have a late morning nap around eleven o'clock or noon. When baby switches to one nap, it will probably be around 2 or 3am. (See related situation on rescheduling the late napper, page 194.)

winding down the reluctant napper

So what do you do if you have followed the suggestions above for cultivating good naptime habits, but naptime is becoming a struggle?

Most babies and children go through stages when it is hard to get them to nap. Yet they still need to sleep, whether they want to admit it or not. Most babies need a morning and an afternoon nap. Most toddlers need at least one nap a day, usually about two hours long. What's more, caregivers need a break. But it's not always easy to get a busy baby or an active toddler to slow down for a nap. They get so involved in fun activities that they don't want to trade playtime for naptime. Yet, without an afternoon nap, they will be cranky and not much fun to be with in the evening. This can be especially upsetting to parents who work outside the home during the day and look forward to spending quality time with their child in the evening. It takes some effort to market the napping concept to a busy toddler, but it's worth it. Here are some tips:

Don't force the naps. If your toddler doesn't seem tired or consistently fights sleep at what used to be his usual naptime, take this as a clue that he is ready to drop that particular nap. If you drop the morning nap because your toddler just isn't settling into it anymore, the afternoon nap will come more easily.

I try not to put her down for a nap unless the tired signals are clearly there. She knows it's naptime but doesn't want to miss anything. She just loves hanging out with us and realizes she's missing something during naps. So, she fights naps.

Nap on the move. Try "moving naps". Put your baby in a baby sling and take a walk. Baby may think he is setting off on a fun adventure with you, but soon the walking motion will lull him into dreamland. This becomes a predictable naptime pattern. When you begin the ritual of putting your baby in the baby sling and starting to walk, baby clicks into the preset pattern of association – first the sling, then the nap. Babies will often stay asleep longer while on the move nestled in a sling.

Or, try buckling your toddler into his car seat and taking a ride around the town until he is fully asleep. Then return home and ease him from the car seat into his bed to complete his nap. If you have a busy day with lots of errands to run, let your child nap in the car seat while you drive home. Martha would often try to time our infants' and toddlers' naps with the afternoon school pick-up. This became a predictable naptime pattern.

The jogging stroller is great because I stay outside the entire time she sleeps, so I can get a good sixty minutes of exercise in. Ditto this for shopping. After two shops she is often ready for a long afternoon snooze in the buggy.

Sometimes if she falls asleep in the car seat, I will just park the car in the drive and lean my seat back and take a nap or relax with a book. Even if I didn't sleep, I still got some rest.

Have an active morning. Fresh air, outdoor play, and socializing with other children will prepare a child for an afternoon nap. Adults sleep better at night when they exercise a lot during the day. Older babies and toddlers are more willing to take an afternoon nap when they have had a busy morning.

Make a nap nook. Some children fall asleep best if they fall asleep in the same place every time. Others can be enticed into napping in a new, special setting. Some children feel lonely in a big bed in a big room. A nap "nest" is cosier and more contained. If you are struggling to get your toddler to nap, you're probably willing to let him nap anywhere, just so long as he sleeps. He may find it easier to let go of fun activities if he gets to nap in the corner behind the family room couch. We would make a *nap nook* for our reluctant nappers by putting a futon or "special bed" wherever the child wanted. The locations they chose included under the piano, in a little tent made of blankets, and in a large cardboard box with a cut out like a cat-door that the child crawled into when she was tired. In a tent or a large box a child can pretend to camp or to be sleeping with a favourite character from a story, or you can tell him, "It's time to put Teddy Bear down to nap." Making these little hideaways capitalizes on children's natural desire to construct their own retreats in nooks and crannies throughout the house.

Naps are never in the place where we sleep at night. I think children regard naps as being different from sleeping at night. Sleeping at night is a "sleep till it gets light" thing. Naptime is a "wake up whenever" thing.

Nap with a "friend". Let your child snuggle up with a toy friend – "It's time to put Teddy Bear down to nap." Your child will likely fall asleep too.

Announce "special time". Naptime does not always mean sleep time for the older toddler or preschooler. Some children can get the rest they need with a *quiet time* in the afternoon when they have to lie down and listen to a tape or story. (Watching videos is too stimulating for a quiet time.) Market this as "special time" when Mummy, Daddy, or another caregiver and the child rest and nest together in a quiet room. Some days this will result in a nap. Other days it will just be a time to rest and relax.

Sometimes I will shut my daughter's bedroom door and lie on her bed and rest while she plays on the floor. Her mattress is on the floor, so she can crawl in with me if she needs a quick hug or wants to nap.

faqs about naps

Naps that are too short, naps that come too late in the afternoon, naps that don't happen at all – there are lots of reasons parents are unhappy with their children's napping habits. Here are some real nap-life situations and some helpful solutions:

Naps too short

Our nine-month-old sleeps brilliantly at night, but when I put him down for a nap during the day he wakes up after only twenty minutes. Has he really slept enough? How can I get him to nap longer?

As a general rule, if your child sleeps well at night and is mostly happy during the day, don't change anything, especially his nap pattern. Be grateful for what you have. If you try to lengthen baby's naps, you could end up with a baby who sleeps less at night.

Is your baby happy and rested after a short nap? That may be all the sleep he needs. Some infants are *power nappers*. They can take a few 15–20 minute naps and be refreshed and happy. If baby wakes up cranky and stays that way, he may not have slept long enough and deeply enough to feel rested. If that's the case, follow the strategies for better, longer napping we've laid out in this chapter. Remember to minimize distracting noises. (Turn off the phone ringer, put tape over the doorbell, close the curtains and the windows.) And, if your baby starts to wake up prematurely, try to soothe him back to sleep before he has a chance to become fully awake. Pat him, talk soothingly to him, offer the breast – whatever you did to get him down for a nap in the first place. If you can anticipate when baby is likely to wake up (check your nap log), you can be right there, on the spot and ready to help him go back to sleep. You may end up lying down with your baby to get him to sleep longer – but hey, you had the first half of baby's nap to do what you wanted to do.

Late nap, later to bed

Our nine-month-old likes to take a late afternoon nap around 4pm, but then he's awake until 10pm. By then, we're exhausted. We'd really like to have some time in the evening to ourselves. How can we change this pattern?

Ah, the dreaded late-afternoon nap. Babies who fall asleep at 4pm or later can keep going and going, on into the nighttime. They bask in their parents' attention and love staying up late with the grown-ups.

Believe it or not, this works out well for some families. When Dad, Mum, or both are gone all day, they may enjoy having baby's company in the evening, and it's a lot more fun to play with a baby who is well-rested. With today's busy lifestyles, the custom of early naps and early bedtimes may be a modern mismatch. A child who takes an early-afternoon nap will be tired and cranky by "happy hour", that pre-dinner hour in the early evening when adults are likely to be pretty crabby themselves. Before you try to change things, you might want to make sure that you really do want your child to go to bed earlier. There's no rule that says babies have to be in bed by 7, 8, or 9pm.

If the late-afternoon nap is truly not working for you, you'll need to turn back your baby's internal napping clock. Some suggestions:

- Try putting your baby down for a nap 15–30 minutes earlier each day. You can gradually work your way back to a regular naptime earlier in the afternoon.
- Maybe your baby is ready to give up a morning nap. This will help him fall asleep earlier in the afternoon. Or try shortening baby's morning nap.
- Start watching for those *need-a-nap signals* in the early afternoon, and try all the nap-inducing tips listed above as soon as you see them. If your baby takes short naps in the late morning or early afternoon, try the tips listed above for lengthening naptime.

- If baby does decide to take a nap at 4pm or later, wake him after 20 minutes or so. A catnap may give him enough sleep to make him pleasant to be around, but not so much sleep that he's then awake until 10pm.

Sometimes skips naps

Our two-year-old is usually a predictable napper, but sometimes he skips naps. How can we keep him on a regular nap pattern?

If there's one thing you can count on with babies, it's change. Just when you manage to get baby on a consistent nap schedule, his sleep needs change and you must make adjustments. Can you do this without throwing baby's bedtime routine out of whack? Here are some suggestions:

When baby misses a nap. This will happen from time to time. Simply watch for baby's next tired time and put baby down for a nap then. But what if this catch-up nap comes too late in the day? Should you skip the nap and try keeping baby awake until bedtime? It's your decision. Maybe you can compromise and let baby take a catnap. Wake him after twenty minutes or so, and he may be rested enough, but not too much.

Giving up a nap. You will see baby's nap routines change as baby gets older. Sometime between his first and second birthday, your baby will probably make the transition from two naps a day to just one. By the age of five, most children give up napping altogether. (There goes your free time!) Some children give up naps as early as age three, long before their caregivers are prepared to enjoy their company *all* afternoon. These changing nap patterns can wreak havoc with regular bedtimes, especially if your child manages to stay active and awake for much of the day, only to crash in the late afternoon and then wake up with enough energy to last until midnight. So what can you do when your child is in this no-man's land? Experiment. Try new naptimes, quiet times, catnaps, earlier times for rising, earlier bedtimes, or even (shudder) later bedtimes to see what works best for you and your child. You may have to help your child through some cranky evenings and even a few late nights before the new nap – or no-nap – pattern settles in.

She's a lap napper

Our two-month-old has no problem sleeping alone in her Moses basket at night, but the only way she'll nap during the day is in my arms or on my lap. I don't mind holding her, for now, but I worry that I am creating a bad habit. Will she outgrow the need to sleep in my arms?

No, you are not creating a "bad" habit, and yes, she will outgrow the need to nap in your lap. After all, your baby is only two months of age and many babies this age still need the security of a womb-like environment to sleep well. Celebrate and enjoy this special closeness, since it will pass all too soon. Like many "problems" in parenting, you can also see this as an opportunity. Take it as a compliment that your baby loves to nestle in your arms. A perk for you of having your baby sleep in your arms is that

this forces you to take time to relax. You certainly need this rest, but unless baby "demands" it, most mothers don't allow themselves the luxury of frequent rest stops during the day.

As your baby gets older, you can experiment with alternatives that will gradually teach her to sleep more independently. Most nappers who need to snuggle up to Mum enjoy co-napping. You might be more comfortable lying down on your bed with your baby and actually falling asleep, rather than sitting up in a chair. Lying down next to your baby also allows you the option of getting up to do your own thing after baby has fallen into a deep sleep. As babies grow, they learn to sleep more soundly and they enjoy having more space in which to stretch out and sleep. Your little lap-napper will gradually sleep in her own space. (For nap props instead of your lap, see suggestions on page 20.)

Sibling naps out of sync

How can I get our six-month-old and our two-year-old to nap at the same time?

It's easy for us to tell the mother of just one child to "nap when your baby naps". But you can't do this with a two-year-old on the loose. Infants and toddlers have different nap needs, as do siblings with different schedules and different temperaments. But if they never nap at the same time, when does Mum get to rest? With two children, you are likely to be doubly tired.

Ideally, you want both children to nap at the same time, at least once a day. Here are some strategies that have worked for us:

Try a nap nook. It's probably easier to get your six-month-old down for a nap than it is to get your two-year-old to fall asleep, so work on the two-year-old's nap first. Try the nap nook idea to sell your older child on the idea of taking time out from her day to sleep. Put the nap nook in your bedroom so that once your toddler is asleep, you can lie down and nap with your baby.

Co-nap. Another idea is to try co-napping with *both* children. Pick a time of the day when all three of you are ready for a rest and snuggle between your baby and your toddler. You can feed and cuddle your baby to sleep in one arm while holding your two-year-old with the other. Sing something soft and monotonous and both children can nod off together.

Wear baby down. Still another alternative is to wear your baby down to sleep in a sling and then settle down with your toddler for a quiet story, a song, or a back rub. Even if your toddler doesn't want to take a nap at that time, you can at least get into the habit of daily "quiet time". When there's a younger baby to compete with, the older sibling welcomes this special cuddle time with Mum when baby is asleep and not bothering "me and my Mummy". You may not get a nap, but at least you can put your feet up for a while and relax.

Play nap. When you really need to get some rest, try making a childproofed play area in your bedroom for your toddler. You can lie down and feed the baby while your toddler plays quietly on the floor. You may not be able to sleep, but you can doze and rest, keeping one ear open for whatever your two-year-old is doing.

Hire nap help. If simultaneous naps aren't working, call in some help. Get someone to play with your two-year-old while you nap with your baby. Have your partner take the older child outside or to the park. Hire a teen to come in after school and play with your toddler while you rest with your baby. Toddlers like young teens, and they're relatively inexpensive to hire.

Time for self during baby's naps

I enjoy napping with my baby, but sometimes I'd like to be free to do things just for myself while she naps. Yet she doesn't sleep very long when I'm not with her. Help!

Just as many babies sleep better at night when a loving parent is close by, they also nap better when they know mother is near. Resting while baby naps is an important thing you can do for yourself, but there may be times when you need to do something more than sleep. Use the sleep science you've already applied to baby's nighttime needs to your advantage at naptime. Wait until your baby is in the deepest stages of sleep before you try to put her down and sneak away. Sleep research has shown that babies usually enjoy longer naps and deeper sleep in the afternoon than in the morning. So, plan your activities during baby's *afternoon* nap (or for whatever time *your* baby seems to sleep the deepest and the longest). Above all, don't try to sneak away when baby is in the REM, or lighter, stage of sleep. (Recognize this by baby's tight fists, flexed limbs, facial and limb movements, and squirming.) Baby will know that you are gone and will wake up, and you won't get to do what you want to do. Wait until baby is obviously in a deeper stage of sleep with a quiet face and relaxed fists and limbs, before you leave him sleeping on his own.

Another solution if she wakes when you leave the room is to see if she'll stay asleep longer if you stay in the room, near her, and still do something for yourself, like read, write letters, catch up on email, make shopping and to-do lists, sew or knit … She'll sense your presence and sleep better than if you are not in the room.

Napping at day-care

Our eight-month-old will soon be going to day nursery part-time. At home she feeds to sleep and we also co-nap. What can we do to get her to nap well at day nursery?

Ask your day nursery to try to match the naptime routine to the one you use at home. Tell them when and how your baby is used to going to sleep. Explain that you want your baby to enjoy going to sleep without you. Ask her to "nurse" your baby to sleep by rocking, singing a lullaby, wearing her down in a carrier, or even lying next to her while she drifts off to sleep. At the very least, expect her to stay by baby's cot and sing or pat her off to napland.

Wearing a baby down to sleep in a baby sling may be a new concept for your day-care provider. So show and tell her how to do it. Show your caregiver how to use the sling. (Carrying your baby in a sling would make it easier for her to walk around and tend to other babies.) Tell her how to recognize when baby is sleeping deeply enough to be put down, and then show her how to ease herself out of the sling and lay baby down in his cot. Most experienced day-care providers realize that babies are happier and easier to manage throughout the day if they are well rested.

Nap safety in a big bed

I lie down with my baby in my bed to help her fall asleep at naptime. Once she's asleep, I get up to go and do other things. But I'm afraid she's going to roll or crawl off the bed when I'm not there with her. How can I keep her safe?

Many co-sleeping parents face this situation. Besides following the safe sleep guidelines in the co-sleeping chapter 5, here are some ways you can keep your mobile infant safe in your bed during naps.

- Use a baby monitor so you can hear baby start to awaken when you are in another room. Check on your infant anytime you hear rustling.
- Put guardrails up on both sides of the bed.
- Take your mattress off the bed frame and put it on the floor. If baby does scoot across the bed or crawl off, she won't have far to fall. Then place cushions on the floor around the bed, so if she falls her landing will be soft.
- Let her nap on a futon rather than in a big bed.
- During playtime, teach baby how to crawl backwards off the bed so she can do it safely by herself when she wakes from a nap.

chapter 10

should baby cry it out?

The dictum to "let your baby cry it out" has been standard advice in childcare books for more than a century. We can trace it back as far as a baby-training book written by Dr Emmett Holt in 1894.

And you'll find that same tired cry it out advice in books published in the twenty-first century. Same advice – just a new package.

Sound familiar? You can't get through those first months of life with a new baby without having someone tell you that this is what you must do if your baby is ever going to learn to sleep well. Letting baby cry it out is regarded as a rite of passage for parents – after a month or two, they must harden their hearts and get tough about crying, for baby's own good, or so the sleep trainers pontificate.

If babies could vote they would all put their little thumbs down on the CIO advice: "I'm just a baby. Please don't *force* me to sleep. Instead, *teach* me to sleep." And in this book, we've given you the tools to do that.

Why does crying it out persist as part of the nighttime parenting advice package? One reason is because it appears to "work", at least for some babies. If no one comes to comfort them, some babies do eventually stop crying. But the fact

that this method works *some* of the time for *some* babies doesn't make it right for *every* baby.

In this chapter we are going to share with you our honest opinion of this method, based on our experience with our own kids, our combined 40 years of pediatric practice, and scientific research on sleep and child development. We are also going to give you some ideas and alternatives to consider if you feel desperate enough to want to try this method with your baby.

what sleep sages shouldn't say

We have read a lot of books about how to get babies to sleep. Frankly, we think that some of them ought to be titled, "How to Train Your *Pet* to Sleep through the Night", because the advice they contain would be better applied to a dog than to a human infant. Dogs can – and should – be trained to do what their masters expect. Human children are more complicated. Yet sleep advisors offer the kind of inflexible rules one would use to train an animal. Here are some sad solutions from popular books about how to train your child to sleep through the night:

- "If your baby cries, don't back down. Let him cry for up to an hour at naptime and for as long as it takes at nighttime."
- "Once your child is in bed, he is there to stay, no matter how long he cries."

- "Don't sing, rock, or feed your baby to sleep. He may get used to it."
- "At nine months of age there is no need to be fed." (Try telling that to a baby who *knows* when he is hungry and when he is not!)
- "Detach yourself from your baby's protests." "Harden your heart …"
- "There is no evidence that babies are harmed when they are allowed to cry."
- "It's okay if he cries so hard he vomits."

This tough love approach assumes that when babies cry they are being disrespectful, defiant, and disobedient like an undisciplined puppy. If your dog defies you, you scold and exclaim "Bad dog!" in your most authoritative voice. Yet a baby is just a baby. Is baby's crying really about defiance? Or do baby's cries express real human needs?

what crying it out really means

"Let your baby cry it out," sounds simple enough. You simply allow your baby to cry until he's all done crying. But what really happens when you follow the "cry it out" (CIO) advice? There's more to this simple phrase than meets the eye – or the ear. Let's analyse the phrase "let your baby cry it out" in order to understand why we believe this phrase has no place in parenting.

"Let … " CIO advocates often talk about night crying as if it's a control issue. According to some CIO advocates, if mother responds to baby's cries, she will give the baby the idea that he is in control – and parents should never ever let their children control them. So instead, parents should abandon their crying baby bit by bit, until she gives up. "Let the baby cry" equals "Let the baby alone". At least, that's how it feels to baby.

"… your …" It's presumptuous for someone who isn't there at 3am, who doesn't know your baby, and who has no biological connection to your baby, to tell a tired and vulnerable mother to let *her* baby cry it out. We believe that the only person who knows if, when, and how long a baby should be left to cry is the person most involved in that baby's care. Usually, this is the person who shared an umbilical cord with the crier: the mother – the person most dedicated to reading and responding to baby's smiles, cues, and complaints.

I was so tired that I tried the cry it out approach since my friends recommended it. Big mistake! It tore me up inside to hear her cry. The next morning my baby was hoarse and I had a hurting heart. She clung to me like a koala for the next couple of days. I will never do that again!

"… baby …" Babies are different from adults. Adults do not need to eat in the middle of the night, but to grow adequately, almost all babies need one or two nighttime feedings in the first six months. They also have a need for close human contact and for comfort when they are in distress – a need that is almost as great as their need for food. Babies who do not get enough touching do not grow well. Babies who are not comforted become anxious and cry more.

When I try to put our usually co-sleeping baby to sleep in a cot, he cries. I believe he's trying to tell me, "Get me out of here!"

Yet the CIO club insists that babies cry at night because they *want* mother's attention, not because they need it. In order for the CIO scheme to pass muster with caring parents it has to downgrade real needs into mere wants. Thus, the CIO philosophy tells parents that a baby cries at night because he *wants* to be held, but the baby doesn't necessarily *need* to be held. Parents shouldn't always respond to *wants*, only to biological needs. Babies' needs do change as they get older, and eventually nighttime crying may have more to do with baby wanting company than needing food or comfort; but once again, we believe that only someone who knows baby very well – a parent – can tell the difference between a need and a want. In young babies – those under four to six months of age, needs and wants are pretty much the same thing. And in older babies, wanting to be held could still be viewed as a need – an emotional need for comfort. Think of it this way. Perhaps your child is crying for help, and if your child could talk would say, "Mummy, *help me learn* how to get back to sleep."

Listen to them when they are young and they will listen to you when they are older.

"… cry …" A baby's cry is a baby's language. It's an attachment behaviour, designed to ensure the survival of the baby by provoking a response from the parents, especially the mother. A baby's cry is a baby's way of saying, "Something is not right. Please make it right!" *Babies cry to communicate, not manipulate*. Mothers know this instinctively. If your natural maternal response to your baby's cry was measured in a laboratory, here's what would happen. The various wires and monitors would detect an increase in blood flow to your breasts. Blood samples would show a sharp increase in the level of oxytocin in your blood, which makes you want to pick up your baby and feed her. Your body might also respond to your baby's cries by producing stress hormones, which rev your body up to pick up your baby and comfort her. Mothers are hormonally wired to respond to, not ignore, their baby's cries. (Fathers, take note: you can't argue with biology!)

I am a speech pathologist who works in early childhood programmes. A cry is a form of communication. Children begin to communicate as soon as they are born, using cries and then differentiated cries. If a parent does not respond to their child's cries, I feel that it lets the child know that their communication is not important to the parent.

"… it …" What really is the "it" in "cry it out"? CIO advisors regard the cry as a bothersome behaviour that needs to be "extinguished". ("Extinction" is a term behavioural psychologists use to describe how you can get someone to stop doing something by not rewarding the

just noise?

With a little imagination, one could hear a baby's cry as actual words instead of just noise. "Mummy, Daddy, I need you. Please pick me up!" Do we as parents ignore an older child when he or she speaks to us? Do we ignore our friends or our partner when they say, "I need you"? Sometimes, but not often. Why should we ignore a baby's language?

behaviour.) Is crying a habit that must be broken? Mothers know differently. Their body's response is a clue that baby's crying indicates a need that must be met. Anthropologists who study the behaviour of human mothers and infants believe that crying is a survival tool. Babies are programmed to cry when they are separated too long from their mother or trusted caregiver. The cry is designed to get baby the help he needs to survive in the world. Make that cry go away by letting baby cry it out, and baby loses a valuable tool for getting the attention he needs to stay safe, grow, and develop into a mature human being. For more on what "it" is, read on.

"… out." What goes "out" of a baby who is left alone to cry? A baby has two choices when no one listens. Either she can cry louder and harder, hoping desperately that someone will finally listen. Or she can clam up, stop bothering everyone, and become a "good baby" (meaning a quiet, undemanding, convenient baby). Either way, what goes out of baby is trust in his ability to communicate with his caregivers and his belief that they will respond to his needs. Parents beware. If you "let your baby cry it out", you may get rid of much more than a simple night-waking problem. What goes out of your baby may be trust, security and the desire to communicate. There's a lot more at stake here than a few hours of sleep.

Get behind the eyes of your baby. Imagine how you would feel if, in the middle of the night, you needed something and you tried your best to communicate that need, but no one listened? No doubt you would feel powerless, unimportant, and angry that no one cared enough to listen and respond to you. Some babies in this situation will give up trying to communicate. They give up on trust and security at the same time. Other babies will cry persistently for hours, night after night. They don't follow the CIO book, which says that crying at night is just a habit that is easy to break. Common sense tells us that a *habit that is not easy to break is really a need*. When babies are left to cry it out, their need for closeness may be extinguished. But as a result, this child may lose something valuable – the desire and ability to achieve *intimacy*. That is the "it" that gets cried out.

Something important also goes "out" of parents, especially mothers, when baby is left to cry it out. Parents lose their sensitivity. When you "harden your heart", as cry it out advisors insist you must do, you ignore your basic biology. You work hard to desensitize yourself to your baby's signals and to your intuitive responses. Mothers we have interviewed who have bought into this method will often confide to us, "My baby's cry no longer bothers me." When I hear this, I think: "That's the problem. Your baby's cries *should* bother you. You're made that way. Why do you want to be less sensitive to your baby?" A mother once told me, "I can't let my baby cry …" I replied, "If you can't, you shouldn't."

Dr Bob relates: friends of ours made the decision to let their baby cry it out, starting around one month of age. The mum honestly felt that this was right for her and her baby, and she was thrilled to report that this system "worked" immediately. When we asked about it,

experience is the best teacher

A young pediatrician friend of ours told us that after she had her first child, she spent a whole year apologizing to her patients' parents for all the "packaged book" advice that she had dispensed during the first few years of her practice – especially the cry it out approach to getting babies to sleep through the night.

however, the mum would state that the baby cried every night for 30 to 60 minutes before falling asleep. Figuring this would diminish over time, the mum decided to continue with this method. At six months of age the baby still cried for 30 minutes every night, and at one year it was still the same. The mother thought the method "worked" simply because the child did eventually go to sleep. At some point he did stop crying himself to sleep (we don't know when – we stopped asking about it). But wow! A whole year of this! That child's cries either didn't bother the mum, or she refused to let it get to her.

Her child is now older and has been diagnosed with ADHD, learning disabilities, and other psychological and behavioural problems. We're not saying that crying it out caused these problems – they may have been "wired" into the baby's brain before birth. But clearly, this baby was trying to tell his mother that he needed help in settling down to sleep. Ignoring his signals did not make the problem go away. Instead, mother missed out on valuable opportunities for teaching her baby how to calm down without crying. Mother and father also missed an opportunity to sharpen their sensitivity skills, which they would later need for his learning and behavioural problems.

how crying it out sabotages the parent-child relationship

What's wrong with this picture? Baby is put down in her cot to sleep. Her parents leave the room. She cries and the crying continues for ten minutes (or whatever time the book or doctor said). Her parents return. Father puts a hand on baby's tummy, says, "It's okay", but does not pick her up. Baby cries even harder as her parents again leave the room.

CIO weakens communication between parents and baby. In this scenario, Mum and Dad are following the instructions in the sleep-training book, which says that their baby has to learn to go to sleep in her cot, not in her parent's arms. CIO advisors tell parents to "reassure" their baby that all is okay, but "don't pick him up". Imagine how this looks from your baby's point of view, down there on the cot mattress. There's Mum, standing over you, mumbling some words that you don't understand. Then Mum walks away. Maybe you know that she is in the next room, or maybe you don't. (Babies don't understand that people continue to exist when they can't see them.) You don't know if this important person will return. When mother finally does come back, she just stands next to your cot, with her arms folded. She says something, but the one

kind of communication you understand – the comfort of being in Mum's open arms – is withheld.

You can see how this would be confusing (and probably enraging) to a baby. Mother has to fight her feelings, too. She wants to open her arms and reach out to her baby, but the book warns her not to. The cry it out advice has somehow come between mother and baby and is sabotaging their natural communication-response network. A distance begins to develop between them.

Remember how the cry-response system is designed to work. Baby senses something is wrong; for example, his tummy hurts because he's hungry, or he is growing anxious and worried because he is alone. He becomes restless, frets, complains, and finally cries. Mother comes to his rescue, picks him up, and tries various ways of comforting him until something finally works. With practice, both mother and baby become more skilled at this cue-response pattern. Mother learns to recognize the early signals and respond to baby's restlessness or complaining, even before he cries. Baby learns that he can depend on his mother to respond, so he works hard at communicating in more subtle ways. Baby learns to "talk" better, and mother becomes able to read her infant's signals more precisely. Eventually she knows when to come running and when she can hold off a bit before she picks baby up. Because baby trusts that mother will come, he doesn't always even *have* to cry to communicate his needs. Mother and baby gradually become more independent of one another, but the close understanding between them remains.

I think rigid sleep-training methods make baby angry with mother.

Let's take a deeper look at how the CIO advice affects parents and babies. While cry it out advisors promise parents that they will have more independent children and more freedom for themselves, the CIO advice actually fails to deliver on these points, because it goes against much of what we know about the attachment between mothers and babies. More importantly, CIO fails to recognize the dangers of CIO to the healthy emotional (and even physical, in some cases) development of babies, who need solid attachment to thrive and grow into emotionally healthy adults.

CIO is biologically incorrect. As described above, a mother's body is programmed to respond to her baby's cries. Responding to the cry not only rescues baby from his misery, it also relaxes Mummy. When you follow your biological signals and pick up and feed your crying baby, you enjoy the relaxing effects of the calming hormones released by breastfeeding. Not only does feeding calm baby, it also helps you become less anxious about baby's cries. Enjoy the benefits of allowing your biology to work for you!

CIO leads to poor quality sleep. Which baby do you think will sleep more peacefully? A baby who goes to sleep held in a parent's loving arms or a baby put down to go to sleep alone, left to face the innate fear that babies have when no one is with them?

To sleep peacefully you have to relax and wind down. A baby who cries furiously before

ninety-five per cent of mothers can't be wrong

We use the families in our pediatric practice as a focus group when we are working on a book. To gather information about nighttime crying and parents' responses, we gave questionnaires to several hundred families. One of the questions was, "What advice do you most commonly get about what to do when your baby wakes up during the night?" The advice most commonly offered to parents was "let the baby cry it out". We also asked parents to tell us how they felt about this advice. Ninety-five per cent of mothers who responded to our survey told us that the cry it out advice did not feel right to them. We concluded: 95 PER CENT OF MOTHERS CAN'T BE WRONG!

falling asleep will sleep in a state of hormonal havoc. Crying releases stress hormones into baby's circulation. Going to sleep should be a relaxing process, a time when stress hormones go down, not up. Frantic, unattended-to crying that escalates in intensity can keep a baby from going to sleep, and when eventually he does drop off to sleep, he may have trouble staying asleep. Then the crying starts all over again. Listening to baby cry also releases stress hormones in the mother that will prevent her from sleeping. As a result, you have two or more *anxious sleepers* in the house.

You cannot force someone to fall asleep. Better to try to create calming conditions which

science says: crying it out can be hazardous to baby's health

In the world of medical science, policies and practices are usually based on sound medical research. Medical professionals generally accept no treatment until extensive research proves it is safe and effective. While experience has shown us that the cry it out approach results in an independent sleeper, research has also shown that the cry it out method could be harmful to babies (see page 23). Science says infants who are separated from parents, routinely endure periods of crying, and don't have their needs responded to are at higher risk for:

Increased risk of Attention Deficit/Hyperactivity Disorder

One study showed children who experienced persistent crying episodes as infants had a 20 per cent chance of ADHD as a child, along with poor school performance and antisocial behaviour. The incidence of ADHD for non-criers was only 2 per cent. Interestingly, infants diagnosed with colic were not high risk. The researchers concluded these findings were due to the lack of responsive attitude of the parents toward their babies.

Decreased intellectual development

Infant developmental specialist, Dr Michael Lewis, speaking on what builds brighter babies, presented research findings at an American Academy of Pediatrics meeting and concluded that "the single most important influence of a child's intellectual development is the responsiveness of the mother to the cues of her baby."

Increased crying during the day and delayed social development

Developmental researchers found that the more a baby's cry is ignored in the first 6 months of life, the more that baby will cry in the second 6 months. Other research has shown that these babies have a more annoying quality to their cry, are clingier during the day, and take longer to become independent as children.

Harmful physiological changes

Research has shown when separated from parents, animal infants and pre-school age human children show unstable temperatures, heart arrhythmias, and decreased REM sleep (the stage of sleep that promotes brain development).

Parents will often report that their baby vomited after being left alone in the cot to cry. Crying so hard that you vomit is physiologically extremely stressful, yet some baby sleep books still condone this practice! Some actually say that babies vomit on purpose, which is why you should leave them that way till the morning, so they'll learn it won't work.

Another medical myth is "crying is good for baby's lungs!" It isn't. Studies have shown that baby's blood oxygen levels go down during prolonged, intense crying. Some infants will even hold their breath so long that they pass out. Prolonged, escalating, unresponded-to crying has absolutely no medical benefits. Again – duh! If an adult vomited or cried that hard, would you not go to them to see what was wrong?

Chemical and hormonal imbalances in the brain

Research has shown that infants who are routinely separated from parents in a stressful way have either abnormally high or low levels of the stress hormone cortisol, as well as lower growth hormone levels. These imbalances actually inhibit the development of nerve tissue in the brain, suppress growth, and depress the immune system.

In reviewing medical research, the logical conclusion is the cry it out method is harmful to the long-term well-being of children. For a list of medical references to the above studies, see Appendix C.

allow sleep to overtake the baby. The baby who falls asleep at mother's breast or in father's arms, rocked and soothed into a peaceful state, will sleep more restfully. What type of sleep memories do you want your child to have? Warmth and comfort before falling asleep or the stress of being left alone?

CIO sabotages parents' sensitivity. When you choose not to respond to your baby's cues, you run the risk that you and your baby will drift apart. Letting baby cry it out can be a lose-lose situation. Both parent and baby are affected. When you go against your biological programming, you lose confidence in your own ability to understand your baby. Your baby loses trust in his ability to make himself understood.

Because the two of you do not communicate as well, you drift apart.

I went to visit my friend and her newborn in their home. While we were talking, her baby started crying in the nursery. Her baby kept crying, harder and louder. Her baby's cries didn't bother her, but they bothered me. My breasts almost started to leak milk! Yet my friend seemed oblivious to her baby's signals. Finally, I couldn't stand it anymore and I said, "It's okay, feed your baby. We can talk later." Matter-of-factly she replied, "No, it's not time for his feeding." Incredulous, I asked, "Where on earth did you get that advice?" "From a baby-training class," she proudly insisted. "I want my baby to learn that I am in control, not him."

This novice mother, wanting to do the best for her baby, had fallen into the wrong crowd of advisors. She was unknowingly starting her parenting career with distance developing between her and her baby. This insensitivity to each other spells trouble for the relationship, now and in the years to come.

CIO can interfere with healthy growth. Above all, ignore anyone who tells you not to feed your baby once you've put him down to sleep. If you feel he's hungry, feed him. If he is telling you that he is hungry, feed him. Studies have shown that babies have a remarkable ability to know how much food they need and when. Trust your baby to know when he is hungry. Trust yourself to know when your baby is hungry. Don't trust a book.

CIO is medically incorrect. Healthcare providers please take note! In our pediatric practice we often see babies whose medical problems have been missed because of the cry it out advice. Someone made the erroneous assumption that baby was crying at night out of habit and that ignoring the crying would make it go away. Instead, a medical problem was ignored, despite the baby's clear signals that something was wrong. See chapter 11 for possible medical problems.

CIO doesn't work in the long run. Studies have shown that most babies who are left to cry it out in the name of sleep training may not become such "good babies" after all. When their cries go unheeded, they learn to "cry it *in*" in ways that are disturbing. They often cling to their parents more, and actually take longer to become independent, or they withdraw, shut down, and become "independent" way too soon. Many parents who have tried this method have told us that it doesn't work, or if it does "work", they feel really bad about it. Sometimes they tell us that it worked for a while and then the child went back to crying and cried louder and harder, because he never really learned *how* to fall asleep.

sensitive sleep-training that does work

We are going to be honest with you. The cry it out method appears to work – at least some of the time, in some families. Many parents have tried it, and some babies have learned to go to sleep on their own fairly quickly, without too many nights of crying. Parents get some much-needed rest, and everyone seems happy.

But it will not work with every baby. It's the easy-going babies who learn to go to sleep on their own with minimal fuss that have made this approach so popular (or it's parents who do it, but don't tell you how awful it was). Because the cry it out approach worked on a neighbour's easy baby, parents naturally want it to work on their own baby, even if their baby has a different temperament. High-need babies with very persistent personalities will probably have a very rough time if they are left to cry it out. They may eventually learn to fall asleep independently, but at a high cost (as we discussed above).

Also, whether crying it out works or not depends upon how you define "works". If you stop responding to a child's nighttime needs, of course she will eventually give up on asking for your attention and go to sleep. But she has not really learned that it's nice to go to sleep by herself. She has learned that she has no other choice. For some parents and infants, this is the beginning of a distant, less sensitive relationship. Crying it out proves to be a bad investment – an apparent short-term gain, but a long-term loss.

Parenting isn't about plans and programmes. It's about relationships. Remember, we are nurturing a little human being, not training a pet. One-size-fits-all methods may work for puppies (or they may not). One-size-fits-all definitely doesn't work for babies and children.

But you wouldn't be reading this book if you didn't want to change something about how your baby sleeps – or doesn't sleep. In this chapter we have spoken out fairly strongly against the cry it out method. But we have also stressed that individual parents know what is best for their baby. So who are we to say that the cry it out method is wrong for your baby? We have never used it on any of our own babies, and we have never told a patient to give it a try. But we know that some of you reading this chapter will try this method. So we want to offer you some guidance on how to individualize a sleep-training approach for your baby (which, as you'll see, is really *not* CIO) – guidance that you may not receive from the people or books that advocate this approach.

A sensitive approach to sleep training means that you adapt the cry it out programme to fit your baby. You don't just follow the recipe in the cry it out cookbook. Instead, you learn to read the signs that indicate that your baby is sleepy. You think about your baby's unique sleep difficulties and find ways to parent him through the process of falling asleep. Remember that sleep-trainers can offer only general advice – what works for some babies. But every baby comes with his own unique personality. No matter how hard or how long you work at it, you may not be able to get your baby to act like the baby in the book. Persisting with a bad experiment will get parents into trouble. Both you and your baby will end up frustrated and angry.

Sensitive sleep training does not mean forcing your infant to sleep. Rather, it should imply creating conditions that make sleep more attractive to baby and teaching baby tools to help himself go to sleep and back to sleep. In toilet training (better called "toilet learning"), you wouldn't lock your child in a bathroom and let him cry until he removed his own nappy and used the toilet. Instead, you would gradually teach him how to listen to his need-to-go signals and what to do. Before you embark on any sleep-training method:

Get connected. It's very important not to begin using any sleep-training method until you feel you are connected to your baby – you know her well, understand her cries, and can usually soothe them. Sleep training is only a small part of how you parent your infant. Parents who start off using as many of the attachment tools – the Baby B's listed on page 66 – as they can, will naturally be more sensitive about sleep training. Of course, because they are sensitive to their infant's needs, they usually decide that crying it out is simply not an option for them, and they will be motivated to experiment with the more sensitive alternatives.

Consider your baby's personality. An easy-going, mellow baby may learn to fall asleep independently without a great deal of fussing. However, if you have a high-need baby, one with a persistent personality who does not give up easily, please don't try the cry it out-alone method. It will be too tough on your baby and on you. Babies with persistent personalities will cry for a long time, and if you don't respond, you risk destroying the trusting connection between the two of you. To help your high need baby sleep more independently, try the sleep tips offered in chapters 1 and 2, as well as the additional suggestions in the Night Weaning chapter and the Fathering chapter.

Realize the difference between CIO and CIOA (cry it out alone). It's the alone part that we have the real problem with. All babies cry, some a lot more than others, and often there's not much you can do about it but hold baby and wait it out – example, teething. And there are those times when you feel it's okay to let a baby cry – but always in the arms of a caring person, such as Dad when Mum is desperate for sleep or when baby is old enough to handle the frustration of not getting what he wants at night.

Consider baby's age. As baby gets older, your response time can lengthen. You don't always need to respond to a nine-month-old as quickly as you would a nine-day-old. But no form of

CIOA is appropriate for a baby at *any* age. And even a nine-month-old, or a 20-month-old, needs to know a person is going to show up fairly promptly. It's what you do after you show up that requires some planning.

Consider medical causes of night waking. Before you try sleep training, go through the checklist on page 213 to make sure that baby's night waking isn't due to a medical problem.

Observe warning signs. Study the warning signs opposite so that you will know whether or not you and your baby are okay with this experiment.

For a sensitive alternative to the cry it out method, see how we guided one of our patients through a difficult situation of night waking and mother burnout, page 94.

Why cry it out is so popular

The cry it out advice is very popular. Yet there is plenty of controversy about it, probably because it goes against many parents' basic instincts. Here are some reasons why CIO is so popular, along with our reasons why we feel such popularity is unwarranted.

It sells! Promote a sure-fire way to get your baby to sleep on a magazine cover, and copies will fly off the newsstand. Books that promise an easy plan to a good night's sleep sell quickly. Even pediatricians and other professionals fall into the quick-fix trap.

It takes time and energy to work through sleep problems, but it is time well spent. You get to know

warning signs!

No one method of helping a baby learn to sleep better works for all babies. If whatever method you are using isn't working, don't persist with a bad experiment. As we have said before, parenting is about building a relationship with your child, not about getting your child to conform to a programme or a plan. Here are some clues that you need a change of direction:

- Your "parent gut" says this isn't right for your baby.
- Baby seems distant and withdrawn during the day.
- Baby seems anxiously clingy during the day.
- A distance is developing between you and your baby.

- Stress signs appear while baby is crying, for example, you or your baby are hyperventilating. Harmful physiological changes are often a clue of underlying stress that needs to be resolved in another way.

extreme warning signs!

If you are doing CIO, these are *extreme warning* signs that you'd better stop:

- Baby vomits while being left alone to cry it out.
- Your milk supply is dwindling. In this case, baby is way too young to even do sleep training.

- Your baby is not gaining enough weight.
- Baby is not making progress toward developmental milestones.

your child better in the process, and your child not only learns to fall asleep more independently, she also develops a healthier attitude toward sleep. The problem is, it's a complicated process, full of twists and turns, successes and false starts – a lot like life in general.

It works! Well, yes it does. For many babies it works very well. It's what it does to babies in order to make it work that we worry about. It works much better for easy-going babies who don't end up needing to fuss too loud for too long. And because it worked for the neighbour's easy baby, everyone on the street wants it to work for them.

Doctors recommend it! Parents choose everything from toothpaste to medications because 4 out of 5 doctors recommend it. This is also true for sleep advice. But here's a little secret. Doctors don't advise CIO because they are taught it in medical school or because they've read it in a medical text. The cry it out advice is not based on sound research into child development. It's simply a quick-fix answer to a complicated problem, and doctors like it because it "works".

GPs receive little or no formal training in handling sleep problems and other parenting dilemmas. So what they tell parents is based on their own reading or experience with their children. Journal articles and sleep-training books for parents written by influential directors of university sleep disorder clinics espouse this method. These sleep trainers have impressive academic credentials, and doctors are inclined to trust them – even if other experts, for example, psychologists who study infant development, do not support crying it out.

There is also a time issue. Parents need to realize that complex problems don't have simple answers. Most doctors find it very frustrating when parents ask about a complicated problem at the end of the allotted time for a routine check-up. When parents ask, "By the way, my baby wakes up a lot. How can I get him to sleep longer?" it's a challenge for any doctor to answer this complicated question in just a few minutes. A doctor is likely to refer a patient to a book that they trust and know will "work". On the other hand, if a patient comes in for a separate appointment to discuss only sleep issues, a doctor is able to put the necessary thought into finding answers specific to that family. In our practice, we do not try to solve sleep problems during regular check ups. We ask patients to come back for an extended appointment where we can spend time going over the problem, causes, and possible solutions.

It is our hope that in the future medical professionals will become more aware of what science says about the cry it out method. Doctors like to consider research when they formulate treatment plans and protocols, and as more and more doctors understand the harmful effects of cry it out, they will begin looking for other solutions.

chapter 11

hidden medical and
physical causes of night waking

When parents tell us that their frequently waking baby seems to be in pain, we take this observation seriously. These parents have often "tried everything" to get their baby to sleep longer and more comfortably at night, but with no success.

Some sleep advisors might dismiss their concerns and suggest to these "overly anxious parents" that a few nights of crying it out will teach their baby not to wake up. But in our practice, we take parents at their word. When babies wake up because they seem to be hurting, there is usually a medical or physical cause for their night waking.

when to suspect a medical cause for night waking

As we have told you in earlier chapters, babies wake up at night for lots of good reasons: they get hungry, they need closeness, and their brains are not mature enough to sleep soundly. How do you tell the difference between normal, baby-will-grow-out-of-it night waking, and night waking caused by a medical problem? Here are some clues that indicate that baby's frequent waking may have a physical cause:

- Baby has not slept well since birth.
- Baby awakens suddenly with colicky-type abdominal pain.
- Baby is restless all through the night.
- Baby seems to gag or choke frequently at night.
- Baby possets frequently day or night.
- A previously "good sleeper" suddenly becomes a restless sleeper.
- Baby has been labelled "colicky".
- Night waking is occurring more rather than less often.
- Baby cries a lot for no apparent reason (not tired, hungry, bored, etc).
- The usual sleep-inducing strategies aren't working.

- Baby seems very cranky or excessively irritable.
- Your "parent gut" tells you your baby hurts somewhere.

Does this sound like your baby? If so, there may be a hidden medical cause behind baby's frequent night waking. This chapter describes common medical causes of night waking in babies and toddlers and what parents can do about them.

gastroesophageal reflux (ger)

Is your baby "colicky"? Suspect gastroesophageal reflux, or GER. GER, also called "acid reflux", "acid indigestion", and "gastroesophageal reflux disease" (GERD), is a painful medical condition caused by the regurgitation of acid-containing stomach contents into the oesophagus. Adults call it "heart burn".

When you swallow, the food travels down the oesophagus into the stomach. A circular band of muscle, called the lower oesophageal sphincter (LES), opens to let the food into the stomach and then contracts again to keep stomach contents in the stomach. If the LES relaxes and remains open, stomach acids can escape back into the oesophagus and irritate the sensitive lining causing a painful burning sensation. This backflow from stomach to oesophagus is called "reflux".

Reflux can cause babies to posset – a little or a lot. In other cases, the stomach contents stay in the oesophagus, so there's no posseting, just pain. Sometimes the stomach acids settle in the back of the throat, causing a sore throat ("throat burn"), choking, gagging, coughing, or in older babies and adults erosion of dental enamel. Sometimes the stomach contents can be aspirated into the lungs, causing wheezing and asthma-like problems. Most babies have some degree of reflux during the early months and most gradually outgrow it during the second half of the first year as the LES matures. Mild reflux may not bother some babies. We call them "happy posseters". In this situation, what you have is a laundry problem, not a medical concern. Other babies are bothered a great deal by reflux, and the pain is worse at night, so that they cannot enjoy restful, peaceful sleep.

Susan, a wise and intuitive first-time mother brought her six-month-old baby, Matthew, to our office for consultation about his "colic". We listened as this exhausted and angry mother related her baby's story:

Matthew has never slept well since birth. I'm up with him three or four times a night, and the only thing that seems to settle him is feeding. An hour after I put him down, he wakes up screaming. The same thing for naps. The only way I can get him to nap longer than 45 minutes is to feed him as he sleeps. He seems fine during the day as long as I keep holding him and feeding him, but as soon as I put him down he screams again. I'm so tired of people telling me I'm spoiling him by holding him so much. I've been to six doctors, and twice we've taken Matthew into the emergency room at night because he seemed to be hurting so much. All these doctors have told me that he's waking up out of habit, and if I would just let him cry and not feed him so much he'd quit waking up. But I know there's a reason that he keeps waking up. I'm not just an anxious, overprotective mother as they keep telling me. I know something is wrong with him …

Susan's intuition was right. After delving into Matthew's history, I suspected he was waking because of severe pain from reflux. The esophagoscopy, a procedure that uses a flexible tube with a miniature camera on the end to examine the inside of the oesophagus, revealed severe GERD, to the extent that Matthew had multiple ulcers – open sores – in the lining of his oesophagus. Obviously, this baby truly did hurt.

When I saw the pictures of these oesophageal erosions, I was angry at the "cry it out" crowd who had failed to take this baby's crying seriously, and who had also failed to listen to the person who knew that baby best, his mother. If this problem had been detected and treated earlier, this baby could have been spared six months of pain, and his parents would not have had to suffer through six months of sleep deprivation. Instead, because the reflux had damaged Matthew's oesophagus, he required surgical treatment, following which he grew better, ate better, and eventually slept better. Because Matthew in those early months had been conditioned to associate sleep with pain, he had to be reconditioned into sleeping more normally. This took nearly six months.

How to recognize reflux

Signs and symptoms of GER vary according to the severity of the problem. Babies may have most of the following signs, or just a few. Clues that indicate that your baby may be waking up from reflux are:

- *An early start.* GER starts in the *first few weeks* of life. If your previously sound sleeper starts waking up in pain at four months of age, it is unlikely to be due to GER.
- *Frequent, painful night waking.* Baby wakes up suddenly, sometimes screeching, triggering your gut feeling, "He's hurting somewhere! It's **that** cry again!"
- *Sleeping position.* Baby sleeps soundly when held upright or semi-upright, but sleeps poorly when lying flat. Or baby may sleep better on his stomach than on his back. (But unless your doctor advises you otherwise, put your baby down to sleep on his back, since this is associated with a reduced risk of SIDS.)
- *Poor quality sleep.* Baby is restless, squirms, arches back, and has frequent jerky movements.
- *Posseting.* Baby possets frequently and forcefully, especially when lying down. Sometimes possets like a "volcano". (Note: some babies with GER do not posset).
- *Daytime colic.* Frequent bouts of inconsolable crying during the day. (Not only in late afternoon/evening which is typical of "colic".)
- *Irregular breathing during sleep.* All young babies show some irregular breathing during sleep, but GER is associated with prolonged stop-breathing episodes during sleep.
- *Throaty noises,* as if baby is "clearing his throat". Noisy swallowing, choking and gagging sounds.
- *Excessive drooling.*
- *"Wet burps".* Milk comes up with the air bubble, most of the time.

- *Sour breath.*
- *General fussiness.* "Seems to be better when I hold her upright or feed her."

Severe reflux can take its toll on the family. One sleep-deprived mother of a frequent night waker once told us, "I'm camping out in your office until you find out what's wrong with my baby." A father in our practice was so disturbed by his baby's incessant crying and night waking that he had a vasectomy, explaining: "I'll never go through that again!"

Why GER is worse during sleep. Normal physiological changes that occur during sleep can aggravate reflux. Saliva production and swallowing frequency diminish during sleep. We often refer to saliva as the body's natural "health juice" because it not only helps digestion, it also acts like a natural antacid and lubricant to soothe the inflamed oesophagus. In addition, saliva contains a healing substance called epidermal growth factor, which helps repair the damaged lining of the oesophagus.

"colic" = reflux

In our experience, "colicky" babies who wake up frequently and painfully at night often have gastroesophageal reflux. Babies who are labelled "colicky" during the day, but who sleep reasonably well at night, probably don't have GER. They want to be held and fed frequently during the day because of their own temperament and need level, not because they are in pain.

GER may also be worse during sleep because it takes longer for acid to pass out of the stomach when the body is sleeping. To add insult to injury, the LES, like most muscles, may relax more during sleep, which makes reflux more likely. And lying flat during naptime or nighttime makes it easier for stomach contents to regurgitate back up into the oesophagus. When baby is upright, gravity helps keep stomach contents down. (However, in some infants and children with reflux, position changes seem to make no difference.)

GER may also affect baby's breathing at night. When a baby falls asleep, the muscles surrounding the airway relax and the airway gets narrower. In babies with normal airway structures and no reflux, this does not compromise breathing. Yet this can be a problem in babies whose airways are already irritated by acid containing throat contents. The inflammation can obstruct breathing, causing baby to wake up frequently, or it can cause wheezing and restless sleep.

How to help a baby with reflux sleep better

As you can see, there are plenty of reasons for a baby with reflux, like Matthew, to cry out for help at night. You can also see that Mum's "medicine" was instinctively right. Frequent holding kept Matthew upright, so that gravity helped keep down the stomach contents. Frequent doses of Mum's milk acted like an antacid to soothe the burning oesophagus. Over our many years in pediatric practice, we have been amazed at how mothers instinctively do what's medically right for their infants and children, even if it means going against professional advice. Because we see many infants like Matthew with medical causes of night waking, we are passionate about teaching parents to respond to their babies' cries and to avoid using cry it out-alone methods of sleep training.

If you suspect that your baby is waking up frequently at night because of GER, start keeping a journal about baby's symptoms to take with you when you visit your doctor. Include in your journal your baby's response to the following ten tips on lessening pain from GER:

Feed smaller amounts more frequently. Here's our rule for reflux feeding:

Feed half as much twice as often

Frequent feedings stimulate saliva production, which, as described above, neutralizes stomach acid and lessens the irritating effects of the acid on the lining of the oesophagus. Smaller amounts of milk and food empty out of the stomach into the intestines more quickly, so there's less opportunity for stomach contents to flow back into the oesophagus. Babies, just like adults, are more likely to have heartburn after a big meal than after a small one.

Breastfeed as often and as long as possible. Studies show that GER is less severe in breastfed babies. Here's why Mum's milk is a magic medicine for babies with reflux: breastfed babies naturally feed more frequently, so they get more frequent doses of this natural antacid. Breastmilk empties from the stomach much faster than food or formula. Breastmilk makes the stools softer and easier to pass, thus lessening the reflux-aggravating effects of constipation. Finally, breastfeeding mothers enjoy the effects of the relaxing hormones during breastfeeding, which helps them cope with the extra doses of mothering a baby with reflux requires. Here's a testimony from a mother in our pediatric practice:

At age five months and after consulting four different pediatricians, Jacob was diagnosed with gastroesophageal reflux. I am forever grateful I did not give up! The goal of one of Jacob's reflux medications was to help digestion so he would not reflux. What could be better for him than the most easily digested food for babies … Mum's milk! When the specialist first met Jacob, he was shocked to see him looking so happy. He told me that most babies with that degree of reflux fail to thrive and are very sickly. I am convinced that Jacob did not fail to thrive because he was breastfed.

Eliminate possible food sensitivities. If you are breastfeeding, it is possible that foods you are eating are getting into your milk and bothering your baby. Follow the steps under "Food Allergies/Sensitivities" on page 219 to eliminate possible culprits.

Use a pre-digested, hypoallergenic infant formula. If you are not breastfeeding, remember the reflux feeding rule: *get the stuff out of the stomach fast.* In "hypoallergenic" infant formulas, the proteins have been pre-digested through processing, which helps the formula move through the stomach faster than standard formulas. Many infants with reflux also seem to be allergic to milk-based infant formulas. The special formula, though more expensive and less palatable, often helps. Ask your GP to prescribe a hypoallergenic formula. Then feed half as much twice as often. Since an infant's tummy is about the size of her fist, place baby's fist next to the bottle and feed her an average of one fistful per feeding. For most infants during the first six months, this will amount to two to three ounces every couple of hours.

Burp better. A tummy full of air aggravates reflux. Burp baby well when switching breasts during breastfeeding. If bottle-feeding, burp baby after every few ounces and use a feeding system that prevents air bubbles from collecting in the bottle.

Keep baby upright and quiet after feedings. Shake up that tiny, full tummy and you're likely to get a splat of spit-up on your shirt. Instead, hold, cuddle, or wear your baby upright in a sling for at least thirty minutes after a feeding. Move gently with your baby. Bouncing around may jostle the stomach contents and trigger reflux.

Pacify baby. Mothers of infants with reflux often report that their babies want to feed constantly. This is because frequent sucking calms babies and increases saliva production. Expect baby to feed for long periods to soothe her sore oesophagus. The "half as much twice as often" idea does not mean that you should shorten your breastfed baby's time at the breast. If you're comfortable with long feeding sessions and they seem to help your baby, then relax and enjoy this soothing time together. If you find that the human nipple or the person attached to it is wearing out, try offering your baby a dummy or a finger to suck on after feedings. Some infants will suck so vigorously on dummies that they swallow air, which can aggravate reflux. You may have to experiment with the dummy to see what keeps your baby most comfortable.

Dress for sleep. Let baby "sleep loose". Avoid clothing that binds baby around the waist, such as tight nappies and sleep suits with tight waistbands. Any increased pressure on the abdomen can aggravate reflux.

Position for sleep. During the first year, it's safest to position your baby to sleep on her back, even though sleeping on the tummy may lessen reflux (see back-sleeping, page 73). For toddlers one year and older, sleeping on the *left* side may reduce reflux. Sleeping on the left side positions the gastric inlet higher than the outlet, which helps gravity keep the food down. Elevate the head of baby's cot at least thirty degrees. If baby sleeps in your bed, try positioning baby on a foam wedge

No smoking, please. Nicotine has a double-fault: it stimulates the production of stomach acids and relaxes the LES, two factors that aggravate reflux. Don't smoke around baby. Don't smoke at all if you breastfeed, since nicotine passes through your milk into baby.

Talk with your doctor about reflux. Try as many of these home remedies as you can and enter what works and what doesn't in your journal. This information will help your child's doctor determine whether or not your infant has reflux, how severe it might be, and what type of treatment is needed. Often working out an individual reflux plan using the above remedies is all that is necessary. If your doctor and you are fairly sure your baby has reflux, and the usual

feeding older children with reflux

Babies often outgrow problems with reflux, but for some it remains a problem – and a cause of night waking – into the preschool years. Here are some tips on feeding toddlers and older children who have reflux.

- Avoid heavy meals just before bedtime. Serve dinner earlier in the evening and make bedtime snacks low-fat, low-fibre foods that empty from the stomach faster.
- Avoid giving your child foods that aggravate reflux, such as: spicy foods, acidic foods (citrus fruits and juices), caffeine-containing beverages, chocolate, fried foods, peppermint and spearmint, and carbonated beverages.
- Raise a grazer. Continue the small, frequent feeding pattern you began in infancy. Offer small, frequent mini meals rather than three big meals. Try the "sipping solution". Encourage your toddler to sip on a fruit and yoghurt smoothie throughout the day. Blended foods empty from the stomach faster.
- Raise a lean child. Obesity tends to aggravate reflux, perhaps due to the increased intra-abdominal pressure from excess abdominal fat.
- Play chew-chew. His mouth is your child's own blender. Encourage him to take small bites and chew his food well. Food chewed into smaller portions empties from the stomach faster, and children who eat more slowly tend to swallow less air.

home remedies aren't working, your doctor will likely prescribe an antacid medication as a trial to see if it helps (see the next point). If the degree of reflux is still suspect, your doctor may choose to have a pediatric gastro-enterologist do some special tests to determine if your baby has reflux and how severe it is.

Get support. Night waking from reflux ranks at the top of the list of causes of family sleep deprivation. As you gathered from the treatment list above, medical treatment usually plays a minor role in helping reflux, and parental remedies play a major role. Support from other parents will help you work out how to help your baby and how to cope yourself. We highly recommend that you contact PAGER (Pediatric/Adolescent Gastroesophageal Reflux Association, www.reflux.org – an American website, which has an on-line discussion group).

food allergies/sensitivities

Rumblings in the gut can keep tiny tummies awake. Because the intestines are richly supplied with nerves, what bothers the stomach also bothers the brain. Ever try to go to sleep with a gassy-bloated abdomen after indulging in an elaborate late-night meal? The same gut feeling happens in babies who are sensitive to certain foods. Clues that food sensitivities may be keeping your baby awake are:

- Baby generally seems windy or bloated after feeding.
- You feel and hear baby's intestines churning and he seems generally irritable after a feeding.
- Baby shows a change in bowel habits, either diarrhoea or constipation, after introducing new foods.
- Baby shows a "target sign" – a red, circular rash around the anus, which is caused by the skin reacting to overly acidic stools.
- Baby shows colicky, abdominal pain, irritability, or diarrhoea following breastfeeding (suggesting baby may be intolerant to something in the breastfeeding mothers' diet.)
- Baby has a rough, raised, red, sandpaper-like rash mainly on the cheeks, but also possibly on the elbows and knees. Also, typical "baby acne" progresses onto the scalp and down onto the shoulders.
- Respiratory symptoms: sneezing, runny nose, wheezing, and a persistent cough.
- Recurring ear infections.
- Puffy eyelids or dark circles under the eyes.
- Persistent night waking and restless, fitful sleep.

Food allergies generally affect four areas: skin, respiratory passages, intestines, and behavioural changes (such as night waking). While it's easy to pin night waking on food sensitivities when you're desperate to find a cause, in our opinion,

if a food sensitivity is severe enough to cause night waking, you'll also notice some of the above clues in baby's skin, respiratory passages, or intestines. If baby has reasonably clear skin, a happy, non-allergic-looking face, no congestion of the nasal and respiratory passages and no digestive problems, it is unlikely (but not impossible) that baby is waking up because he is hurting from food sensitivities. About 90 per cent of food allergies in infants are caused by these nine foods (known as the "nasty nine"):

- Dairy products
- Wheat
- Shellfish
- Soy
- Egg whites
- Tree nuts
- Peanuts
- Corn
- Tomatoes

Other suspects are strawberries, chocolate, and citrus fruits. The only food sensitivity that has been scientifically correlated with night waking in a breastfeeding mother's diet is dairy products, yet many mothers have reported their babies getting colicky, with facial and respiratory symptoms and night waking, when they eat lots of wheat-containing foods. Caffeine-containing foods, such as coffee, tea, chocolate, and soft drinks may bother some babies. Also, beware of the caffeine in some over-the-counter cough remedies. Usually, but not always, a breastfeeding mother must consume a lot of caffeine to keep her baby awake. Very spicy foods usually do not bother most breastfeeding babies, but these foods should still be on your elimination list. Some mothers report that gassy foods, such as broccoli, onions, Brussels sprouts, cabbage, and cauliflower (usually only in the raw state) may make their baby windy and cause night waking. It's hard to scientifically explain how gassy vegetables eaten by a breastfeeding mother can cause wind in her baby, yet this does occur.

In many breastfeeding mothers and infants, the food sensitivities are dose related: your baby may wake up a lot if you drink two glasses of milk that evening, but not if you have a small dish of yoghurt.

Tracking down foods that could cause night waking

Blood tests to detect food allergies are notoriously inaccurate, especially in the first year. Better to rely on your own observations. Here are some steps to become your baby's fuss-food detective:

Step 1: Make a fuss-food chart. From the above list, select the foods that are the most likely culprits. Next, list the signs and symptoms that you relate to food sensitivities, and then note your baby's change after you eliminated the foods. It may take up to two weeks or more to see a change, especially if your baby is older when you are doing this. As we advised above, true food sensitivities usually show up not only as night waking, but also in other symptoms, such as skin, breathing, and GI tract.

Step 2: Eliminate suspect foods. Choose the most likely suspects and eliminate as many of these foods as you can for ten days. Using the sample chart below, record changes, if any.

Step 3: Gradually reintroduce the suspect foods one at a time. If you've eliminated all of the above most common allergenic foods and your baby gets better, but you're not sure *which* foods were causing your baby's night waking, add one food at a time back into your diet in gradually increasing doses. If the symptoms reappear, put that one on your forbidden food list.

Avoid the suspected foods for a few months and, unless your baby has severe food allergies, reintroduce one food at a time in gradually increasing doses. Most food sensitivities

sample chart

Suspected Food	Signs and Symptoms	Change after Elimination
Milk	Facial rash, diarrhoea, and night waking with wind	Facial rash much less, stools firmer, and sleep less restless.

completely or partially subside by two to three years of age.

Step 4: The Desperation Diet. If you've tried eliminating the most common foods, but baby still isn't doing well, you can eliminate "everything" all at once from your diet and spend two weeks just eating 6 foods that are virtually guaranteed not to bother baby. These are turkey (or lamb), potatoes (white or sweet), squash, rice (or millet – another grain), pears (or pear juice). Use rice milk (which isn't milk at all – it should be called rice water) as needed. Rice comes in many forms – flour, cakes, cereal, bread (from nutrition stores). Do not use soy. Oh, and drink lots of water. Eat, drink, and take absolutely nothing else (including vitamins and any other natural supplements). If you are on any medications, ask your doctor if you can safely go off for a brief time.

Sounds fun huh? Fill your fridge and cupboard with these delights and enjoy for two weeks. You may feel quite hungry at first but you learn to eat more of these foods and be creative with them. The deprivation is worth it when you see that your baby hurts a lot less. If baby gets much better, then you can slowly add in your favourite foods (one food every 4 days) and keep a list of anything that bothers baby (and, obviously, don't eat that food for a few months). Martha's foods to avoid were dairy, wheat and corn. Our daughter-in-law could eventually eat anything but bananas.

formula intolerance

If your formula-fed baby is waking up frequently and is showing some of the signs of food sensitivity listed above, suspect that your baby's formula is the culprit. Here are the formula changes you can try, in this order, to solve the problem. Allow each formula about a 1 to 2 week trial to see if it works. If baby significantly worsens sooner, then move on to the next step right away. While you can try these changes without consulting your doctor, we suggest you do let your health visitor know if you end up making a formula change long term.

Change the "form" of formula. If you are using powdered formula, change to the same brand in liquid form. If using liquid, try the powder.

Change the brand, but not the type. Whatever type (milk-based, soy, or other) of formula you are using, try a different brand of the same type. If on a milk-based formula, try a different brand that is still milk-based, since the protein formulation may be more comfortable on baby's tummy.

Change the type of formula. If baby is on a milk-based formula, try changing to soy. If on soy, milk. If neither works, try a hypoallergenic formula.

Consult your health visitor. If this doesn't work, consult your health visitor or GP. If you do find a "happy" formula, let them know at your next visit.

stuffy noses

Tiny babies prefer (even need) to breathe through their noses rather than their mouths, so even a slight bit of stuffiness in already narrow infant nasal passages can lead to difficulty breathing and consequent night waking. Even previous long sleepers often wake up more during a cold. The more severe the cold and the congestion of the respiratory passages, the more frequent the night waking.

Our 15-month-old got a very bad cold and started waking up crying a couple times a night. A month later he is still waking up at least once a night. How can we get him back to sleeping through the night?

It's common for children who once slept for long stretches to revert back to frequent night waking following an illness. An illness throws off a child's sleep rhythms, and once they start waking up, they seem to temporarily forget how to get themselves back to sleep. Also, when a child is sick, parents are naturally sympathetic and nurturing, especially at night, so waking up has its rewards. Your child got used to, and enjoyed, the extra tender loving care at night, and now it's hard to go back to the other way of sleeping. It's sort of like going back to real food after enjoying lots of ice-lollies and ice cream while you had a sore throat. Expect at least another month of retraining your child to sleep through the night. In addition to the sleep-inducing strategies we mentioned on page 28, try what worked for you to help him sleep longer stretches before he got sick. (See home remedies for un-stuffing little noses, page 224.)

ear infections

Ear infections are one of the most painful causes of night waking. The same fluid draining from baby's snotty nose collects in the middle ear and causes pressure on the eardrum (especially if baby lies with the affected ear down). Clues that an ear infection could be causing your baby's night waking are:

- Your baby's cold worsens and the discharge from her nose becomes thick and snotty, also accompanied by yellow drainage from both eyes.
- Baby's sleeping patterns suddenly change and she wakes up with painful cries.

Ear infections seem to bother infants and toddlers more at night for two reasons: the middle ear fluid presses on the eardrum when baby is lying with the affected ear down (Hold baby upright a while to relieve ear pain, or encourage your toddler to sleep with the suspect ear up). And at night there are no distractions from the sensations of a painful ear. Babies vary tremendously in their sensitivity to ear pain. Some are bothered by a slight bit of fluid in the middle ear, others are not. Usually, but not always, if an ear infection is severe enough to cause night waking, baby will have others signs of a cold.

Fevers that accompany colds and other infections can also trigger night waking, mainly because of the overall bodily discomfort caused by the fever and the infection. Rarely is it necessary to awaken a sleeping child to take her temperature or administer fever-lowering medicines. Simply kiss her forehead to check the temperature.

environmental allergies

Allergens in the bedroom (animal dander, dust, and mould) can congest baby's breathing passages and cause night waking. Remove possible allergens from baby's bedroom. Try a HEPA-type air filter and put out the dogs and cats. (For detailed instructions on how to allergy-proof your baby's bedroom, see www.askdrsears.com) Perfumes and hairsprays may give off fumes that act like nasal irritants, causing a stuffy nose in a co-sleeping baby. Above all, no smoking in baby's bedroom.

Dry air, especially during the winter months of central heating, can cause the normal secretions in baby's respiratory passages to thicken and impair breathing. Try to keep the humidity in baby's bedroom around fifty per cent by using a cool-mist humidifier. If baby's nose is stuffy, try a warm-mist vaporizer. Since hot vaporizers pose a burn hazard, be sure to place it safely beyond baby's reach. As an extra perk, the steam from vaporizers can act as an extra heat source, allowing you to turn down the temperature in baby's bedroom.

Try to put your baby to bed with a clear nose and breathing passages. To do this, try Dr Sears' two home remedies: a "nose hose" and a "steam clean". Sprinkle a few drops of saltwater nose drops (to loosen secretions) available at your pharmacy as "saline nasal spray" or make your own by adding a quarter teaspoon of salt to eight ounces of water. Using a nasal aspirator (veteran parents call this handy gadget a "snot snatcher"), gently remove the loosened secretions from baby's nose. Steam up the bathroom with a hot shower. Then sit in the bathroom and read to your baby before bedtime. Steam loosens the thickened secretions in baby's airways.

anaemia

We have seen many babies who had a low haemoglobin (detected by one drop of blood by a quick finger prick during baby's check up) and restless sleep. After a month or two of increasing the iron content of their diets, mothers reported their babies slept better. A low iron level not only bothers the blood, it bothers the brain, leading to poor quality sleep. Iron deficiency anaemia is most common between six and twenty-four months of age. You might want to mention this possible cause of night waking to your baby's GP.

pinworms

Occasionally, the itching caused by pinworms can awaken a child. At night the pregnant pinworm crawls out of the rectum to lay her eggs around the anus. All this wormy activity around the anus may itch. The child scratches the itchy area and picks up eggs under his fingernails, sucks his fingers or shakes the hand of a friend and the eggs travel from mouth through intestines where they hatch and repeat the cycle.

Here's how to be a home pinworm detective. Suspect pinworms if your child has scratch marks on his bottom or complains of an itchy bottom. Sometimes you can shine a flashlight around your child's anus at night and see the pinworms. They look like tiny pieces of white thread about a centimetre long. If you can't see the worms but still suspect your child has them, place a piece of tape (sticky side out) on an ice lolly stick and capture the eggs by pressing the sticky tape on the skin around the anus. Best time for the tape test is in the morning just before your child awakens. Take the tape to your doctor's office or a laboratory where it can be examined under a microscope to look for eggs. If present your doctor can prescribe treatment.

sleep apnoea

Our three-year-old snores and is a very noisy and restless sleeper. He often falls asleep at nursery. Should I be worried?

While your child could simply be a noisy sleeper, sometimes loud and persistent snoring is a clue of a structural problem in the nose or throat that partially obstructs the breathing at night. During sleep, the muscles that keep the airway open during the day relax at night, allowing the airway to become narrower. The air passing through narrowed airways causes vibration of the tissues around the airway, producing the sound called "snoring". Sometimes snoring is a clue to a condition called sleep apnoea in which the compromised breathing also compromises your child's sleep, resulting in a restless night and a tired child the next day. Here's how you can tell if your child has sleep apnoea. Video record your child's sleep during the first couple of hours, especially when he is snoring the loudest. In sleep apnoea, the child will breathe very noisily with periods of noiseless stretches of 10–15 seconds where he doesn't breathe, followed by a loud catch-up breath. This sleep apnoea pattern usually results in a tired and cranky child the next day and, if present in an older child, usually compromises their behaviour and school performance.

The most common cause of sleep apnoea is large tonsils. During the day, the tonsils do not compromise the airway, but at night the airway passages relax, become more narrow, and require more effort to move enough air through them, causing the noisy breathing associated with sleep apnoea.

Have your child's nasal passages and throat examined by your GP. If your doctor says the nasal passages are clear and the tonsils are not obstructively large, show your doctor the video recording. If the above pattern is not present on your recording, you can rest assured that snoring is not a sign of sleep apnoea and no surgical treatment is needed.

To lessen snoring, have your child experiment with various sleeping positions, such as tummy or side sleeping. Be sure your child's sleeping environment is free of allergens, including dust collectors or animal dander, which can cause nighttime stuffiness and result in abnormal breathing. Put a HEPA-type air purifier in your child's bedroom to remove nasal irritants from the air.

If you and your child's doctor suspect sleep apnoea, the next step is a referral to an ear, nose, throat (ENT) specialist.

Take sleep apnoea seriously. It interferes with the child's overall health and well-being. When children's airways are partially obstructed during sleep, they often partially awaken with a startle from lack of air. This causes an adrenaline rush and revs up the child's nervous system at night, interfering with sleep. Incidentally, sleep apnoea is a common hidden cause of bedwetting because this adrenaline rush causes the bladder to empty. So, as an added perk, your previously bedwetting child may enjoy nighttime dryness once those tonsils and adenoids are in a hospital pickle jar.

irritating sleepwear

Several mothers in our practice went through the checklist of causes of night waking on page 229 and discovered their babies were sensitive to polyester sleep suits. Once they changed to 100 per cent cotton clothing, their babies slept more comfortably. (Flame-retardant cotton sleepwear is now available.) Other babies don't like the sensation of fabric on their feet. A clue to this irritation is when baby starts pulling off his socks and pulling at the footie of the PJs. (See "Sleepwear – How to Dress Your Baby Safely and Comfortably for Sleep", page 72.)

teething

As those pearly whites push their way through sensitive gums, teething pain can cause frequent night waking, especially in babies between four and seven months. Even though you may not see or feel the teeth until six or eight months, teething discomfort may start as early as three or four months as witnessed by the tell-tale signs of increased drooling, a drool rash on the face, constant finger chewing, and wet bed sheets. Also, the increased saliva production ("drool") can collect at the back of the throat, causing normal gurgly breathing sounds and coughs that may sometimes awaken a sleeping baby. Beginning at six months of age, expect a tooth to erupt around once a month until two to two and a half years of age. Theoretically, teething pain could cause night waking throughout this teething time. Tiny teethers often enjoy a few restful weeks between dental eruptions.

It would be nice if a tiny tooth fairy could comfortably usher those teeth in, yet this is a fairytale. If you suspect your baby is waking because of teething pain, in consultation with your baby's doctor, give an appropriate dose of paracetemol (or ibuprofen, which may last longer) just before bedtime for a few nights, and repeat every four hours if baby wakes up. Also, let your tooth-sore baby gnaw on your knuckle when she wakes up. This readily available hard comforter may help her go back to sleep. While during the day cold comforters, such as a frozen banana, may soothe sensitive, swollen gums, this home remedy is likely to awaken baby even more if tried at night. Babies often intensify their feeding – day and night. During teething times is when babies often become all-night suckers, and it's also the time to bring in more "pacifiers". Sometimes, teething triggers the opposite of increased feeding – a feeding strike.

growing pains

While we think of growing pains as a cause of night waking in older children, parents often report their babies seem to wake up more when going through growth spurts. Since growth occurs most at night (that's when growth hormone is secreted), it's theoretically possible that the changing biochemistry and physical growth could cause enough discomfort to awaken baby. Some babies will go on five-night feeding marathons to get the extra nutrition they need to fuel these growth spurts. That's one time it's best to give in and feed that often to supply the growing body's increased demand. (See related section on growth spurts, page 59.)

We have noticed that babies often wake up when going through major motor milestones, such as sitting to crawling, and crawling to

is it teething or is it an ear infection?

In our pediatric practice we have an inside joke we call "the five-month ear check". Baby starts teething and night waking, and is pulling on the ears during the day. Parents rush baby in to check the ears (hoping the night waking is something we can then fix). This scenario is almost never an ear infection. How can you tell at home without seeing your doctor? If baby has no cold symptoms and no fever, then it is likely to be simple teething. If baby does have cold symptoms and a fever, then it could be an ear infection.

walking. A half-asleep baby may sit up to "practise" his newly found motor skills and crawl into the wooden rail of the cot. Or, he becomes a cot sleepwalker, stumbles, and wakes himself up

To explain these nighttime developmental quirks, perhaps baby is dreaming about crawling or walking and tries to practise his skills while partially asleep. He falls, startles, awakens, and quickly summons his favourite comforters – Mum or Dad.

nappy irritation

Since babies are used to the feeling of wet or soiled nappies, this is an unlikely cause of night waking. If your baby sleeps through wet or soiled nappies, there is no need to awaken him for a change. Yet, if baby has one of those "power poops", he may need a nappy change. If baby is going through a nappy rash stage, the protective skin barrier is broken down when wet or soiled, allowing the nappy contents to more easily irritate baby's sensitive skin. In this case, slather a generous amount of a zinc-oxide-containing barrier cream over the rash as a protective barrier to irritating nappy contents. This may help baby sleep through a wet or soiled nappy without a change. Yet, if she wakes up, try to do the quick-change method as described on page 10.

baby too hot or too cold

Infants are creatures of consistency, and a stable bedroom temperature and relative humidity helps babies sleep. See page 11 for how to maintain a consistent and sleep-conducive temperature and relative humidity in baby's bedroom.

bedroom noise

Tiny babies are used to sleeping amidst the ambient sounds of a busy family, which is why older children seldom need to be advised to tiptoe around a sleeping baby. Yet, some babies are more noise sensitive than others, especially if they are already going through a night waking stage. Tighten and oil loose joints on a squeaky cot, especially if your toddler moves around a lot at night. Oil the hinges on the bedroom door.

Close the window if there is a lot of outside noise, such as middle-of-the-night or early-morning rubbish pick-ups. If baby does seem to be noise sensitive, try the white noise sounds listed on page 22.

separation anxiety

How can anxiety be a physical cause of night waking? If you've ever been anxious, you know that you'll recognize the intense physical discomforts – sweating, fast heartbeat, muscle tension, etc. – that comes from feeling anxious. Add to that the release of stress hormones that turn on the waking switch, and it's no wonder you rush in to see your crying, sweating baby standing up rattling his cage to get out. Many babies seem to have two developmental stages when they are particularly sensitive to separation anxiety: six to nine months and fourteen to eighteen months. We believe there is a natural, in-born developmental reason for this curious quirk.

When baby develops the motor abilities to crawl or run away from the security of caregivers, the mind acts as a safety regulator that discourages aloneness. It's like the body says, "go", but the mind says "no". When baby wakes up alone in a quiet, dark room, aloneness is naturally upsetting to him and he protests. Those with persistent personalities protest louder. Babies with easier temperaments can often self-soothe back to sleep. At some time or another, most of us have awakened with varying degrees of anxiety. Remember how comforting it

possible medical and physical causes of night waking

If you are having difficulty pinning down why your baby is waking up, go through this checklist:

- separation anxiety
- change in family routine
- hunger
- gastroesophageal reflux
- stuffy nose
- sleep apnoea
- irritating sleepwear
- teething
- nappy rash
- too hot
- too cold
- fever
- a cold

- food formula sensitivity
- nasal irritants:
    - perfume
    - powder
    - hairspray
    - animal dander
    - cigarette smoke
    - dust
    - mould
- squeaky cot
- bedroom or outside noises
- pinworms

is to have someone who loves you sleeping right next to you? Have you ever found it more difficult to go back to sleep when you awaken and your partner is on a business trip and you are alone in bed? A baby doesn't yet have all the adult self-help mental mechanisms to soothe himself back to sleep. When a baby wakes up anxious, his simple mechanism is, "Something is not right here, and my parents can make it right."

Separation anxiety intensifies during a major change in family routine, such as a move, divorce, or the absence of one parent. Many parents have told us that their baby seems to be more separation sensitive at night when they themselves have had a bad day.

chapter 12

nighttime parenting in special situations

As you live, so shall you sleep. When babies have special needs or families are going through changes, parents may face more challenging sleep problems. Here is a guide for families with special sleep situations.

night waking after mother returns to work

More and more mothers are continuing to breastfeed after returning to work. This is a big nutritional plus for these babies. Breastfeeding's benefits multiply the longer mothers feed.

Pumping your breasts while you are away from your baby helps maintain your milk supply. Just as important to pumping enough milk is feeding your baby frequently during the time you are together. Babies, who are very smart about things as important to them as breastfeeding, make up for their time away from Mum by wanting to feed more often when she is there. Even though they are drinking Mum's own milk from bottles when they are with their substitute caregiver, babies miss the real thing.

Be prepared for your baby to wake up more often at night after you return to work, to make up for the feeding and touch time he missed during the day. Night waking and increased night feeding is a reflection of the physiological principle that babies will do what they need to do in order to thrive. Babies need mother's milk and touch to thrive, and so they are literally going to "milk" those night feedings for all they can get. Some babies seem to reverse their days and nights after mother returns to work. They nap more and feed less during the day when she is gone, and then breastfeed very frequently during the evening and through the night. While this sounds exhausting (and sometimes it is), mothers we have interviewed who succeed at combining breastfeeding and working consider this reverse-cycle feeding a plus. Breastfeeding at night helps them unwind, relax, sleep better, and most important enjoy their baby more. It also keeps up their milk supply. The challenge is to find enough energy to work during the day and to satisfy baby's need to feed at night. In our pediatric practice we give mothers who plan to return to work a crash course on working and sleeping. Here's what these mothers have told us helps them the most.

Co-sleep. Sleeping with your baby brings a double perk to working mums: it makes up for the milk baby has missed during the daytime and for the missed "touch time". If you are already co-sleeping, you have no doubt discovered that co-sleeping babies feed more frequently. Most working and breastfeeding mothers consider this a plus. They can feed the baby several times at night and still get enough sleep themselves. Even mothers who weren't co-sleeping prior to returning to work may end up discovering that co-sleeping is best for themselves and their babies. If you haven't already mastered the art of co-sleeping, it may take you and your baby a while to get used to it. Read chapter 5 on co-sleeping, especially the benefits of, page 109. Also read about how to make night-feeding easier (page 134), since it will be important for you to find ways to get enough sleep when you are breastfeeding several times a night.

Enjoy an early morning feed. Add 20–30 minutes of early morning feeding to your getting-ready-for-work routine. Feed your baby as soon as you awaken, before you get out of bed and shower and dress. Then feed baby once more before you leave home or before you leave him at the caregiver's.

One month before going back to work, I started getting up about one and a half hours before he woke up. Sometimes I'd wake up on my own from the engorgement of very full breasts or my partner would wake me up. I would pump off what I had and freeze it. By the time my baby woke up, I'd have plenty of milk for him to drink. This approach also made the first feeding more pleasant. I didn't have painful breasts to feed him with. By the time I went back to work, I had a big milk bank stored up.

Adjust baby's nap schedule. When you were home on maternity leave, your baby may have had an early afternoon nap and an early bedtime. Yet, most working mothers find it works better for baby to have a late afternoon nap and a later bedtime. This allows you to enjoy more quality time with your baby during the evening, as well as to get in an extra feeding before bedtime.

Enjoy a happy feeding reunion. Ask your caregiver not to feed baby during the hour before you arrive. Call ahead if you're going to be early or late. As soon as you arrive home, sit down and feed your baby. Make this relaxing reunion a priority.

My baby loves to be fed as soon as I get home from work. It also helps me unwind after a tense day at work and fighting the rush-hour traffic. Toward the end of our feeding session, I feel so relaxed.

Plan weekend tank-ups. To build up your milk supply, breastfeed more often on weekends and other non-working days. Feed and nap with your baby to catch up on your sleep and to boost your milk production. Working mothers often notice that even if their milk supply dwindles by Friday, a weekend of feeding ensures that they will make extra milk on Mondays and Tuesdays.

Be flexible. Your baby's sleep patterns will change when you return to work. They may also be affected by changes in the care giving situation or in your work schedule. Try to understand these changes from your baby's point of view and then be flexible about finding ways to cope. Realistically, you won't be able to do much more than work, breastfeed, and care for your baby and yourself. Avoid other commitments during this time.

Get help! If you are going to continue to produce both milk and income, you are going to need help. When Mum works outside the home, Dad must share in both the baby-care and the running of the household (see "Twenty-three Nighttime Fathering Tips", page 166). Delegate as many of the non-baby-related chores you can, and hire help for the house, if possible.

night waking in a premature baby

We're just about ready to take our eight-week premature baby home from the hospital and wonder what type of sleep patterns we should expect.

A general principle of infant behaviour that we have followed during our years as pediatricians is that babies do what they do for basic biological reasons. This principle explains the different sleep patterns of premature babies. In the first few months, preemies may sleep for more total hours (16–18 hours a day) than term babies, but they also awaken more frequently. Here's why.

As you learned on page 53, there are two main states of sleep: active sleep (also called REM sleep) and quiet or deep sleep (called non REM sleep). The younger the human being, the greater the percentage of active sleep. The pre-born baby's sleep may be nearly 100 per cent active sleep; premature infants (especially micro preemies) may have nearly 90 per cent; and term infants 50–70 per cent. By the time children are two years old, 25 per cent of their sleeping time is spent in active sleep. Adolescents and adults spend around 20 per cent of their sleep time in active sleep. This shift to a more mature sleep pattern as babies get older is one of the reasons they sleep "better" (that is, wake up less) the older they get.

Why do preemies and younger babies spend so much time in active sleep? They are doing what they do for biological reasons. The last months in the womb and the first months of life are a time of rapid brain development, and sleep researchers believe that REM sleep helps the brain develop. The brain rests during quiet sleep, but is busily at work during REM sleep. Blood flow to the brain increases during REM sleep, particularly in the area of the brain that automatically controls breathing. During active sleep the body also increases the manufacture of certain proteins that are the building blocks of the neurons in the brain. So, in a nutshell, all this active sleep is helping preemies' brains grow.

Because of these normal and developmentally beneficial differences in sleep patterns, you should expect your preemie to wake up more frequently than a baby. It may also take longer for your baby to reach sleep maturity. If your baby was eight weeks early, then in theory, you could expect him to continue to wake up frequently eight weeks longer than you would expect of a term newborn.

Now that you understand your preemie's unique sleep patterns and developmental needs, you can see that you have some nighttime challenges ahead of you. It is especially important for the parents of premature infants to develop a nurturing style of nighttime parenting.

Early sleep training – not for preemies. While it's wise for all parents to shun the cry it out crowd, especially during the early months, this caution is particularly important for preemies. In fact, our general advice of "don't let your baby cry it out" becomes a double-don't for premature infants. Crying wastes energy, oxygen, and food – and preemies need more of all of these things to grow. You may hear someone say, "Crying is good for his lungs." Nonsense. Crying is hard on term babies, and it's doubly difficult for preemies. Excessive crying lowers a baby's level of blood oxygen, which is already marginal in most premature infants. Babies waste a lot of energy in crying, energy that is needed for catch-up growth. Finally, crying leads to posseting or reflux. Preemies are prone to reflux and need to keep that food in their tummy.

Consider co-sleeping. Newborns enter the world with disorganized physiological systems. The brain's control over breathing patterns, heart rates, and waking and sleeping is far from perfect. Preemies are even more disorganized than term newborns. So co-sleeping, which helps organize baby's physiological systems, has got to be good for growth. What helps preemies grow? More milk, more touch, and less wasted energy. That's exactly what co-sleeping provides. Here are reasons why co-sleeping is particularly beneficial for premature infants:

• *Preemies grow better.* Levels of prolactin, the milk-making hormone, are higher during sleep. There is lots of milk available to co-sleeping babies in the middle of the night. Mothers often produce milk that is higher in fat at night, particularly in brain-building omega-3 fats. Co-sleeping enables you to deliver more "smart milk" and "grow milk" to your preemie.
• *Preemies sleep safer.* Preemies are prone to irregular breathing patterns and stop-breathing episodes, called apnoea. You probably learned about apnoea and apnoea monitors while your baby was in the hospital, and you may be using an apnoea monitor at home. The co-sleeping mother is like a human apnoea monitor. Her presence helps to keep baby breathing. Many parents of preemies in our pediatric practice have reported their babies seem to breathe more regularly and show fewer apnoea alarms when monitored during co-sleeping.

When my baby was discharged from the hospital, I was told to have her sleep alone in a cot with an apnoea monitor. The monitor went off all night long and it became a nightmare for our whole family. After a while, I left the monitor on her but put her next to me in bed. We both slept wonderfully side by side, and the monitor alarm never sounded. I strongly feel that my presence stimulated her to breathe until she outgrew her stop-breathing tendencies. My touch and closeness was all she needed.

sleep training – not for preemies

Ban the baby trainers from your home and bookshelf if you have a premature infant. The dictums of baby trainers are: scheduled feedings, not holding baby so much for fear of "spoiling", and letting baby cry it out so that baby learns to sleep through the night. All three of these techniques carry risks for term babies, but they are downright hazardous to the health of preemies. Rigid baby training keeps preemies from thriving and Mummies from thriving. Here's why:

Rigid three- or four-hour feeding schedules, as recommended by most baby trainers, will not work for a preemie. Because preemies have tiny tummies, immature digestive systems, and tire easily during feedings, they need smaller, more frequent feedings. We've mentioned above how the cry it out advice keeps babies from thriving. It also keeps mothers from thriving by desensitising them to the needs of their baby. You need to care for your baby in ways that build up your sensitivity, not tear it down. Baby training makes no physiologic sense, especially in the care and feeding of premature infants.

- *Sleeping close to Mummy delivers therapeutic touch.* Increased touch helps babies grow, probably for two physiologic reasons: touch stimulates the release of growth hormone and lowers the level of energy wasting stress hormones.
- *Co-sleeping babies sleep more peacefully.* Videotape studies by sleep researcher Dr James McKenna revealed that solo sleepers squirm and seem more restless at night than co-sleepers. Instead of wasting energy squirming, you want your preemie to put that energy into growing.
- *Mothers sleep better.* Research has shown that co-sleeping babies do night feed more frequently. Premature babies need to night feed even more frequently. Naturally, co-sleeping is the answer for easier night feeding. Remember the perk of breastfeeding acting like a natural tranquillizer? Feeding your preemie frequently at night naturally stimulates the release of relaxing hormones that help you sleep.

twins and multiples

We have newborn twins on the way and my friends who also have twins are always complaining that they don't get enough sleep. Are there things I can do to get more sleep but still meet their nighttime needs?

Being blessed with two babies doesn't necessarily mean you will get half as much sleep. If anything, mothers of twins need more sleep than mothers of singletons. Here are some strategies to try to avoid mother-of-twin burnout.

Consider co-bedding. Since they were "womb mates" for many months, your babies are used to sleeping together. Neo-natologists have long observed that twins placed together in the same incubator or Moses basket tend to breathe better and grow faster. In a study reported in 2002 in *Clinical Pediatrics*, researchers placed apnoea monitors on eleven sets of pre-term twins and compared the readings when the twins slept together in the same Moses basket and slept separately. The co-bedding twins showed significantly fewer episodes of apnoea.

Another perk is that co-bedding helps get twin babies on similar sleep schedules, which is particularly helpful if one baby seems to be a "sleeper" and the other one a "waker". You can also try a bedside co-sleeper (see illustration, page 123) and have your babies sleep right next to you.

Sometime between four and six months of age, when your babies start moving around and flailing their limbs during sleep, you may decide it's time to try separate sleeping, so that the babies don't wake each other. As they grow, cot-mates may become playmates, and it's time to separate them at night. You'll want to keep them apart if one is teething or wakeful for other reasons. Yet since they're used to sleeping next to a person, this is a good time to get each one a safe "comforter" so they don't feel they are waking up "alone".

Consider co-sleeping. Twins benefit from co-sleeping just like single babies. In fact, they may need the therapeutic touch and other growth-stimulating effects of co-sleeping more, since twins are often born a bit early (see co-sleeping with preemies above). Is it possible to co-sleep, night-feed , and still get enough sleep yourself? It has worked for many mothers of twins. Try putting your babies down on their backs in your bed and sleeping between them. A king-size bed is a must. If bed space is still a problem, consider using a bedside co-sleeper. Co-sleeping is particularly helpful in those early months of marathon night-feeding during frequent growth spurts.

In the morning I would move the twins from their co-sleeper into bed with me, one snuggled up on each side. With the warmth and presence of Mummy, they just relaxed and slept more soundly, and so did I. It was really easy to feed one baby while lying on my side then roll over and feed the other one.

Double the nighttime parenting. While many mothers of single babies consider nighttime help from their partners a luxury, for mothers of multiples, it's a necessity. Dad can do everything at night that mother can do, except breastfeed. And remember, Dad can "father nurse" a fussy but full baby back to sleep. (See the many tips on nighttime fathering, page 176).

Both were bottle-fed and we each took an assigned baby for the night. That way each of us got up only half the night. Then, as one of them started sleeping through, we changed to being the parent on-call all night. With this arrangement, we each got to sleep every other night.

Try for the same sleep schedules. "Do everything together" will be your survival motto. Just as you try to get both babies on approximately the same feeding schedules, try to get them on the same sleeping schedule. This may not be possible if they have very different sleep temperaments, yet one twin will often take a sleep cue from the other one. If the one who fights sleep sees the easy baby drifting off to sleep, he may imitate his twin. Or he may see this as a chance to get one-on-one time with parents and may try all the harder to stay awake. This is where it really helps to have two sets of arms to get two babies down to sleep at the same time.

Give yourself a break. "Once our twins were four weeks, I would occasionally pump a little bit before the normal feeding around 6pm and then I'd run to bed. My partner would give them a bottle and play with them in the evening. I would wake up and feed them again at 10pm, and then we would all go to sleep."

Do high-needs shift work. Most mothers of twins report that one or the other of their babies will go through a high-need stage and want to be held or fed more than the other. You may find that sometimes you can put the easier baby to sleep in a cot and then snuggle down with the needy one.

Get double help during the day. If you've got to double the energy you spend holding and feeding your babies, you've got to cut the time you spend doing non-baby-related chores in half. Hire help or delegate the cooking, cleaning, and tidying up to your partner, friends, older children, or willing relatives. Your local Mothers of Twins Club should be able to give you some practical sleep advice. (Helpful organisations are: TAMBA (Twins and Multiple Births Association) www.tamba.org.uk). For helpful tips on co-sleeping and night feeding see La Leche League's book, Mothering Multiples (www.laleche.org.uk)

I would get all set up with pillows while my partner changed one nappy, brought the first baby to me, then changed the second and delivered the second to me. He'd go back to bed while I fed them at the same time for 20 to 30 minutes. I cherished the silence, two little nuzzling heads, just the three of us in our little circle. Then my partner and I would put the twins back into their shared cot. We'd just stand over their cot and watch for a few minutes with tears in our eyes. I love our time together like that!

when child is sick

Children often have difficulty sleeping when they are sick. Pain or discomfort gets worse when you're alone in the dark, so children's misery prefers company. When sick, children often cling to their favourite source of comfort and healing, Dr Mum. Children who usually sleep alone may lobby for sleeping with you in your bed. If illness is zapping their energy, they may take longer naps, fall asleep earlier at bedtime, and then wake up in the wee hours of the morning and be unable to go back to sleep. Just what you need, right?

We have noticed how much more quickly children seem to get better when a parent sleeps close to them. It's that therapeutic power of touch again. Hospitals are recognizing the healing power of parents by routinely providing a camp bed so that parents can sleep next to the child's hospital bed.

During the writing of this book, we had to hospitalize three-year-old Madison because of severe asthma. Sandy, an intuitive mother of five, had been down this road many times and knew what worked. She spent many hours a day, and much of the night, snuggling next to Madison in her hospital bed. The nurses, the mother, and we pediatricians all noticed that the alarm that was supposed to sound when Madison's blood oxygen levels fell went off much less when Mum slept next to her. That made sense, since sleep relaxes the whole body, especially those wheezy breathing passages.

Dr Bill recalls: the therapeutic effects of relaxing sleep are most evident in the child with croup. One of my most memorable hospital moments was the night I stood by the bedside of nine-month-old Tony, worrying as his croup was getting worse. He was barking like a seal while he struggled to get a breath. I called the ENT specialist and put the operating room on standby, fearing that Tony would need a tracheotomy, a tube in his neck that would bypass the swollen vocal cords to help him breathe. I told Tony's mother, "If only he could go to sleep, his croup might get better and he wouldn't need the operation." She said, "Let me try one more thing." She snuggled next to Tony in the tiny bed and fed him through the opening in the oxygen tent. Tony breastfed himself to sleep, his breathing relaxed, and the surgery was not necessary. Now that he is a teenager, I remind him, especially when he's a little rough on his Mum, about how his mother saved him from having a hole in his neck.

when travelling

Children are creatures of habits and routines, and these are disrupted when you travel. Different time zones, different beds, different noises, and different activities can all make it hard to get to sleep. Try these travel tips to help your child sleep better when away from home:

Strive for safety and sameness. New places and new faces are the reason you travel, but try to keep some things the same for baby. New and exciting activities during the day, meeting new family members, and sleeping in a different bed all make it hard for babies and toddlers to wind down at bedtime. Stick to your usual bedtime routine, if possible. Take along a bit of "home", such as baby's favourite "cuddly" or blanket. If baby is a cot-sleeper, be sure that your hotel or holiday place has a suitable and safe cot. (See safe cot sleeping, page 76.) If baby is a confirmed co-sleeper, be sure the adult bed is safe. (See safe co-sleeping, page 74.)

Our baby was used to sleeping in his cot at home. On holiday we stayed in an apartment

travel tip

To block out the ray of sunlight peering through the slit in the curtain-shades, bring along some metal clips and clip the edges together before you go to bed at night. That may get you an extra hour or two of sleep in the morning. We have found that while most hotels have opaque curtain shades, they leak rays of sunlight in the morning and need to be clipped together.

that didn't have a cot, so he slept with us. Now that we're home, we can't get him out of our bed. Smart baby!

Plan ahead for time-zone changes. While some infants adjust better than adults to time zone changes, others are upset by them. It often helps to plan ahead and let baby go to sleep and wake up at the new times starting a few days before your trip. Of course, even if you try your hardest to manipulate baby's sleep schedule, she may still outfox you and wake up when the first ray of sunlight comes through the window at 6am. To avoid spending your first day of holiday sleep deprived, be sure the bedroom is dark.

moving

Moving to a new home can be stressful for the whole family, infants and toddlers included. This is not usually a good time to make major changes in sleeping routines. With all the excitement and exhaustion involved in moving, your child will need you more during the night, not less. This is not the time to suddenly eject the toddler from your bed and make him sleep in his own. On the other hand, it might be an opportune time to introduce your child to his very own bedroom or a new "big boy" bed. Just don't expect him to sleep there until he feels safe and secure in his new surroundings.

when dad travels

My partner travels a lot, and when he's away our three-year-old is restless and often comes into my room in the middle of the night. How can I get her to sleep better during these times?

A change in family routine, especially one as upsetting as a parent being gone, often disturbs children's sleep. If you are a closely attached family and your child spends a lot of time with her father, she is going to be upset when he is gone. Also, when Dad is away, Mum is often tense and tired, and children can sense this.

It's natural for your child to feel anxious when your partner is out of town. In fact, separation anxiety is often considered a psychological strength rather than a weakness. It's the more securely attached infants and toddlers who are often bothered the most by the absence of a parent. Try these extra doses of daytime and nighttime security when one parent is away:

- *Explain the absence.* If one or both parents are away, the child under three may not fully understand that Mummy or Daddy will be back in "two days". When one or both of us travelled, we softened the separation anxiety by helping our children understand when we would come back. Your child may not comprehend the concept of "two days" or "Daddy will be back on Friday." Use concrete terms she can understand: "Today we'll go to the store and visit granny and then go to sleep. Tomorrow we'll play with your friends. One more bedtime and then Daddy will come home." Make a chart or a picture and cross off the events as they happen.
- *Leave a bit of yourself behind.* When you travel, leave a picture of yourself by your child's bedside or a tape-recording of your voice reading a favourite story, singing a bedtime song, or just saying, "I love you. Goodnight."
- *Stay connected while apart.* Send your child email about what you are doing on your trip. Include pictures of yourself, if you want to get fancy. Your child can dictate replies to send back to you. Phone frequently. Speaking in word pictures, let your child know what you are doing: "Think about Daddy giving a talk to a whole crowd of people and showing pictures. Imagine me going to bed thinking all about you." Planting these mental images in your child's mind helps her make you a part of her day and night.

Our children used to take advantage of me being on the road and use it as an opportunity to enjoy a family bedroom again. Martha would welcome them to snuggle with her or put a futon or sleeping bag at the foot of our bed and let them enjoy this "special bed" when Daddy was away.

I have a hard time getting our little girl who is almost three to go to sleep. Her Navy dad is sailing again after being home for the first three years of her life. What can I do?

Prolonged separation from military Dad on deployment is bound to keep any three-year-old awake, and it is hard on Mum, too. This is not the time to be tough on your daughter. She needs the security of knowing you are there for her, night and day. Many military mums find it's best to have their infant or preschool child sleep in their room, or even in their bed, while Dad is away. Lie down together on your bed until your child falls asleep and then get up to resume your evening activities. When you retire for the night, you can leave her in the bed, move her onto a mattress at the foot of your bed, or carry her to her own room.

Beware of the "sleep trainers" who advise you to let her cry it out. Your child has reason for nighttime insecurities right now, and if you respect them you'll both probably sleep a lot better while Dad is away.

"feeding" baby to sleep during childcare

Our one-year-old will be attending day nursery when I go back to work. He's so used to feeding to sleep, especially for naps, that I'm worried he won't know how to go to sleep for someone else, especially day nursery. Help!

Since your baby loves to nap-feed, you're going to need some creative strategies to get your baby to accept someone else putting him to sleep. First, try to get baby used to naptime alternatives at home (see alternative naptime strategies, page 192). Next, be sure your substitute caregiver has a parenting mindset like yours. Watch out for red flags, such as, "I see he's spoiled and can't go to sleep on his own …" There are enough changes going on already once you go back to work. This is certainly not the time for a less-than-nurturing caregiver to enter the picture. As a clue, ask a perspective nanny, childminder or day nursery how they feel about the "let baby cry it out" advice. You certainly don't want your baby to be put in a cot and left to cry himself to sleep. Again, remember that "nursing" implies comforting, not just breastfeeding. Also, if baby gets a bottle during childcare, be sure to give your caregiver the bottle-feeding advice listed on page 173.

On the other hand, it may be helpful for baby to get used to novel sleep associations. If you have a sensitive and nurturing caregiver, you may wish to let her devise her own sleep plan. If it's working, stick with it.

Play show and tell. Tell your caregiver that you feel strongly about your baby being rocked, sung, or worn off to sleep. Show her how to wear your baby in a sling as soon as the signs of *tired time* appear. Let her know what your baby's usual drowsy signs are. (See related sections: "Wearing Down", page 19; "and "Napping at Day-care", page 198.)

single parents – two different beds

Depending on the child's age, night waking from night fears may occur more often when children are bounced between two beds in separate homes. The child may get used to a primary sleeping arrangement in the home of the custodial parent, yet have to sleep in a different arrangement in the home of the other parent. Or, in cases of dual custody, some children may spend half their time in one bed and half their time in another. Depending on the age and sleep temperament of the child, this may or may not be a problem. If a child is used to sleeping in one arrangement, such as co-sleeping with Mum, that child may have difficulty solo sleeping at Dad's house. On the other hand, some more adaptable, older children have no trouble sleeping in two different beds, and some even enjoy the novelty. It's important that both parents respect their children's individual nighttime needs and not let custody squabbles keep their children awake.

Agree on an approach to nighttime parenting. It helps for both parents to know what bedtime rituals work. If you have found one that works for you, share it with the other parent, and encourage him/her to do likewise. As long as your child is parented to sleep and not just put to sleep, your child may actually enjoy two different nighttime parenting styles and rituals. For the sake of your child, try to agree on a nighttime parenting philosophy as much as possible.

A common custody squabble in the United States that often leads to a legal squabble is when a toddler is still night feeding, yet Dad wants overnights with his child. This is a sensitive situation which luckily has not yet happened in the UK, but is probably only a matter of time. Few judges understand a toddler's need to night feed and may misinterpret co-sleeping and night feeding as fostering a dependency, or as a ploy to keep Dad from enjoying overnights with his child. La Leche League International has a wealth of information gleaned from cases in the US that professionally discusses this sensitive situation and offers you some helpful guidelines, while in the UK the various other voluntary organisations, like The National Childbirth Trust (NCT) 0870 444 8707, Breastfeeding Network (BfN) 0870 900 8787 and Association of Breastfeeding Mothers (ABM) 0870 401 7711 would also support you in any custody and breastfeeding situation. We have personally been involved as consultants in such custody squabbles.

The bottom line is: what's in the best interest of the child?

nightmares

Our three-year-old recently began having nightmares. How can I help him through these?

Nightmares occur most commonly in children between two and five years of age. Dreams distort reality. The harmless cartoon character turns into a monster in a child's dream, and this scary image frightens the child awake. Nightmares occur during the light state of sleep, or REM sleep, so children tend to awaken easily from bad dreams. Other sleep disturbances, such as night terrors (also called sleep terrors), sleepwalking, and bedwetting, occur during deep sleep, or non-REM sleep, and usually these don't awaken the child.

Scary dreams can become even more terrifying after a child wakes up, because young children are not yet capable of distinguishing fantasy from reality. It's harder for them to understand that the monster in the dream is not real and is not lurking in a corner of the bedroom. The scary details of the dream linger in the child's mind, and it's hard to go back to sleep.

A principle that's good for parenting – and good for life – is that problems can be turned into opportunities. Parenting your child through nightmares gives you an opportunity to star as a trusted and helpful resource in your child's emotional life. You'll reap the benefits for many years to come. Here's how:

Comfort your child. When a nightmare strikes, be there to help your child sort out what's real and what's not. Your presence, your touch, your soothing voice will help your child get through his fear and get ready to go back to sleep. Try to keep your child from being overwhelmed by his fears. Otherwise, the child may become afraid to go to sleep.

Explain nightmares to your child. Help your child understand that dreams are not real. They're just "pictures in your brain". Practise telling what's real and what's pretend during the daytime. As your child matures, he will be able to understand that dreams are not real, so he won't be so terrified by them. And, he will be old enough to understand that "monsters" don't really exist.

Minimize scary daytime experiences. Do some detective work to find out what triggered the nightmares. Ask your child to explain the content of the dreams to see if you can pinpoint the trigger. Take inventory of any new, and possibly scary, events in your child's life, such as a recent move, starting a new school, or squabbles with friends. In our pediatric practice, we've heard about preschool children who have nightmares after hearing their parents argue in the evening (don't always assume those little ears are totally asleep).

Martha notes: when Lauren was ten, she revealed to us that when she was little she could hear us arguing: "You thought I was asleep, but I heard you being mad at each other …" Ah, a teachable moment. As soon as Lauren shocked us with her revelation, Bill turned this problem into an opportunity. He told her, "When Mummy and Daddy are angry at each other we have a deal. We always make up and never go to bed angry." We believe children are likely to remember how their parents *solved their problems* rather than only the problems.

Play self-soothing music. If nightmares are a frequent occurrence, try playing a continuous-play tape recording of your child's favourite lullabies during the night. When he awakens,

hearing a familiar lullaby may calm him enough that he can get back to sleep on his own.

Unplug scary TV and other upsetting media images. Obviously, young children should not watch scary, violent movies and television programmes. Watch out for other frightening images in the media. The picture of a bleeding soldier on the front page of the paper, or a story on the TV news, can trigger nightmares. You cannot completely protect your child from learning about the scary things that happen in our world. But children do not need to linger over the details. Children need to be children. They need to know that the adults in their lives love them and will keep them safe.

Provide a secure sleeping environment. Nightmares are especially terrifying when preschoolers wake up alone. During this nightmare stage, try letting your child sleep in your bed, on a toddler mattress or "special bed" in your room, or with a sibling. Studies have shown that children who sleep with siblings tend to have fewer nightmares.

Have a peaceful day. Anything that can trigger a change in the circuits of the brain, such as a fever or a disruption of the child's normal sleep patterns, can trigger nightmares or sleep terrors (described opposite). The best way to lessen nightmares and sleep terrors is to help your child have a peaceful day and fall asleep peacefully at night.

sleep terrors

Our 2½-year-old daughter wakes up screaming several times a week, but she's not really awake. What's going on, and how can we help her?

These episodes are called sleep terrors. While sleep terrors can be frightening for parents to witness, they are less unsettling for the child than nightmares. Children remember nightmares. Even if they don't remember the details, they remember being gripped by fear. Unlike nightmares, which occur during REM or light sleep, sleep terrors happen during non-REM or deep sleep. Consequently, sleep terrors do not fully awaken the child. Children with sleep terrors don't remember this bizarre behaviour because they aren't awake during the episodes. Children with sleep terrors don't seem to be sleep-deprived the next day and they don't develop a fearful attitude about going to sleep. Parents may feel sleep-deprived the next day, but sleep terrors seldom bother children, and they go away with age.

Here's what a typical sleep terror episode looks like. A child suddenly sits up in bed, lets out a piercing scream, looks terrified, and stares straight ahead with eyes wide open. You come running to see what's wrong, and the child continues to cry and breathes heavily. You may feel her heart pounding, her pupils may be dilated, and she may perspire profusely. If you try to wake her, she seems confused and totally disconnected from what's going on. She is oblivious to your attempts to help her. Don't take it personally, but she may try to push you away when you try to hold her. In fact, trying to help may hinder the process of getting through the sleep terror, as some children become more upset if you bother them during these episodes. Sleep terrors may last from five to ten minutes, after which the child – who was never really awake – falls into a deep, calm sleep. The child seems none the worse for wear, but you may be a wreck.

During a sleep terror episode, a child may bolt out of bed and dart out of the bedroom. Because children can hurt themselves during sleep terrors it's important to stay with and protect your child until she falls calmly back to sleep. Accident-proof her bedroom, so if she sleep walks during the terror, she does not trip and hurt herself.

Sleep terrors are considered a quirk in the mysterious neuro-circuitry in the brain. Unlike nightmares which occur toward the end of the night when the brain is busy dreaming, sleep terrors tend to occur earlier. Sleep terrors usually occur during the first or second deep sleep state of the night, a couple hours after the child goes to sleep. Keep a log of when they occur and you may be able to find a way to prevent them. A time-honoured trick for preventing night terrors is to *fully awaken your child just before the usual time the night terror occurs,* and then cuddle him back to sleep. This helpful parental intervention resets the sleep cycles, which will often prevent an episode of sleep terrors.

Sleep disorder clinics report that the most common trigger of sleep terrors is *sleep deprivation.* Ensuring that your child gets enough quality sleep is the best home remedy you can offer. Stress can contribute to sleep

the difference between sleep terrors and nightmares: how to tell

Feature	Sleep Terrors	Nightmares
Age of child	May occur in toddler hood, but more common in school-age children	Most common from 2–5 years of age
When they occur	First few hours of night	Last few hours
Sleep cycle	Occurs during non-REM, non-dreaming, deep sleep	Occurs during REM, or dreaming, light sleep
Consciousness	Not awake, terrified	Fully awakens
Activity during	May bolt out of bed and dart out of room	Usually stays in bed
Memory of event	No memory, or fuzzy recollection	Recalls vivid details
Comfort needed	None or little	Reassured by your comfort
Parental help	Hands-off	Hands-on
Danger of injury	High possibility	Usually none
Sleepy next day	Usually okay	Tired

deprivation. This explains why sleep terrors are more common during illnesses and family upsets that affect your child's sleep pattern. Several children in our practice have experienced sleep terrors during or shortly after a traumatic hospital experience. Also, avoid caffeine-containing drinks, such as colas, that may disturb your child's usual sleep patterns.

Help your child have peaceful days, and encourage active outdoor play that will help her sleep better at night.

It is not always easy to tell the difference between nightmares and sleep terrors. More important than knowing exactly what's happening is what you do to help your child. Remain as calm as possible while helping your child resettle. Often, just being there and issuing a reassuring, "It's okay …" is enough to get your child back to sleep. Once your child senses that you are not afraid, he is less likely to be afraid.

chapter 13

eleven tips to help parents sleep better

Most of the sleep tips in this book are designed to help your baby or child sleep better. If your baby sleeps better, you will probably sleep better, too. You can't always control your baby's sleep pattern, but you can control your own sleep choices. The tips in this chapter are designed to help *you* enjoy a more restful night's sleep, even when your baby is not.

1. make sleep a priority

When you are working around the clock to meet the needs of your baby, it's easy to forget to take care of yourself. Yet parents who do not get enough sleep may not always be effective parents. Your baby needs to sleep well to thrive, and so do you. Remember, your baby needs a reasonably well-rested mother. This means that you must make getting enough sleep a priority – for your own sake and for your baby's.

When a new baby joins the family, parents, especially first-time parents, are often in for a rude awakening – literally. A baby upsets parents' previously predictable lifestyle, especially sleeping routines. It's important to be realistic about this. During that first year or two of parenting you're going to need to make some adjustments in your lifestyle to get enough sleep.

Basically, I was the sleep problem. When I slept better, our baby slept better and woke up a lot less. I learned to nap during the day. I let the housework go. I needed sleep more than the house needed to be cleaned. If baby went to bed, I did, too!

Unclutter your daytime life. With a baby to care for, you can't expect to accomplish all the things you used to be able to do in a day and still have time left over to get enough sleep. You will need to set some priorities for your daytime life and let go of what's less important. Read some tips on how to accomplish this, page 63.

Go to bed earlier. It's tempting to use those few hours between baby's bedtime and your own bedtime to "finally get something done" or to relax with your partner. The sense of freedom you feel with baby finally down in bed can entice you into staying up much too late. Try to go to bed at least eight hours before baby's usual morning awake time. If your baby routinely wakes up about 6am, you should be in bed by 10pm. The deep and most restful stage of sleep occurs in the first third of the night. If you go to bed at midnight, and your baby (who went to bed at eight) wakes up at one, you are not going to feel very rested in the morning, because this deep sleep stage has been interrupted. Going to bed earlier will yield more high-quality sleep time for you at the beginning of the night.

Nurse yourself to sleep after you nurse your baby to sleep. After you have fed your baby to sleep, you may be tempted to shake off that drowsy, relaxed feeling you get from breastfeeding and get up and do something else. But making your escape from the bedroom prevents you from taking advantage of the breastfeeding hormones that can help you sleep better. While your baby is feeding, your level of prolactin, a sleep-inducing and relaxing hormone, rises and peaks 45 minutes after breastfeeding. This makes it easy to fall asleep. Take advantage of this biological perk and use it to help you fall asleep soon after feeding baby.

The older kids can wait. Permit us to get on our soapbox for a minute. Today's kids are overbooked, overstuffed, overfed, and over coddled. Just say no! When a new baby comes into the home, older children have to learn the meaning of the word "wait!" This is a time when they learn that Mums need to be taken care of too, and that Mum can't always come running whenever anyone needs her. It helps for Dad to call a family council together and tell the older children: "This is what Mum needs …" and then help children respect Mum's needs. Learning that family relationships involve both giving and receiving is an important life lesson. Twenty years or so down the road your child's future partner will thank you.

If the "older" children in the family are still very young, asking them to wait or to solve their own problems may not be appropriate. Toddlers of one, two, or three years of age still need lots of hands-on care and attention, especially when a new baby enters the family. This is a time for Dad to pitch in and help with the older child, so that Mum can rest. Another strategy to give Mum a break from the demands of an active young sibling is to hire a teenager to come in a couple afternoons a week and entertain the toddler while Mum and baby take a nap.

Martha notes: realize that to be a good Mum you don't have to operate on all eight cylinders all the time. You can function on six, or even five. I call this the "Mum zone" – not bright-eyed and bushy-tailed, but not zombied-out either, though you may be both of those from time to time. In the Mum zone you have plenty of energy to love your child, but not enough to read Shakespeare or balance your chequebook. You have the energy to read another story, bake a batch of biscuits, or maybe cook two vegetables for dinner (but not three), yet not all in the same day. The laundry can wait

sleep deprivation – hazardous for mums

The health hazards of sleep-deprivation are vastly underrated. New mothers (and fathers) who don't get enough sleep put their health and their ability to care for their family at risk. Here are the most concerning effects of chronic sleep deprivation:

Can make you sick

Sleep deprivation depresses immunity by reducing white blood cells that circulate throughout your body on search-and-destroy missions against invading germs. Being sick all the time makes the energy draining first year of your child's life much harder. Staying healthy helps mothers and fathers maintain a positive attitude toward the stresses of parenting.

Reduces your ability to pay attention

When you don't get enough sleep it's hard to concentrate, especially during boring and routine tasks such as driving. Falling asleep at the wheel is a common result of sleep deprivation. Also, sleep deprivation slows your reaction time, which also increases the risk of traffic accidents.

Lessens the enjoyment of your new baby

It is hard to care about things when you are tired all the time. Sleep deprivation dampens your enthusiasm for parenting and keeps you from enjoying special moments with your baby. When you are sleep-deprived, it is more difficult to tune in to your parenting intuition and make those on-the-spot decisions about what your baby needs or why she is crying. It may even affect your judgment and ability to handle emergencies.

Keeps you from enjoying life

Being sleep-deprived will affect your relationship with your partner, your performance on the job, and your outlook on life in general. Babies need happy, well-rested parents in order to be happy themselves.

Repay your sleep debt

As often as you can, or at least once a week, try to arrange a night to get an eight or nine hour stretch of sleep. Hire help, delegate household responsibilities to your partner, or do whatever it takes to get out of sleep debt. Even the most bankrupt sleepers find they can get out of sleep debt with one un-fragmented night's sleep.

another day or three, but your mate and your child will get enough to go around – just maybe not as much as they'd like – that day. The Mum zone doesn't go on endlessly. There will be bright and bushy days again. And that thought can keep you cheerful enough to enjoy the feeling at the end of the day that you've been a good-enough mother.

A sleep note for dads: help your partner get out of sleep debt. A sleep-deprived mum becomes a burned-out partner, and the whole family suffers. Yet, it's amazing how a relaxing day and one un-fragmented night's sleep can restore her well-being. Once a week arrange for her to have an afternoon at the spa or "just for me" time. Hire help or take over the household chores and as much of baby-care as you can. Setting your partner up for a few hours off-duty can help restore her well-being, and the whole family benefits. Don't just suggest this to your partner, do it: "I've made an appointment for you at the spa. I've already paid for it and I can't get our money back. I'll drive you there." This set-up is especially important to a mother who is of the mindset: "I don't have time to take care of myself because my baby needs me so much."

2. eat to sleep

What and when you eat can affect how you sleep. Some foods work like natural sleeping pills, helping you relax and drift off to sleep. The food/mood connection is vastly underrated. As neurobiologist Michael Gershon, M.D., points out in his book, *The Second Brain,* (Harper Collins, 2000) 95 per cent of the body's serotonin (the relaxing hormone) is found in the bowels. On page 40 of this book you'll find which foods are sleepers and which are wakers. Wakers are junk-carbohydrate foods that send the brain on a sleepless roller coaster ride due to rising and falling blood sugar levels, triggering stress hormones. Carbohydrates that are partnered with protein, fibre, and fat are much better sleep inducers than foods that contain little more than sugar.

Don't dine after nine. Best to eat the evening meal at least three hours before bedtime. It is harder to fall asleep if your gut is working overtime digesting a heavy meal. The intestines are richly supplied with nerves, and if these nerves in the gut "brain" are revved up, the brain that is trying to fall asleep will be revved up too. Your body will rest better if your intestines are at rest. Yet don't go to bed hungry. The hormones released when blood sugar is too low can rev up your brain and keep you awake as well.

If you suffer from gastroesophageal reflux (also called acid reflux or heartburn), research shows that early eaters produce less stomach acid compared to late diners.

Eat easy-to-digest foods. Especially if you suffer from reflux or heartburn, avoid foods that are slow to digest, including foods that are high in fat, spicy foods, and those that you know give you wind. If you are sensitive to certain foods or substances in food, such as the monosodium glutamate (MSG) found in Chinese cooking and other processed foods, be particularly careful to avoid these foods before bedtime.

dr bill's before-bed smoothie: sleep-ade

Try our Sears' smoothie recipe, which is a blend of the sleep-inducing nutrients tryptophan, calcium, magnesium, and healthy carbohydrates:

- 1 cup of milk
- 1 banana
- ½ cup yoghurt
- 100g tofu

- 1 tbsp. ground flaxseed meal
- 1 tsp. cinnamon

Blend and enjoy an hour or so before bed.

Take inventory of your nutritional status. In the first six months after giving birth, your body is replenishing nutrients that were depleted during pregnancy. Also, breastfeeding makes additional nutritional demands on your body. Be sure to continue to take any prenatal vitamins and minerals prescribed by your doctor. B-vitamins help your brain use the sleep-inducer tryptophan, so that you can sleep better. Iron deficiency anaemia, one of the medical causes of night waking in infants and toddlers, can create a state of hyper-anxiety in mums, leading to sleeplessness. Be sure your doctor checks you for anaemia during your postnatal check-up.

Beware of crash diets. Many women can't wait to return to their pre-pregnancy weight, but there are many good reasons not to go on a crash diet during the postpartum period. Hunger itself can release hormones that can keep you awake. Be sure to avoid very low-carbohydrate diets (those that throw the body into a state of chronic ketosis), as they are not healthy for the postpartum mum. Chronic ketosis can cause tiredness and irritability during the day and

keep you awake at night. Also, you need carbohydrates in the bloodstream to partner with the sleep inducer tryptophan and help usher it into brain cells.

Decaf your day. Watch your caffeine intake while your baby is learning how to sleep better and you are adjusting your own sleep habits. Caffeine can stay in your bloodstream for eight hours or longer. Even one cup of coffee in the morning can interfere with your afternoon nap and may even contribute to sleeplessness at night. If you are using large amounts of caffeine during the day (more than the equivalent of five cups of coffee), there may be enough caffeine in your breastmilk to interfere with baby's sleep. Caffeine sensitivity is extremely variable. If you are a caffeine-sensitive person, it is best to avoid it entirely at this stage of your parenting.

Avoid alcohol. For most adults, an occasional glass of wine with the evening meal won't adversely affect sleep, but drinking too much, too close to bedtime can interfere with your natural sleep cycles. Specifically, alcohol

what about sleeping pills?

We advise that you avoid all over-the-counter and prescription sleeping medications during the time that you are working on getting everyone in the family a good night's sleep. Sleeping medications can be habit forming, so it may eventually become difficult to fall asleep without medication. Many sleep-inducing drugs (for example, alcohol) interfere with the natural stages of sleep. They may help you to fall asleep, but you don't get the same quality of sleep as you would without the drug. Also, some sleep medications may diminish a mother's awareness and sensitivity to her baby's needs at night. There may be medical circumstances that warrant the short-term use of sleep medication for some mothers, but these medications should not be used routinely.

Co-sleeping warning

It's unsafe to sleep with your baby in your bed if you take prescription sleeping medications.

Some over-the-counter allergy and headache-relief medications contain substances that rev up the system and cause hyperirritability and sleeplessness. Read labels carefully and avoid medications that contain caffeine. Before taking any over-the-counter or prescription medicine ask your pharmacist or GP about possible effects on sleep.

As an alternative to prescription sleep medications, in consultation with your doctor, try these sleep-inducing natural remedies:

- Chamomile tea
- Valerian root extract (Do not take with sleeping medications or for longer than two weeks at a time.)
- Tryptophan supplements: 500 mg. to 2,000 mg. taken with fruit juice an hour before bedtime.

In consultation with your doctor, try taking tryptophan for three nights each week. Since tryptophan levels accumulate in the bloodstream, it's safest to give the body a few days off this extra supplement. Tryptophan supplements should be taken only with carbohydrates (such as juice or fruit) since carbohydrates usher the tryptophan into the brain. Don't take with protein foods since the amino acids in the protein compete with the tryptophan and lessen the amount that gets into the brain. Or, try the tryptophan/carbohydrate combination foods listed on page 40. As a perk, sleep research has shown that taking extra B-vitamins may increase the sleep effect of tryptophan.

You can get between 500–1,000 milligrams of tryptophan naturally in a before-bedtime snack by enjoying our smoothie recipe opposite.

decreases the amount of time you spend in deep sleep, thus decreasing the overall quality of your sleep. In the morning, you may feel like you are in a fog – which is no way to begin the day with a needy baby.

Don't smoke. Nicotine releases stress hormones. It revs up the body by increasing your pulse and blood pressure and revs up the brain because it is a neurostimulant. Besides harming your health and your sleep, nicotine is hazardous to your baby's health, increasing the risk of nearly every major disease, especially SIDS (Sudden Infant Death Syndrome).

3. dress for sleep

Cotton clothing is cooler and breathes better than synthetics. Wear a cotton nightgown or pyjamas to bed. In warm weather try cotton sheets. In cold weather, try flannel ones. (If you're co-sleeping and night feeding, see helpful hints on sleepwear, page 76.)

Sears' Sleep Tip: Sleeping and Working. If you are a sleep-deprived mum who works outside the home, try having the babysitter arrive a couple hours early one or two mornings a week. The sitter can care for the kids while you grab an extra hour or two of sleep. (This is also a good way for partners to help out!) During the day, try taking a 20-minute power nap during your lunch break.

4. exercise for sleep

Exercising at least an hour a day – in addition to chasing after a busy toddler – can improve the quality of your sleep at night. How does this happen? It's those hormones again! To relax your mind and tone your muscles, enrol in a Yoga, Pilates or Tai Chi class. Strenuous exercise improves the quality of deep sleep by stimulating the release of relaxing endorphins and growth hormones, which are natural sleep inducers. Try these tips for getting more exercise every day:

When to exercise? Steal whatever time you can during the day for exercise you enjoy. While exercising anytime during the day can help you sleep better, sleep researchers have found that exercising five to six hours before bedtime has the best effect on sleep. Early-morning exercise will have less impact on how well you sleep, since the hormonal effects wear off during the day. If you exercise vigorously an hour or two before bedtime, you may be too revved up and energized to wind down easily.

Sears' Sleep Tip: Walk and Wear. A tip we frequently offer new parents is something we have dubbed *walk and wear.* Many babies have their fussiest period between 4 and 6pm. Before this "happy hour" strikes, put your baby in a baby sling and take a vigorous walk that lasts at least a half hour. This late afternoon walk will help you de-stress, and it will calm baby, too. Exercising with Mummy and enjoying the great outdoors often reduces late afternoon fussiness and helps both mothers and babies sleep better at night.

How much to move? Try to get between a half hour and one hour of aerobic exercise at least four or five days a week. Work out at a pace that raises your heart and breathing rate enough that you find it slightly taxing to carry on a long conversation while exercising. Exercise options include a brisk walk, time on the treadmill or stair stepper, a fast swim, or repeatedly going up and down stairs. Some mothers like to put on a CD and dance energetically while baby watches.

5. enjoy a before-bed bath

Sitting in a warm bath not only relaxes the body but also relaxes the mind for sleep. Twenty minutes in a hot bath will make your body temperature go up. Then shortly after you go to bed your body temperature falls again. This rise and fall in body temperature releases sleep-inducing hormones.

6. turn off the tube

Studies show that children who watch more TV have more problems with sleep disturbances, especially children who have TV sets in their bedrooms. Television may have similar effects on many adults. Late-night news shows are enough to keep anyone awake. The rapid change of images and artificial light patterns on the TV screen rev up the brain and disrupt the process of falling asleep.

Sears' Sleep Tip: Wake and Write. If you just can't get off to sleep or wake up and can't get back to sleep, this is a good time to log the events of the day, especially pleasant ones. Using the technique called "restful visualisation", visualize scenes that you know relax you and help you sleep. Keep a list entitled "Scenes to Sleep By", and fill your mind with instant replay of these scenes to relax the brain off to sleep.

7. don't worry, be happy!

Remember, sleep is not a state you can force yourself into. But you can create a physical and mental environment that allows sleep to overtake you. In that last hour or so before you go to bed, choose quiet, relaxing activities, such as listening to music, reading a not-too-interesting book, meditating or writing, or quietly conversing with your mate. This is a time to think about what went right with your day, not what went wrong. When it's time to turn out the lights, turn your mind to "happy thoughts" – perhaps recollecting happy moments from your life (or just from your day) or visualising pleasant scenes such as a walk along the beach. Try not to muddle your mind with disturbing thoughts.

Late evening is not the time to argue with your partner, balance the chequebook, or discuss disturbing family matters. Once your mind gets occupied with difficult problems, it's hard to shut off the worrying and fall asleep. Anxiety and anger release stress hormones. The unresolved tension keeps you awake, sometimes for hours, and affects the quality of whatever sleep you do get. Once your mind gets full of disturbing stuff, you then "try" to go to sleep, which only adds to the difficulty of falling asleep. An hour or two later the tension escalates and you're still awake. Drifting off to sleep is the time to focus on what went right during the day, not what went wrong. Re-programme yourself that at least an hour or two before you go to bed is going to be happy hour, a time engaged in pleasant conversation and happy thoughts.

Avoiding conflict and tension late at night is easier said than done, since many new parents find that the only time during the day that they can talk to each other is after the baby and the older children are in bed. Perhaps you and your partner can schedule specific times during the week – perhaps a weekend breakfast or a Sunday afternoon walk – to discuss family business. When you are both tired and need to talk at night, use your best communication skills to avoid arguments and upset feelings.

Another mental obstacle to getting a good night's rest is what sleep researchers call the "*on-call syndrome*". We remember experiencing this during our early years of medical training – we had trouble sleeping on the nights we were on-call for emergencies. Even while we slept, some part of our brains was alert, listening for the wake-up call, and this led to a lot of fragmented sleep. Anticipating that baby is going to wake up can have the same effect on parents' sleep. Even on the occasional night when baby sleeps longer stretches, mother may feel like she's on-call. She wakes up even when baby doesn't and does not sleep as soundly as she could. When you go to bed, try not to think about the night ahead, since those worries are likely to keep you awake. Don't anticipate every peep or cry your baby is going to make during the night. Concentrate on what you need to do, which is to relax and benefit from sleep.

Some night training was necessary for me. I had to train myself to go to the bathroom or count to twenty before I went to him, because most times he was able to settle back to sleep without me and I wanted to encourage that behaviour.

Sears' Sleep Tip: When you go to bed, don't think about how soon your baby is going to wake up. Fretting about baby's night waking ("Is this going to be another night of waking up every two hours?") will make it harder to cope with it. Instead, reflect on the joyful blessings you experienced during the day and the precious little person who also needs you at night.

8. sleep more the first month

Many mums enter motherhood already sleep-deprived, thanks to the discomforts and middle-of-the-night trips to the bathroom that are common during the last weeks of pregnancy. Add to this sleep lost during all-night labours, birth, and the euphoria that follows, and you have a new mother who badly needs to catch up on her sleep. Unfortunately, during this first month postpartum, newborns often have their days and nights mixed up, and they sleep long stretches during the day (like they did in the womb) and less at night. This is a time for you to sleep "like a baby", even if this means you sleep long stretches during the day yourself. After you've repaid a bit of sleep debt and built up your sleep bank account during the first month, you'll be better able to cope with your baby's daytime and nighttime needs. As your newborn eases into day/night sleep maturity, you will be able to get more of the sleep you need at night, though you may still need an afternoon nap.

9. enjoy a before-bed ritual

Babies and children aren't the only ones who enjoy bedtime rituals. Adults are creatures of habit, too. Develop your own sleep-inducing routine to help you unwind: a warm bath, massage, music, and stories – night-night! Your bedtime ritual may be very similar to your child's: wind-down activities. Bedtime sex is a time-honoured and very effective sleep inducer, but as we discussed on page 126, many new mothers are too tired to enjoy sex after a long day of infant care. Morning or mid-afternoon sex is more realistic during that first year with a new baby.

10. nap when baby does

Easier said than done? Not if you follow tip 1: make sleep a priority. Naps are a necessity for new mothers whose sleep is regularly interrupted by night feedings. Don't be concerned that napping during the day will make it harder for you to sleep at night. Sleep researchers have found that people who nap usually sleep better at night. If you know you can look forward to a nap during the day, you'll worry less about losing sleep at night and just having that reassurance may help you sleep better.

"But", you say, "I just *can't* fall asleep during the day." Just like at bedtime, you have to create the conditions that allow sleep to overtake you. One way to do this is to work with your body's natural rhythms. Whether you're awake or asleep depends on two systems in the brain: the arousal system (the "on" switch) and the sleep system (the "off" switch). Letting sleep overtake you is basically letting the "off" switch overcome the "on" switch. Your brain is wired to allow the "off" switch to predominate over the "on" switch at different times through a 24-hour day. Sleep researchers have found that during the day the "off" switch is most likely to win the competition between one and three o'clock in the afternoon. Take advantage of this natural drive to sleep and nap during that time. If you lie down with your baby and breastfeed, the breastfeeding hormones will also help to switch off the part of your brain that wants to stay awake.

11. make nighttime mothering more restful

Can you actually make waking up at night more restful? Yes, you can. Again, make sleep your priority. Put your energy into getting the sleep you need rather than into fretting about not sleeping. Do everything you can to make your sleeping environment quiet, comfortable, and welcoming. Care for your baby's needs in ways that allow you to get back to sleep quickly. For more ideas to help make nighttime parenting more restful read:

- "Fifteen Ways to Make Night Feeding Easier", page 134.
- "Twenty-three Nighttime Fathering Tips", page 166.
- "Music to Sleep By", opposite.

What helped me get back to sleep was to develop a pleasant ritual that I always did after waking up and tending to baby. Rather than toss and turn, I would get up and rub lotion on my feet to help me drift back to sleep.

Surround yourself with darkness. The glow of an alarm clock or the glare from a streetlight outside your window can be very annoying in the wee hours of the morning. Eliminate light sources that bother you. Turn off computers, put a washcloth over an illuminated alarm clock, use blackout shades, and clip the curtains together to block out the early morning light.

Sears' Sleep Tip: Setting Your Body Clock for Bedtime. Consistent bedtimes are just as important for Mums and Dads as they are for children. Try to go bed at about the same time each evening. This will programme your body to fall asleep at a predictable time and in a predictable place. Resist the temptation to lie down on the couch in the evening to just take a rest. If you're tired, go to bed. Chilling out on the couch or in your favourite chair won't get you the high-quality rest you need. As soon as you and your baby wake up in the morning, open the blinds or curtains and let natural light come in. Sleep researchers have found that exposure to natural light in the morning sets the body to "awake mode" and helps it transition into "sleep mode" when darkness comes.

Decorate your bedroom the way you like it. Take the money that you would otherwise spend on decorating a fancy nursery and buying an ornate cot (which your baby won't appreciate anyway) and spend it on your sleep sanctuary. Upgrade your bed to king-size, with a good-quality mattress. Buy soft, comfortable bedding in quiet, soothing colours. Make your bedroom into a restful environment. Eliminate clutter and stacks of paper that you don't want to look at or think about in the middle of the night.

appendix a

music to sleep by

Bizet, 'Adagietto' from *L'Arlésienne*, incidental music Suite I for orchestra

Beethoven, 'Adagio sostenuto' from Piano Sonata no. 14 in C sharp minor (*Moonlight*), Op. 27

— 'Andante' from Piano Concerto no. 4 in G major, Op. 58

— 'Andante cantabile' from Symphony no. 1 in C major, Op. 21

Chopin, 'Larghetto' from Concerto for Piano and Orchestra no. 2 in F minor, Op. 21, CT 48

Debussy, 'Clair de Lune' from *Suite Bergamasque* for piano, L. 75

— *Preludes* and *Suite Bergamasque* for piano

— *Prelude to the Afternoon of a Faun*

Delius, orchestral works

Fauré, *Pavane* for orchestra and chorus ad lib in F sharp minor, Op. 50

Mendelssohn, 'Notturno' from *A Midsummer Night's Dream*, incidental music, Op. 61

Mozart, 'Andante' from Symphony no. 40 in G minor, K. 550

— 'Andante' from Piano Concerto no. 21 in C major (*Elvira Madigan*), K. 467

— 'Romance' from Serenade no. 13 for strings in G major (*Eine kleine Nachtmusik*), K. 525

Pachelbel, 'Canon' from Canon and Gigue for 3 violins and continuo in D major

Rachmaninov, 'Vocalise', song for voice and piano, Op. 34

Satie, *Gymnopédies* for piano

Tchaikovsky, 'Andante' from *Swan Lake*, ballet, Op. 20

— 'Chant sans paroles' ('Song without words') from *Souvenir de Hapsal* for piano

The above selections can be found on: *Night Music, Vol. 1: Classical Favourites for Relaxing and Dreaming* (boxed set) by the NAXOS label.

Other selections:

Bach, Brandenburg Concerto no. 3

— *The Well-Tempered Clavier*, Parts I and II

Debussy, *Dances Sacred and Profane*, piano preludes

Dvořák, *Serenade for Strings*, opus 22, second movement

Haydn, string quartets

Mozart, Symphony no. 17 in G Major, K. 129, first movement
— string divertimenti, early symphonies
Ravel, *Pavane for a Dead Princess*
— piano works

New Age music is also very good for sleeping:

Yanni (most of his albums are suitable)
John Tesh, *Winter Song* album
Drew Tretick, *Serenata*, *Romantica*, and *Summer Serenade*

appendix b

bedtime books to sleep by
– for toddlers and pre-schoolers

Davis, Lee, *Time for Bed, P. B. Bear* (Dorling Kindersley, 2001).

Berenstain, Stan and Jan, *Bears in the Night* (Collins, 1981).

Butterworth, Nick, *Thud!* (Picture Lions, 1998).

— *When It's Time for Bed* (Collins Baby & Toddler, 1994).

Carle, Eric, *Little Cloud* (Puffin, 1998).

— *The Very Hungry Caterpillar* (Puffin, 2002).

Crebbin, June, *The Train Ride* (Walker Books, 1996).

Dale, Penny, *Ten in the Bed* (Walker Books, 1998).

Dunbar, Joyce and Gliori, Debi, *Tell Me Something Happy Before I Go to Sleep* (Corgi Children's Books, 1999).

Eastman, P. D., *Are You My Mother?* (Picture Lions, 2005).

Grindley, Sally, *Shhh!* (Hodder Children's Books, 1999).

Hill, Eric, *Time for Bed, Spot* (Ladybird, 2004).

Hoban, Russell, *Bedtime for Frances* (Red Fox, 2002).

Krauss, Ruth, *A Hole is to Dig* (HarperCollins, 1952).

McBratney, Sam, *Guess How Much I Love You* (Walker Books, 2001).

Mosel, Arlene, *Tikki Tikki Tembo* (Holt, 1989).

Munsch, Robert N., and McGraw, Sheila, *Love You Forever* (Red Fox, 2001).

Murphy, Mary, *I Like It When* (Heinemann Young Books, 2001).

Piper, Watty, *The Little Engine That Could* (Platt, 1961).

Waddell, Martin, *Owl Babies* (Walker Books, 1994).

Waddell, Martin and Firth, Barbara, *Can't You Sleep, Little Bear?* (Walker Books, 2001).

Wells, Rosemary, *Max's First Word* (Collins, 1989).

Wise Brown, Margaret, *Goodnight Moon* (Campbell Books, 2001).

Wood, Audrey, *The Napping House* (Harcourt Brace, 2000).

Zion, Gene, *Harry the Dirty Dog* (Red Fox, 1996).

appendix c

references

chapter 1: five steps to get your baby to sleep better

1. Butler, S. R., *et al.* 1978. "Maternal behavior as a regulator of polyamine biosynthesis in brain and heart of developing rat pups", *Science* 199: 445–447.

2. Kuhn, C. M., *et al.* 1978. "Selective depression of serum growth hormone during maternal deprivation in rat pups", *Science* 201: 1035–1036.

3. Coe, C. L., *et al.* 1985. "Endocrine and immune responses to separation and maternal loss in non-human primates", in *The Psychology of Attachment and Separation*, ed. M. Reite and T. Fields, 163–199. New York: Academic Press.

4. Ahnert, L., *et al.*, 2004. "Transition to child care: associations with infant-mother attachment, infant negative emotion, and cortisol elevations", *Child Development* 75(3): 649–650.

5. Kaufman, J., Charney, D., 2001. "Effects of early stress on brain structure and function: implications for understanding the relationship between child maltreatment and depression", *Developmental Psychopathology* 13(3): 451–471.

6. Teicher, M. H., *et al.*, 2003. "The neurobiological consequences of early stress and childhood maltreatment", *Neuroscience Biobehavior Review* 27(1–2): 33–44.

7. Wolke, D., *et al.*, 2002. "Persistent infant crying and hyperactivity problems in middle childhood", *Pediatrics* 109: 1054–1060.

8. Perry, B., 1997. "Incubated in terror: neurodevelopmental factors in the cycle of violence", in *Children in a Violent Society*. New York: Guilford Press.

9. Schore, A. N., 1996. "The experience-dependent maturation of a regulatory system in the orbital prefrontal cortex and the origin of developmental psychopathology", *Development and Psychopathology* 8: 59–87.

10. Karr-Morse, R., Wiley, M., 1997. Interview with Dr Allan Schore, *Ghosts from the Nursery*, 200: Grove Press/Atlantic Monthly Press.

11. Brazy, J. E., 1988. *Journal of Pediatrics* 112 (3): 457–61.

12. Ludington-Hoe, S. M., 2002. *Neonatal Network* 21(2): 29–36.

13. Leiberman, A. F., Zeanah, H., 1995. "Disorders of attachment in infancy", *Infant Psychiatry* 4: 571–587.

14. Rao, M. R., *et al.*, 2004. "Long-term cognitive development in children with prolonged crying", *Archives of Disease in Childhood* 89: 989–992.

15. Stifter and Spinrad, 2002. "The effect of excessive crying on the development of emotion regulation", *Infancy* 3(2), 133–152.

chapter 5: the joys of co-sleeping with your baby

1. Blair, P. S., Fleming, P. J., Bensley, D., *et al.* 1999. "Where Should Babies Sleep – Alone or With Parents? Factors Influencing the Risk of SIDS in the CESDI Study", *British Medical Journal* 319 : 1457–1462.

2. Butler, S. R., *et al.* 1978. "Maternal behavior as a regulator of polyamine biosynthesis in brain and heart of the developing rat pups", *Science* 199: 445–447.

3. Carpenter, R. G., *et al.* 2004. "Sudden Unexplained Infant Death in 20 Regions in Europe: Case Control Study", *Lancet* 2004; 363: 185–191.

4. Coe, C. L., *et al.* 1985. "Endocrine and immune responses to separation and maternal loss in non-human primates", in *The Psychology of Attachment and Separation*, ed. M. Reite and T. Fields, 163–199. New York: Academic Press.

5. Crawford, M., 1994. "Parenting Practices in the Basque Country: Implications of Infant and Childhood Sleeping Location for Personality Development", *Ethos*, 22, 1: 42–82.

6. Davies, D. P., 1985. "Cot Death In Hong Kong: A Rare Problem?" *Lancet* 2: 1346–1348.

7. Drago, D. A. and Dannenberg, A. L. 1999. "Infant Mechanical Suffocation Deaths in the United States, 1980–1997", *Pediatrics* 103, no. 5 (1999): e59.

8. Elias, M. F., 1986. "Sleep-wake patterns of breastfed infants in the first two years of life", *Pediatrics* 77: 322–329.

9. Field, T., ed. 1995. *Touch in Early Development*. Mahway, New Jersey: Lawrence Earlbaum and Assoc.

10. Forbes, J. F., *et al.* 1992. "The Co-sleeping Habits of Military Children", *Military Medicine,* 157: 196–200.

11. Fukai, S. and Hiroshi, F., 2000. "1999 Annual Report, Japan SIDS Family Association", Sixth SIDS International Conference, Auckland, New Zealand, 2000.

12. Heron, P., 1994. "Non-Reactive Co-sleeping and Child Behavior: Getting a Good Night's Sleep All Night, Every Night", Master's thesis, Department of Psychology, University of Bristol.

13. Hofer, M., 1982. "Some thoughts on 'the transduction of experience' from a developmental perspective", *Psychosom. Med.* 44: 19.

14. Hofer, M., 1983. "The mother-infant interaction as a regulator of infant physiology and behavior", in *Symbiosis in parent-offspring interactions,* ed. Rosenblum and Moltz. New York: Plenum.

15. Hofer, M. and Shair, H., 1982. "Control of sleep-wake states in the infant rat by features of the mother-infant relationship", *Devel. Psychobiol.* 15: 229–243.

16. Kuhn, C. M., *et al.* 1978. "Selective depression of serum growth hormone during maternal deprivation in rat pups", *Science* 201: 1035–1036.

17. Lee, N. P., *et al.* 1999. "Sudden Infant Death Syndrome in Hong Kong: Confirmation of Low Incidence", *British Medical Journal* 298: 72.

18. Lewis, R. J. and Janda, L. H., 1988. "The Relationship Between Adult Sexual Adjustment and Childhood Experience Regarding Exposure to Nudity, Sleeping in the Parental Bed and Parental Attitudes Toward Sexuality", *Arch. Sex. Beh.,* 17: 349–363.

19. McKenna, J., *et al.* 1993. "Infant-parent co-sleeping in an evolutionary perspective: Implications for understanding infant sleep development and SIDS", *Sleep* 16: 263–282.

20. McKenna, J., *et al.* 1994. "Experimental studies of infant-parent co-sleeping: Mutual physiological and behavioral influences and their relevance to SIDS (sudden infant death syndrome)", *Early Human Development* 38: 187–201.

21. Mosenkis, J., 1998. "The Effects of Childhood Co-sleeping on Later Life Development". Master's Thesis, Department of Cultural Psychology, University of Chicago.

22. Mosko, S., *et al.* 1994. "Infant sleeping position and CO2 environment during co-sleeping: The Parents' contribution", *Pediatr. Pulmonol.* 18: 394.

23. Nelson, E. A. S., *et al.* 2001. "SIDS Global Task Force Child Care Study", *Early Human Development* 62 : 43–55.

24. Nelson, E. A. S., *et al.*, 2001. "International Child Care Practice Study: Infant Sleeping Environment", *Early Human Development* 62 (2001): 43–55.

25. Reite, M., and Capitanion, J. P., 1985. "On the nature of social separation and social attachment", in *The Psychobiology of Attachment and Separation*, ed. M. Reite and T. Fields, 228–238. New York: Academic Press.

26. Richard, C., *et al.* 1996. "Sleeping Position, Orientation, and Proximity in Bedsharing Infants and Mothers", *Sleep* 19: 667–684.

27. Sankaran, A. H., *et al.* 2000. "Sudden Infant Death Syndrome and Infant Care Practices in Saskatchewan, Canada", *Programme and Abstracts, Sixth SIDS International Conference*, Auckland, New Zealand, February 8–11, 2000.

28. Sears, W., 1985. "The protective effects of sharing sleep. Can it prevent SIDS?", paper presented at the International Congress of Pediatrics, Honolulu.

29. Sears, W., 1995. *SIDS: A Parents' Guide to Understanding Preventing Sudden Infant Death Syndrome*. New York: Little Brown.

30. Sears, W., *et al.* 1993. "The effect of co-sleeping on infant breathing – implications for SIDS", paper presented at the 11th Apnea of Infancy Conference, Rancho Mirage, California.

index